Herbs and Spices - New Processing Technologies

Edited by Rabia Shabir Ahmad

Published in London, United Kingdom

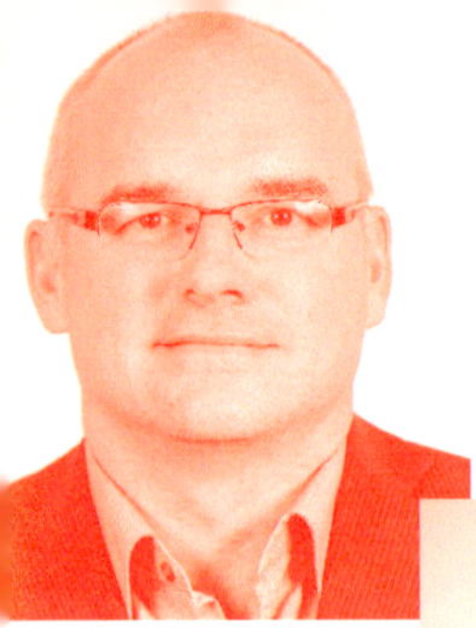
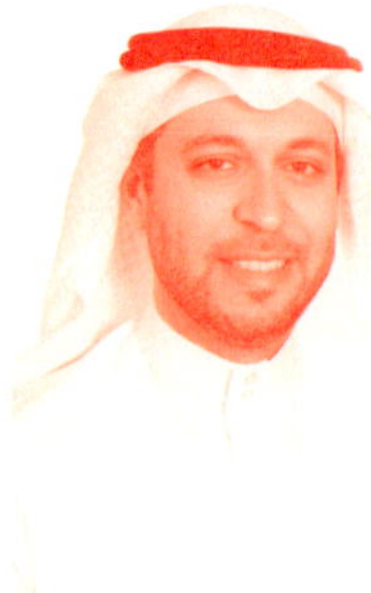
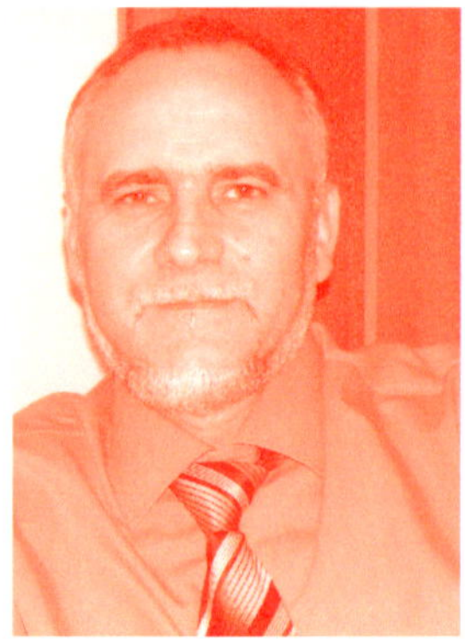
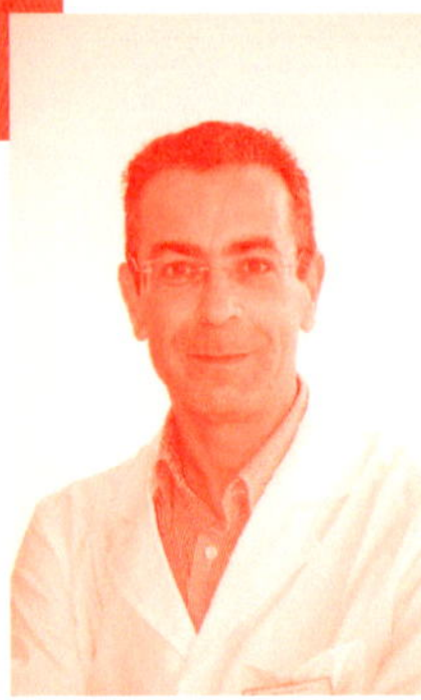
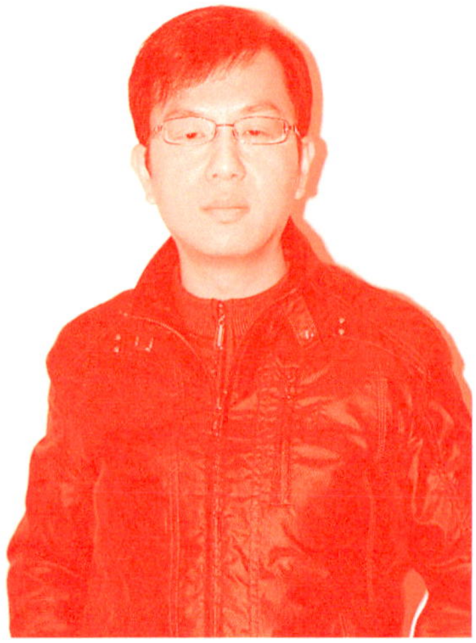
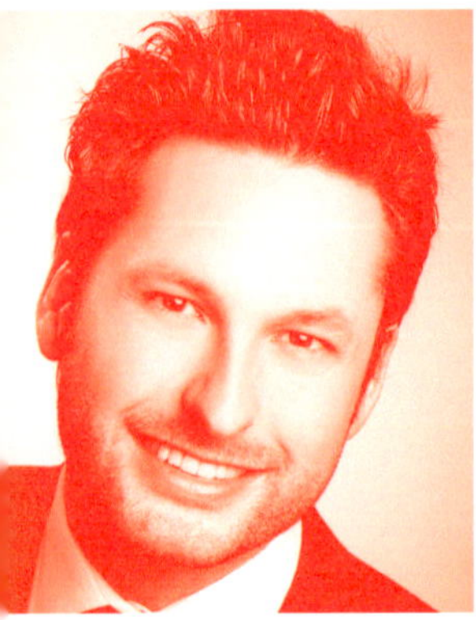
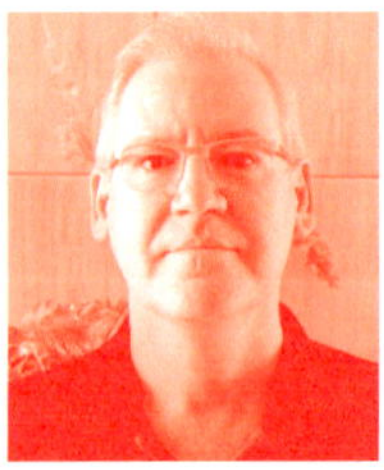

IntechOpen

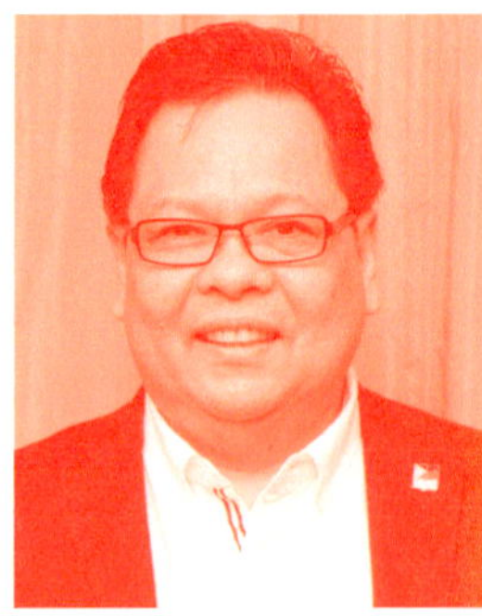
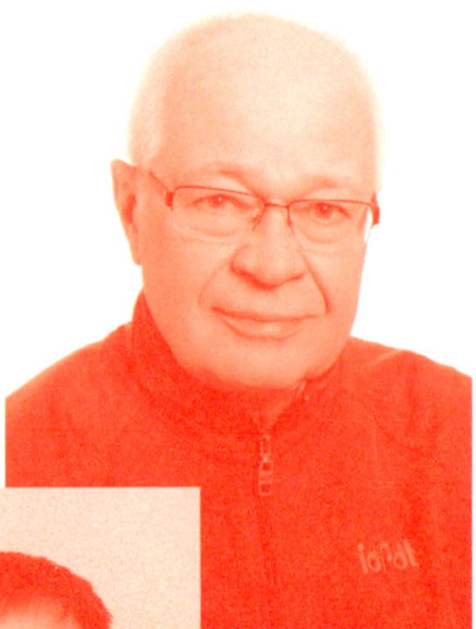
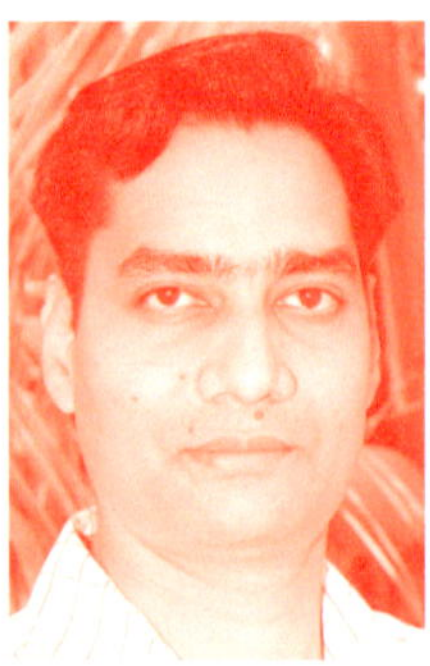
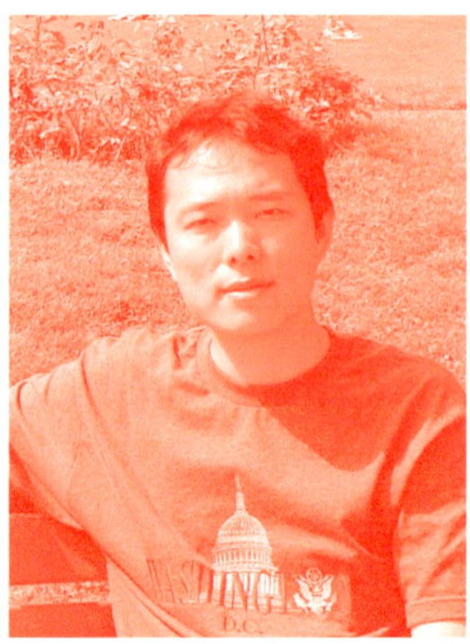
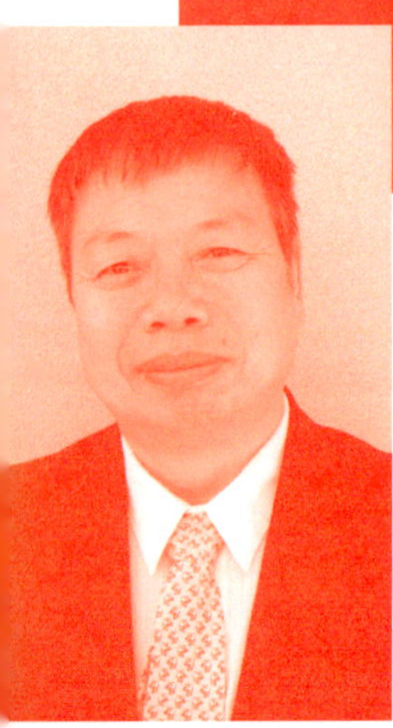
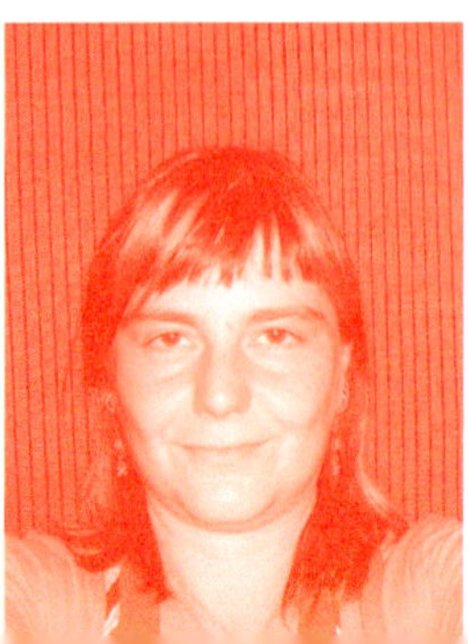

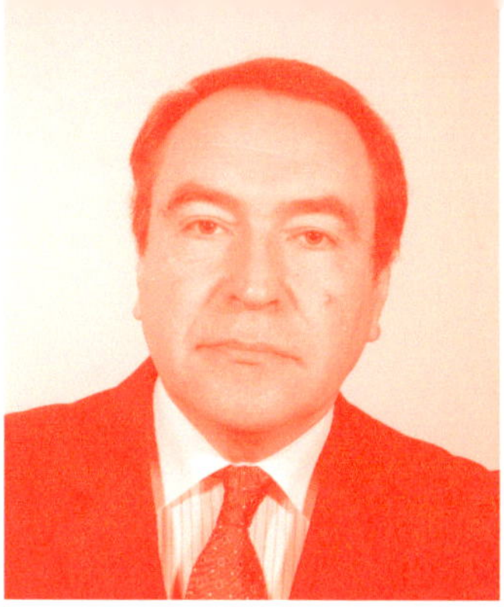

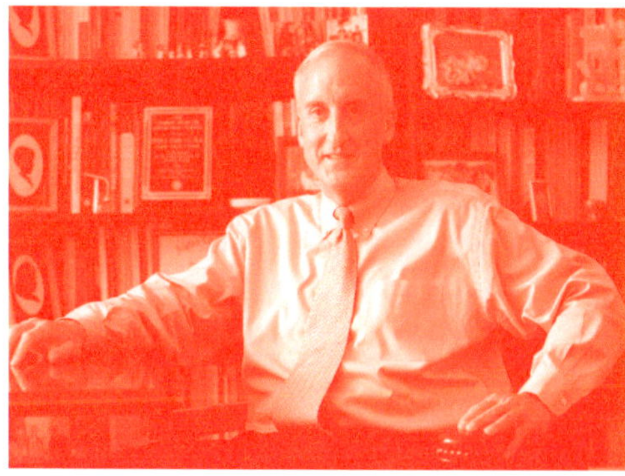

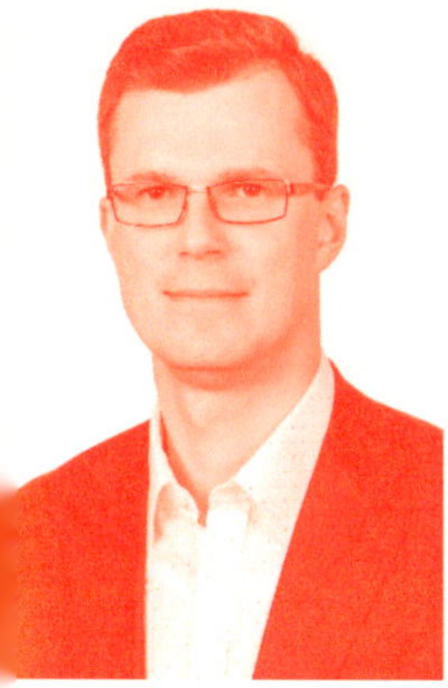

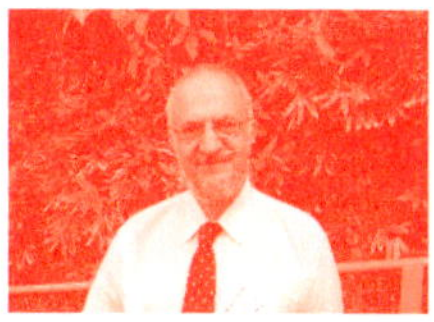

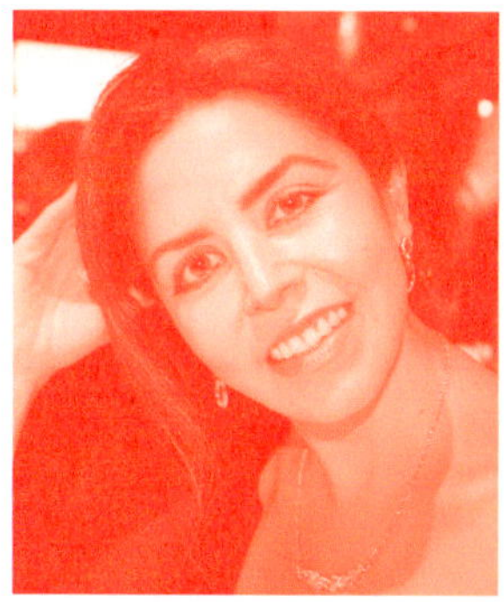

Supporting open minds since 2005

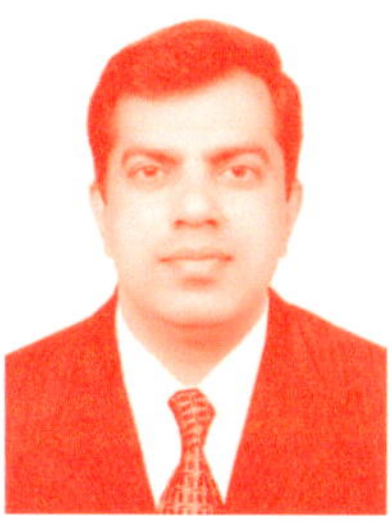

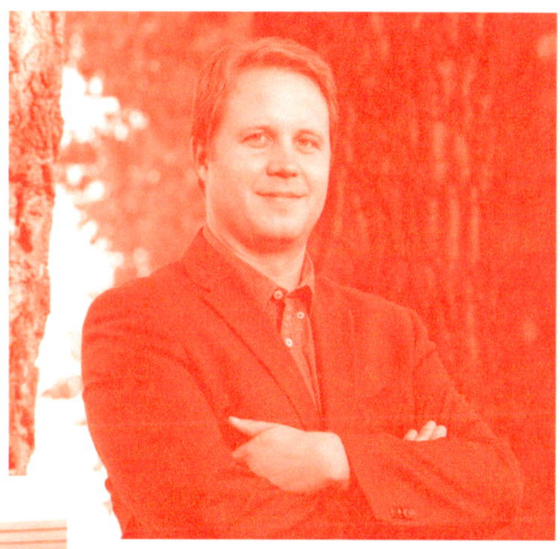

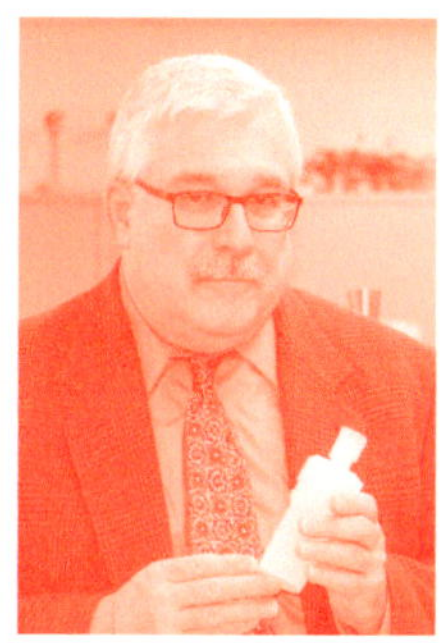

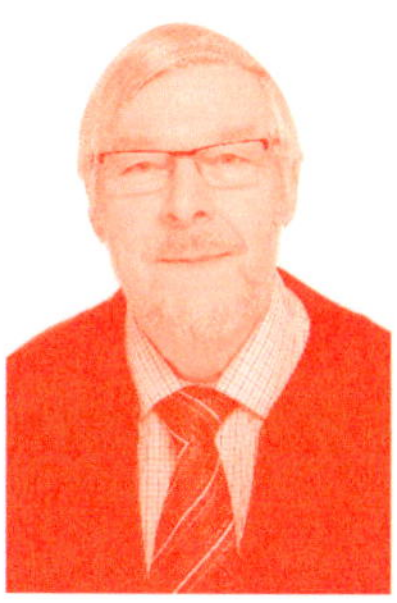

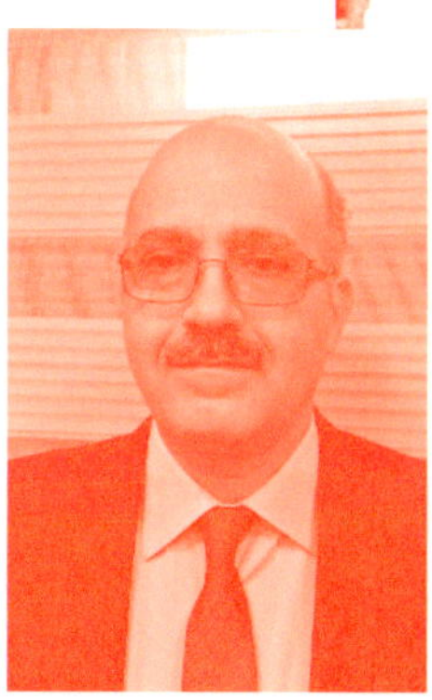

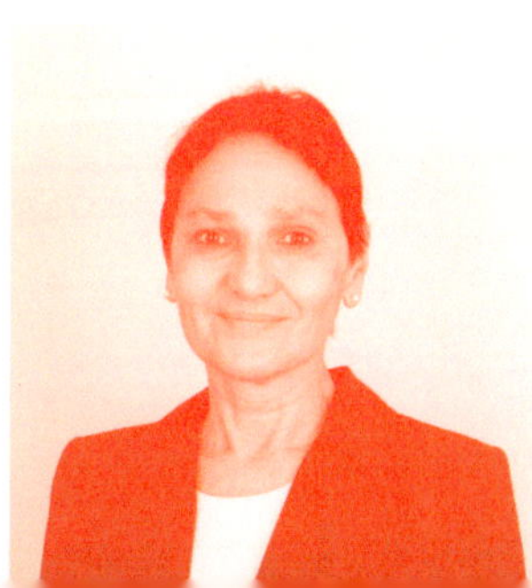

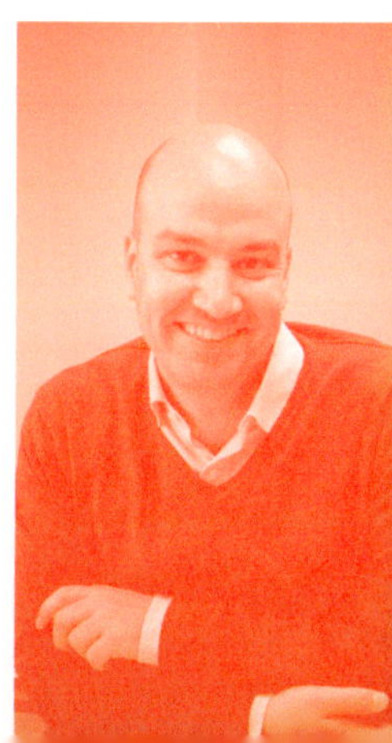

Herbs and Spices - New Processing Technologies
http://dx.doi.org/10.5772/intechopen.95216
Edited by Rabia Shabir Ahmad

Contributors
Nikhat Farhana, Eva Ivanišová, Vikrant Kumar, Deepak Mishra, Mukesh Chandra Joshi, Priyanka Mishra, Megha Tanwar, Prashant Kaushik, Rubi Gupta, Adeyemi Ojutalayo Adeeyo, Mercy Adewumi Alabi, Tshianeo Mellda Ndou, John O. Odiyo, Rachel Makungo, Erinfolami Motunrayo Enitan, Hosana Dumisani Mkoyi, Daniso Beswa, Diego Prado Vásquez, Rasmus Munk, Nabila Rodríguez Valerón, Vinod Kumar Paswan, Chandra Shekhar Singh, Garima Kukreja, Durga Shankar Bunkar, Basant Kumar Bhinchhar, Minoo Divakaran, N.T. Fathima Rafieah, Vinod Kumar Joshi, Apurva Joshi, Santosh Kumar Kar, Sitabja Mukherjee, Mavra Javed, Waqas Ahmed, Abdul Momin Rizwan Ahmad, Rehan Mian, Abebe Ayele Haile, Hency Rose, Yamini S, Aman Rathaur, Rabia Shabir Ahmad, Muhammad Sajid Arshad, Huda Ateeq, Muhammad Abdul Rahim, Muhammad Imran, Muhammad Kamran Khan, Muhammad Haseeb Ahmad, Miroslava Kačániová, Tatsiana A. Savitskaya, Dmitry D. Grinshpan

First published in London, United Kingdom, 2021 by IntechOpen
IntechOpen is the global imprint of INTECHOPEN LIMITED, registered in England and Wales, registration number: 11086078, 5 Princes Gate Court, London, SW7 2QJ, United Kingdom
Printed in Croatia

British Library Cataloguing-in-Publication Data
A catalogue record for this book is available from the British Library

Additional hard and PDF copies can be obtained from orders@intechopen.com

Herbs and Spices - New Processing Technologies
Edited by Rabia Shabir Ahmad
p. cm.
Print ISBN 978-1-83969-608-4
Online ISBN 978-1-83969-609-1
eBook (PDF) ISBN 978-1-83969-610-7

For EU product safety concerns:
IN TECH d.o.o., Prolaz Marije Krucifikse Kozulić 3, 51000 Rijeka, Croatia, info@intechopen.com or visit our website at intechopen.com.

Meet the editor

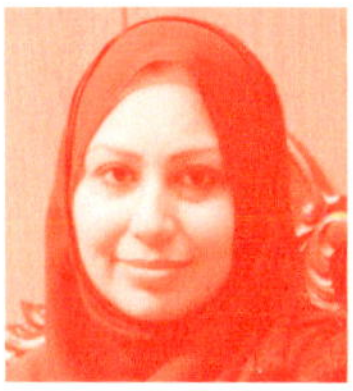

Dr. Rabia Shabir Ahmad has a strong background in academics, teaching, and research. She successfully completed doctoral research funded by the Indigenous Fellowship Program, Higher Education Commission (HEC), Pakistan. During her academic career, Dr. Ahmad was awarded and successfully completed a Start-Up Research Grant Program (SRGP) and National Research Program for Universities (NRPU) project from the HEC as Principal Investigator in the area of functional foods. Along with her teaching and research supervising responsibilities, Dr. Ahmad is also a journal reviewer. She has published numerous research papers in international and national journals and edited several books.

Contents

Preface

This edited volume contains an assortment of research and review articles relating to the latest developments in herbs and spices. Its focus is on plants containing bioactive components and the utilization of novel processing technologies for developing functional products. The book consists of four sections and fourteen chapters written by authors who are highly qualified and dedicated to their research work. Topics discussed include commonly used herbs and spices in food preparations and their therapeutic potential as well as newly developed technologies for adding value to various herbs and spices.

Rabia Shabir Ahmad
Department of Food Science,
Government College University,
Faisalabad, Pakistan

Section 1

Introduction

Chapter 1

Introductory Chapter: Herbs and Spices - An Overview

Rabia Shabir Ahmad, Muhammad Imran, Muhammad Kamran Khan, Muhammad Haseeb Ahmad, Muhammad Sajid Arshad, Huda Ateeq and Muhammad Abdul Rahim

1. Introduction

Herbs and spices have been an essential part in human life for thousands of years that is used at a domestic and industrial level as flavoring, preservation, and coloring agent in nutraceutical, pharmaceutical, and cosmetics products [1]. Spice crop is being affected by insect pests, fungal, and nonpathogenic diseases causing production constraints. Therefore, the quality of spices is very low. For this purpose, agrochemicals are used to improve the quality and production of spices [2].

Most of the known herbs and spices originate from Europe, Africa, and Asian countries. Spices and herbs are obtained from non-woody and flowering plants. Spices are obtained from the dry part of the plant, such as creeping rootstalk, twigs and leaves, fruits, vegetables, nuts, flower buds, whole and ground seeds, and outermost layers of stems and roots, while herbs are always derived from the leaves. Moreover, spices and herbs are playing a significant role in the preparation of new food products. It provides a delectable, distinctive aroma, and taste to food products [3].

Most commonly spices and herbs are used in the preparation of different processing products like pickles, flavor sauces, salad dressings, bakery products, vinegar, beverages, meat products, and sausages. Furthermore, spices and herbs are excellent sources of phenolic and polyphenolic compounds with bioactive functions and phytochemicals [4–7]. Over the past few decades, there has been a significant increase in research into their health benefits, protect the spice crop, and ways to use them in the diet, as many herbs and spices have possessed properties associated with reducing the risk of chronic diseases [8].

2. Classification of spices

The spices and herbs are classified on the basis of botanical analogies or families or parts of the plant. Chili or hot pepper, dry white and black peppercorns, ginger root, mustard seeds, and cilantro belong to the category of hot spices. Aromatic spices include Pimenta, myrtle pepper, *Elettaria*, Chinese cinnamon, *Cinnamomum*, clove, fenugreek, and white and black cumin. Moreover, herbs include estragon, dill weed, Mediterranean herbs, and sweet basil [9]. These spices are most commonly used in the food processing for different purposes on a domestic and large scale [10].

3. Production of quality spices

The production of pest-free, high in quality, and clean spice crops is very important for international globalization. Therefore, organic spice crops are produced that cost 20–50% more than traditionally grown spices. These crops are good in quality, free of pesticides, and chemical residues. Moreover, appropriate agricultural techniques are adopted to reduce pathogens and non-pathogens diseases. In processing industries, quality assurance procedures such as HACCP must be applied as well as suitable packing material and storage practices for maintaining spice quality [11].

3.1 Beneficial microbe

People all over the world are becoming increasingly aware of the health risks associated with eating crops contaminated with pesticides. Every year, it is predicted that a large number of people become ill by the use of pathogen and pest-contaminated spices [12]. Therefore, the promotion of a farming approach that incorporates environmentally sound-evoked plant prevention measures and organic waste management can go a long way toward restoring soil health and lowering pesticide residues in farm products. Various helpful microorganisms, such as propagules, beneficials, and soil bacteria, are playing a significant role in improving the quality of crops and control pathogenic diseases while leaving no chemical residues on plants [13].

3.2 Irradiation process

Radiation processing is used to improve the shelf life of spices and also improve their quality and microbiological safety without altering their inherent flavor characteristics [14]. This method is most commonly used in North America and Europe for imported spices. Major spice-producing countries have also started setting up facilities for radiation processing of spices [15]. On the other hand, irradiated methods such as sterilization, pest control practices, UV irradiation, electron beam irradiation, and microwave irradiation are still widely used all over the world while most are in Asian countries. The delicate scent and flavor ingredients in spices are not affected by using these methods because it is a cold procedure. Irradiating wrapper or container spices has reduced the potential of chemical treatment [16]. High doses of irradiation cannot be assisted to prevent germination in ginger, onions, and other plants as compared to low doses. A medium-dose spray removes harmful bacteria and food microbes, whereas a high dosage application sterilizes food for particular needs and oxidative stability goods without refrigeration as shown in **Table 1** [15, 17].

3.3 Different packaging materials

Spices are hygroscopic in nature, because they are very sensitive to moisture, if they absorb too much moisture, they can cause caking, decolonization, hydrolytic rancidity, mold growth, and insects. Furthermore, heat, light, inadequate packing, and environmental factors are caused by the deterioration of fragrance and flavor components in spices during storage intervals. Therefore, the packaging material for spice packaging should be sterilized and standard so as to reduce contamination during storage [18]. Capsicum, cardamom, turmeric, and saffron contain natural coloring pigments that require light protection. Moreover, spices powders containing highly volatile sulfur compounds, such as onion and garlic, require special

Spices	Irradiation dosage		Reason
	Minimum	Maximum	
Garlic	0.04	0.13	Prevent germination
Shallots (small onion)	0.03	0.14	Prevent germination
Ginger	0.03	0.16	Prevent germination
Onion	0.03	0.08	Prevent germination
Spices	6.2	13.7	High-level sterilization

Table 1.
Radiation dosage for some spices.

protection to prevent flavor loss or absorption [19]. The essential oil components found naturally in most spices are oxidized by oxygen in the air, resulting in off-flavors, especially at high storage temperatures. The factor's effect on spice oils and oleoresins packaged in epoxy-coated metal drums and plastic lab bottles is inhibited. Moreover, aluminum and food containers are utilized for the low-oxidative stability of oils and oleoresins. Polyethylene terephthalate (PET) bottles and food-grade high-molecular-weight high-density polyethylene (HMHDPE) containers are used to store essential oils and oleoresins, which have excellent smell barrier qualities [20, 21]. The pericarp and the natural antioxidants found in it protect most whole spices, so they do not need as much protection as ground spices [22].

3.4 Source of natural colors

A few centuries ago, spices are used to dye food products because they are an excellent source of natural color pigments and safe for humans [23]. For years, the food processing industry has been using synthetic food colorants that increase the risk of many diseases in humans, such as cancer, asthma, allergy, hyperacidity, and hypothyroidism [24]. Nowadays, the food industry is currently returning to natural colorants as a result of changes in laws and customer demand. Natural colors are used sparingly in food processing because of their poor stability (to changes in pH, oxygen, heat, and light), low solubility, off-flavor, and expensive cost. These issues can be solved by employing enzymes, microbes, supercritical carbon dioxide, membrane separation, and microencapsulation methods to improve solubility and stability [25, 26]. Most commonly chili, saffron, turmeric, and others were utilized in Indian dishes before synthetic colors were invented. The food organization has devised a method for producing natural food colors such as kokum (red) and chilies (red). Kokum is a natural color source for acidic food since it contains 2–3% of anthocyanin. Polyisoprenylated chalcone is a fat-soluble yellow component found in the dried skin of the Garcinia indica; hence, it is in food products up to 0.3% level to give a satisfactory color to the product [27–29].

3.4.1 Saffron

Saffron provides a beautiful golden color and nutraceutical properties to a functional food, but it is most commonly used in soups, stews, bread, and rice dishes around the world because of its strong and unique flavor. Saffron is considered a fancy and costly spice, so its use in cuisine is limited. Carotenoids are responsible for the intense color of saffron. Saffron also contains small amounts of alpha- and beta-carotene, lycopene, and zeaxanthin [30–32].

3.4.2 Curcumin

Turmeric is a golden yellow component that is naturally present in curcumin, which is considered a pure color with relatively little flavor. It is not easily dissolved in water; it must be mixed in a solvent with a suspension of tween 80. It dissolves in an acidic pH solution. It appears a strong lemon-yellow color. It is mostly used in a concentration of 5–20 ppm [33, 34]. It is present in two forms such as curcumin powder and oleoresin, both of which are utilized as food coloring and natural food preservatives [35]. It is also used in confectionery, ice cream, and dairy industries as a natural color pigment, as well as other natural colors such as annatto and beetroot red [36].

3.4.3 Paprika

Capsanthin and capsorubin are responsible for their color, which makes up 60% of the total carotenoids in paprika. Some other color components such as carotenoid, lipophilic compound, xanthophyll cycle, the precursor of ABA, and beta-carotene are also present in the paprika. Capsanthin and capsorubin are the essential components found in the skin of paprika. The oleoresin of paprika is orange in color, which is not desired in the worldwide souk because it is insoluble in water and more soluble in lipids. Moreover, oleoresin contains up to 50% of capsorubin. It is most commonly used in confectionery, dairy products, meat products, salad dressings, bakery products, and snacks as a coloring agent [37].

3.5 Spices as sources of natural flavors and essential oils

In previous years, many food industry countries have become more interested in using natural flavors in the preparation of various food products [4]. The major flavor components are found in spices given in **Table 2**.

The oleoresin and oils can be extracted from different spices, as well as the key distinctive components found in the spices. Various methods such as hydrocarbon extraction, separation process, supercritical fluid extraction, pressurized solvent extraction, metabolic process, chemical, and enzymatic treatment process are used

Spice	Flavor compounds
Black	Piperine, S-3 Carene, b-caryophyllene
Chili	Capsaicin, dihydrocapsacin
Allspice	Eugenol, b-caryophyllene
Clove	Eugenol, eugenyl acetate
Mustard	Ally isothiocyanate
Ginger	Gingerol, shogaol, neral, geranial
Saffron	Safranal
Oregano	Carvacrol, thymol
Basil, sweet	Methylchavicol, linalool, methyl eugenol
Spearmint	1-carvone, carvone derivatives
Dill	d-carvone
Cinnamon, cassia	Cinnamaldehyde, eugenol

Table 2.
Flavor profile of spice.

to extract oils and oleoresins from spices [38]. On a commercial basis, supercritical fluid extraction from solid botanicals is currently being used. In this process, protic solvents, monoterpenes, and improved black keys are not produced in essential oils. On the other hand, the biopolishing process and fermentation of raw materials increase the efficiency and quality of extracted essential oil. Moreover, *in vitro* manufacture of lactones, acetone, and further flavoring compounds has recently been achieved using genetic engineering and recombinant DNA technology. Flavorist can also profit from cloning and single-cell culture procedures [39].

4. Function of spices in food products

They are used in food products for various purposes. The antioxidant properties of herbs and spices act as food preservatives against oxidative degradation and also improve the stability of products. The use of herbs and spices as natural preservatives is gaining more attention. Ground black pepper, for example, has been shown to prevent oxidative degradation in processed meat. Antioxidants also help the body to fight cardiovascular disease, some types of cancers (epithelial), and other ailments including arthritis and asthma [22]. Phenolic compounds of black pepper, oregano, thyme, and marjoram are used to protect against heart disease and Crohn's disease. The phenolic compound in ginger is a gingerol that works against intestine intoxication and enhancer of pharmacological activity. Capsaicinoids found in chili peppers are an anti-inflammatory that is utilized in both medicine and nutraceutical. Trigonella foenum-graecum, allium cepa, and allium sativum are all good for lowering cholesterol. Antimicrobial activities have also been discovered in a variety of spices [40].

Author details

Rabia Shabir Ahmad*, Muhammad Imran, Muhammad Kamran Khan, Muhammad Haseeb Ahmad, Muhammad Sajid Arshad, Huda Ateeq and Muhammad Abdul Rahim
Faculty of Life Sciences, Department of Food Science, Government College University, Faisalabad, Punjab, Pakistan

*Address all correspondence to: rabiaahmad@gcuf.edu.pk

References

[1] Dini I. Spices and herbs as therapeutic foods. In: *Food Quality: Balancing Health and Disease*. Cambridge, Massachusetts, United States: Academic Press; 2018. pp. 433-469

[2] Sarma YR, Anandaraj M. Diseases of spice crops and their management. Indian Journal of Arecanut, Spices and Medicinal Plants. 2000;**2**(1):6-20

[3] Peter KV. Handbook of Herbs and Spices. Cambridge, United Kingdom: Woodhead Publishing Limited; 2004

[4] Chi SP, Wu YC. Spices and seasonings. In: *Handbook of Fermented Meat and Poultry*. Hoboken, New Jersey, United States: Wiley-Blackwell, John Wiley & Sons; 2014. pp. 79-88

[5] Embuscado ME. Spices and herbs: Natural sources of antioxidants–A mini review. Journal of Functional Foods. 2015;**18**:811-819

[6] Embuscado ME. Bioactives from culinary spices and herbs: A review. Journal of Food Bioactives. 2019;**6**:68-99

[7] Rathore MS, Shekhawat NS. Incredible spices of India: From traditions to cuisine. American-Eurasian Journal of Botany. 2008;**1**(3):85-89

[8] Jiang TA. Health benefits of culinary herbs and spices. Journal of AOAC International. 2019;**102**(2):395-411

[9] Van Wyk BE. *Culinary Herbs and Spices of the World*. Chicago, Illinois, United States: University of Chicago Press; 2014

[10] Peter, K. V., & Shylaja, M. R. Introduction to herbs and spices: Definitions, trade and applications. In *Handbook of Herbs and Spices*. Cambridge, United Kingdom: Woodhead Publishing Limited; 2012. pp. 1-24

[11] Mellor J. Globalization and the traditional role of agriculture [w:] Trade Reforms and Food Security: Conceptualizing the Linkages. In: *Commodities and Trade Division Food and Agriculture Organization of The United Nations, Rome*. Rome, Italy: Publishing Management Service, FAO division; 2003

[12] Zweifel C, Stephan R. Spices and herbs as source of Salmonella-related foodborne diseases. Food Research International. 2012;**45**(2):765-769

[13] Schweiggert U, Carle R, Schieber A. Conventional and alternative processes for spice production–a review. Trends in Food Science & Technology. 2007;**18**(5):260-268

[14] Sjöberg AM, Manninen M, Pinnioja S, Honkanen E, Latva-Kala K. Irradiation of spices and its detection. Food Reviews International. 1991;**7**(2):233-253

[15] Chmielewski A, Migdał W. Radiation decontamination of herbs and spices. Nukleonika. 2005;**50**(4):179-184

[16] Chauhan SK, Kumar R, Nadanasabapathy S, Bawa AS. Detection methods for irradiated foods. Comprehensive Reviews in Food Science and Food Safety. 2009;**8**(1):4-16

[17] SádECká J. Irradiation of spices–A review. Czech Journal of Food Sciences. 2007;**25**(5):231-242

[18] Voelker AL, Sommer AA, Mauer LJ. Moisture sorption behaviors, water activity-temperature relationships, and physical stability traits of spices, herbs, and seasoning blends containing crystalline and amorphous ingredients. Food Research International. 2020;**136**:109608

[19] King K. Packaging and storage of herbs and spices. In: *Handbook of Herbs*

and Spices. Cambridge, United Kingdom: Woodhead Publishing Limited; 2006. pp. 86-102

[20] Herath LSR. *Development and Evaluation of Low Density Polyethylene-Based Antimicrobial Food Packaging Films Containing Natural Agents* (Doctoral dissertation. Australia: Victoria University; 2010

[21] Peter, K. V. (Ed.). *Handbook of Herbs and Spices*. Cambridge, United Kingdom: Woodhead Publishing Limited, Elsevier; 2012

[22] Yashin A, Yashin Y, Xia X, Nemzer B. Antioxidant activity of spices and their impact on human health: A review. Antioxidants. 2017a;**6**(3):70

[23] Jessica Elizabeth DLT, Gassara F, Kouassi AP, Brar SK, Belkacemi K. Spice use in food: Properties and benefits. Critical Reviews in Food Science and Nutrition. 2017;**57**(6):1078-1088

[24] Sadar P, Dande P, Kulkami N, Pachori R. Evaluation of toxicity of synthetic food colors on human normal flora and yeast. International Journal of Health Sciences and Research. 2017;**7**:110-114

[25] Galaffu N, Bortlik K, Michel M. An industry perspective on natural food colour stability. In: *Colour Additives for Foods and Beverages*. Cambridge, United Kingdom: Woodhead Publishing Limited; 2015. pp. 91-130

[26] Rodriguez-Amaya DB. Natural food pigments and colorants. Current Opinion in Food Science. 2016;**7**:20-26

[27] Houghton JD, Hendry GAF. *Natural food Colorants*. Berlin, Heidelberg, Germany: Springer Science & Business Media; 2012

[28] Kumar V. Seven spices of India—From kitchen to clinic. Journal of Ethnic Foods. 2020;**7**(1):1-16

[29] Ravindran PN, Johny AK, Nirmal BK. Spices in our daily life. Satabdi Smaranika. 2002;**2**:102-105

[30] Cardone L, Castronuovo D, Perniola M, Cicco N, Candido V. Saffron (Crocus sativus L.), the king of spices: An overview. *Scientia Horticulturae*. 2020;**272**:109560

[31] De Monte, C., & Cesa, S. (2021). Use of saffron as a functional food and saffron nutraceuticals. In *Saffron* (pp. 241-273). Cambridge , Massachusetts, United States: Academic Press

[32] Gohari AR, Saeidnia S, Mahmoodabadi MK. An overview on saffron, phytochemicals, and medicinal properties. Bangalore, India: Pharmacognosy Reviews. 2013;**7**(13):61

[33] Chaitanya Lakshmi G. Food coloring: The natural way. Res J Chem Sci. 2014;**2231**(8):606X

[34] Henry BS. Natural food colours. In: *Natural Food Colorants*. Boston, MA: Springer; 1996. pp. 40-79

[35] Abdeldaiem MH. Use of yellow pigment extracted from turmeric (Curcuma longa) rhizomes powder as natural food preservative. American Journal of Food Science and Technology. 2014;**2**(1):36-47

[36] Manoharan A, Ramasamy D, Dhanalashmi B, Gnanalashmi KS, Thyagarajan D. Studies on sensory evaluation of Curcumin powder as natural color for butterscotch flavor ice cream. Indian J Drugs Dis. 2012;**1**(1):2278-2958

[37] Peter, K. V. (Ed.). *Handbook of Herbs and Spices: Volume 3*. Woodhead publishing; 2006

[38] Roohinejad S, Koubaa M, Barba FJ, Leong SY, Khelfa A, Greiner R, et al. Extraction methods of essential oils from herbs and spices. In: Essential Oils

in Food Processing. Chichester, UK: John Wiley & Sons, Ltd; 2017. pp. 21-55

[39] Darriet A. Herbs, spices and essential oils. In: Handbook of Food Products Manufacturing. New York: Wiley; 2007. pp. 205-220

[40] Kurian A. Health benefits of herbs and spices. In: *Handbook of Herbs and Spices*. Woodhead Publishing; 2012. pp. 72-88

Section 2

Therapeutic Prospectives

Chapter 2

Medicinal Herbs: Important Source of Bioactive Compounds for Food Industry

Eva Ivanišová, Miroslava Kačániová, Tatsiana A. Savitskaya and Dmitry D. Grinshpan

Abstract

Medicinal herbs accompany people throughout life – from birth to the grave. Almost every day they come to our table as a part of food in various forms, many are used for technical and bioenergetics purposes, and there is also a large group of plants used in medicine, pharmacy and food industry. In the last decade, the consumption of herbs and spices has increased. They grow spontaneously and free of chemical additives, and some studies have shown higher nutritional value, often more significant compared to other common food plants. Medicinal herbs become increasingly important due to its potential beneficial health effects related to its nutritional composition, such as the presence of vitamins, phenolic, anthocyanins, flavonoids, tannins, among others. These raw materials are considered to be promising, economically and ecologically advantageous for the food industry. In this chapter will be describe selected medicinal herbs from *Lamiaceae* family – bioactive compounds and possibility for using in food industry.

Keywords: herbs, spices, food technology, bioactive compounds

1. Introduction

Medicinal herbs have been used for many centuries especially in traditional folk medicine. Plants are very good source of bioactive compounds for functions including activity to inhibit insects, antimicrobial and antifungal activity and positive effects for animals and humans. Several groups of phytochemicals with biological activity have been identified in medicinal plants – polyphenols, natural colorants, essential oils, mineral compounds, vitamins and many others [1]. Humans have a long tradition for using medicinal and aromatic plants in their lifestyle [2]. Culinary herbs are primarily used for enhancing the flavor of foods including meats, milk products, sauces, vegetables, cereal products and desserts. They can be used as a replacement for salt and sugars, colorants and flavorings agents [3].

The main bioactive compounds presented in medicinal and culinary herbs are polyphenols (especially phenolic acids and flavonoids). These compounds are well known for their biological activity such as anticancer, antioxidant, antimicrobial, neuroprotective, antidiabetic, cardio protective and many others positive effect to human body. It is important to determine their safe intake and dosage in health, gastronomy and food industry [3, 4].

The cooking methods in gastronomy include baking, frying, boiling, roasting, steaming and use of microwave ovens can enhance the textural and sensory properties of the food material but can cause chemical changing of natural phytochemicals especially polyphenols. The amount of phenolic compounds can decrease due to water-soluble phenols loosing during the cooking water and it can be visible also structural changes of these compounds that occurs during cooking process. In addition, thermal processes also produce new bioactive compounds by the Maillard and carbonyl-amine reactions [5].

Prevention of food products from chemical, physical and microbial damages has been a vital concern in the food industry. Nowadays, consumers are interesting for partial or complete substitution of chemical agents due to their possible negative health effects. These benefits has guide to an increasing consciousness in developing more friendly and natural label on processed foods. Incorporation of fresh, dried and powdered medicinal and culinary herbs to foods can enhanced sensory properties, technological properties and increase amount of bioactive compounds in these products [6].

In this chapter are summarized medicinal herbs (spices) as important source of bioactive compounds for food industry especially kinds from *Lamiaceae* family: oregano (*Origanum vulgare* L.), sage (*Salvia officinalis* L.), lavender (*Lavandula angustifolia* L.), mint (*Mentha piperita* L.), lemon balm (*Melissa officinalis* L.) and rosemary (*Rosmarinus officinalis* L.). The family of *Lamiaceae* consists of about 230 genera and 7100 species worldwide. Many species from this family are considered of high importance because of their uses in medicine, culinary, cosmetics, smoking, production of essential oils, repellents, fragrances and charm [7].

2. Oregano (*Origanum vulgare* L.)

Oregano (*Origanum vulgare* L.) is an aromatic, perennial herb with hairy stem, creeping roots, branched woody stems, up to 50 cm high, oval leaves. The flowers are in corymbs with reddish bracts, a two-lipped pale purple corolla and a five-toothed calyx. It grows in arid, sunny meadows and rocky places, widely distributed in Europe and Asia, especially in the Mediterranean region. In moderate climates, the flowering period extends from late June to August. Each flower produces, when mature, four small seed-like structures. The foliage is dotted with small glands containing the volatile or essential oil that gives the plant its aroma and flavor [8, 9]. Oregano is rich for γ-terpinene, p-cymene, thymol and carvacrol methyl ethers, thymol and carvacrol acetates; also compounds such as p-cymenene, p-cymen-8-ol, p-cymen-7-ol; thymoquinone and thymohydroquinone are also present [9]. Oregano contains significant amounts of the vitamin E, especially α,β,γ, and δ-tocopherol, which are involved with the antioxidant capacity. In fresh leaves are presence 45 mg of vitamin C, 0.07 mg of thiamine, 0.81 mg carotene also higher values of B_6, riboflavin, niacin, folate panthotenate and biotin. From mineral compounds are dominant iron, copper, sulfur, iodine, selenium, calcium (310 mg in fresh leaves), magnesium (53 mg in fresh leaves), phosphor (39 mg in fresh leaves), zinc (0.9 mg in fresh leaves) and manganese (0.3 mg in fresh leaves). Amount of potassium is 33 times higher than sodium [10]. Flavonoids – apigenin, luteolin, quercetin, scutellarein and phenolic acids – mainly rosmarinic acid are the main types of phenolic compounds present in oregano [11].

Oregano has ability to increase appetite in human tomato dressing in a pasta meal seasoned with 0.27% of oregano increased the palatability and the intake of food compared with an unseasoned control food. But concentration of oregano is very important – doubling the amount reduced the food intake and eating rate [10].

The dried light green leaves are available whole, flaked or ground. Essential oil is obtained by steam distillation of the dried flowering herb. The oil is a yellow to dark-brown mobile liquid, yield 1–2%. Aroma of oregano is strongly, camphoraceous. Flavor is slightly bitter and pungent, musty, hay and minty notes [2]. Oregano as raw material as well as oregano essential oil is used in meat, sausages, salads, stewings, dressings, soups, alcoholic beverages, baked goods, meats and meat products, condiments and relishes, milk products, processed vegetables, snack foods, and fats and oils. It is the most common spice for pizza. Addition of 5% dry oregano powder increase antioxidant activity (DPPH method – 36.28 mg TEAC/g – TEAC Trolox equivalent antioxidant capacity), total polyphenol (288.46 mg GAE/g – GAE – gallic acid equivalent) and total ash content (0.77%) of Linz biscuits with compare to control variant without addition (DPPH – 3.10 mg TEAC/g; 86.01 mg GAE/g; 0.71%). These biscuits were also very good evaluated from sensory point of view [12]. Oregano is a common ingredient of dressings and a good substitute for table salt. It increases aroma of vegetable dishes as pea soup and other pea dishes, squash and stews made from mixed vegetables, mushrooms and asparagus. Oregano essential oil can be added into edible films in order to prolong the shelf-life of sliced bread and bakery products, due to the antimicrobial activity against some foodborne pathogenic and spoilage microorganism. The oregano essential oil could be used as supplementation on a lamb diet, improving the antioxidant activity which had influence on retarding the lipid meat oxidation during refrigerated and long-term frozen storage. This process could be explained by carvacrol and thymol action on the permeability off cell membrane and by the transformation of lipid and hydroxyl radicals into stable products [9, 13].

3. Sage (*Salvia officinalis* L.)

Sage (*Salvia officinalis* L.) is a plant from *Lamiaceae* family and can be found in Europe around the Mediterranean, in Southeast Asia, and Central and South America. This plant grows in the form of an outcrossing, perennial evergreen subshrub up to 80 cm high. The leaves are opposite silver oval, shiny, covered with fine hairs and large attractive violet flowers 2–4 mm long from the pedicel. They bloom from March to July depending on habitat and climatic condition [2, 14]. The major phenolic acids in sage are rosmarinic acid, caffeic acid and its derivatives, salvianolic acids, sagernic acid and lithospermic acids. From flavonoids are dominant hispidulin, luteolin 7-O-glucoside, apigenin, cirsimaritin, kaempferol and quercetin. The major constituent in essential oil are α-thujone (15–43%), β-thujone (3–9%), camphor (4–24%), 1,8-cineol (10%) camphene, α-pinene, β-pinene, limonene, α-humulene, β-caryophyllene and borneol. The oil is clear, colorless to pale yellow mobile liquid, with yield 2–3.6%. From mineral compounds are dominant in dry matter of sage leaves potassium (14.9 g/kg), calcium (10.1 g/kg), magnesium (4.1 g/kg), iron (885 ppm), zinc (145 ppm), sodium (91 ppm), manganese (52.7 ppm) and copper (6.9 ppm) [15]. The most abounding carbohydrates described in this plant are arabinose, galactose, glucose, mannose, xylose, uronic acids and rhamnose. One teaspoon (0.7 g) of ground sage contains 10% of the reference daily intake of vitamin K and 1.1% of vitamin B_6 [2, 16].

Salvia has long been known for its culinary values, and it also has the potential to be used as a natural preservative in food applications. Leaves are strongly aromatic, sweet, herbaceous, and spicy. The taste is bitter, fragrant warm and astringent. The young leaves and flowers can be eaten raw, boiled, pickled or used in sandwiches. The flowers can also be sprinkled on salads to add color and fragrance. Yang leaves are eaten fresh in salads and cooked in omelets, fritters, soups, yeast breads and rolls, marinades, sausages, meat pies, and poultry stuffing. They are also used in cooking with liver, beef, pork, veal, lamb, fish, poultry, duck, goose, artichokes, tomatoes, asparagus, carrots, squash, corn, potatoes, eggplant, beans, leeks, onions, cabbage and lentils. Sage tea is made from the fresh or dried leaves, it is said to improve the digestion. An essential oil obtained from the plant is used commercially to flavor ice cream, sweets, and bakery products [2, 17]. Addition of 5% dry sage powder increase antioxidant activity (DPPH method – 38.16 mg TEAC/g – TEAC Trolox equivalent antioxidant capacity), total polyphenol (250.29 mg GAE/g – GAE – gallic acid equivalent) and total ash content (0.76%) of Linz biscuits with compare to control variant without addition (DPPH – 3.10 mg TEAC/g; 86.01 mg GAE/g; 0.71%). These biscuits were also very good evaluated from sensory point of view, especially spicy-bitter taste and aftertaste [12]. Several researches have shown that sage efficacy is comparable to that of synthetic preservatives and can thus be used in as a natural preservative. Consequently, sage have potential to be as antioxidants and against spoilage microorganisms such as *Pseudomonas aeruginosa* and *Bacillus cereus* strains. Sage essential oil (0.05–0.1 μL/g) exhibited activity against microbial growth in fresh pork sausages to improve the safety of the meat product during storage. The addition of this essential oil reduced the microbial growth in fresh pork sausages and it had no negative effect on sensory properties of this meat product at 0.05 μL/g [17]. The whey protein concentrate coating incorporated with 4000 ppm of sage extracts on pistachio kernels inhibited *Aspargillus flavus* growth totally [18]. Due to antioxidant and antibacterial properties sage essential oil and sage ethanol extracts may be recommended as an auxiliary factor to prolong the storage stability of frozen, vacuum-packed low-pressure mechanically separated meat from chickens [19].

4. Lavender (*Lavandula angustifolia* L.)

Lavender (*Lavandula angustifolia*, L.), is an evergreen perennial plant native to the Mediterranean region but grown in many other countries of the world, including Slovakia. Lavender grows to a height of 40–60 cm and forms compact, regular clumps. The lower part of stem is woody, while the upper part is green, leaves are linear or lanceolate with curled edges and a highly branched fibrous root system. Silver-green lavender leaves are covered with tomentum, which protects them from strong sunshine, wind, and excessive water loss. The pale violet flowers grow in spikes, arranged in circles (3–5 flowers per circle) in the top part of the stem [2, 20]. Lavender contains anthocyanins, phytosterols, sugars, coumaric acid, glycolic acid, valeric acid, ursolic acid, herniarin, coumarin and tannins (5–10%). Essential oil (1–3%) containing more than 100 constituents including linalyl acetate, linalool, *cis*- and *trans*-β-ocimene, terpinen-4-ol, lavandulol, lavandulyl acetate, 1,8-cineole, limonene. From mineral compounds is possible to find in dry matter of lavender leaves potassium (17.7–23.9 g/kg), calcium (2.13–10.5 g/kg), magnesium (1.40–3.60 g/kg), sodium (0.11–0.15 g/kg), zinc (23–106.27 mg/kg), copper (7.2–11.1 mg/kg) and manganese (9.6–18 mg/kg) [2, 20, 21].

Lavender has a very floral fruity and herbaceous aroma. It has a sweet, floral refreshing, pleasant balsamic-woody undertone. Lavender flowers in the food industry are used as a natural flavoring for beverages, ice cream, candy, chocolates, bakery products, vinegars, sparingly in salads, syrup and jellies. They are used in baked goods, soft candy, gelatin, frozen dairy, pudding, and alcoholic and nonalcoholic beverages. Lavender essential oil could be used as a growth promoter in broiler nutrition with potential improvements in breast meat quality [2, 22]. Addition of lavender in amount 0.1–1% prolonged shelf life of hamsi kaygana (traditional food in the Black Sea Region of Turkey), and confirmed that this products can be transported to wider markets, by increasing its durability and longer-term preservation and easy transportation with different packaging techniques [23]. Addition of 5% dry lavender powder increase antioxidant activity (DPPH method – 19.33 mg TEAC/g – TEAC Trolox equivalent antioxidant capacity), total polyphenol (146.35 mg GAE/g – GAE – gallic acid equivalent) and total ash content (1.17%) of Linz biscuits with compare to control variant without addition (DPPH – 3.10 mg TEAC/g; 86.01 mg GAE/g; 0.71%). These biscuits were also very good evaluated from sensory point of view, especially flower taste and aftertaste [12].

5. Mint (*Mentha piperita* L.)

Mentha is a genus belonging to the family of *Lamiaceae*, whose plants are among the most aromatic and spread in diverse environments worldwide. The plant is indigenous to Europe and widespread in cultivation throughout all regions of the world. It is found wild occasionally with its parent species. It is an invasive species in Australia, the Galapagos Islands, New Zealand and United State. Mint has simple, characteristic leaves with pleasant scent. Mint is a perennial hardy branched plant with bright green, lance shaped sharply toothed leaves, quickly spreading underground runners and white flowers clustered in the form of spikes. Leaves are sessile, lanceolate, or ovate-lanceolate, smooth above and glandular below. The flowers are sharply pointed, long and narrow. The plant is from 25 to 75 cm high [2, 23, 24]. Mint contains menthyl acetate (2–11%), isomenthone (2–8%), essential oils (yield 1–3%) composed of menthol (33–60%), menthone (15–32%), eucalyptol (5–13%), menthofuran (1–10%), limonene (1–7%), menthyl acetate (5%), isomenthone, menthofuran and piperitone. The oil is pale yellow to pale olive-green mobile liquid. Leaves contain 19–23% of polyphenols, which include iriocitrin and rosmarinic acid (59–67%), luteolin 7-orutinoside (7–12%), hesperidin (6–10%), rutin, caffeic, chlorogenic acid; betaine, choline, tannins, α- and γ-tocopherols and α- and β-carotenes [2, 25]. From mineral compounds is dominant calcium (255 ppm), sodium (147 ppm), potassium (15.56 ppm), magnesium (3.9 ppm), iron (2.03 ppm), copper (0.88 ppm), zinc (0.79 ppm), selenium (0.26 ppm), and cobalt (0.25 ppm) [26]. In 100 g of fresh leaf is present approximately 31.8 mg of vitamin C, 0.129 mg of vitamin B6 and 212 μg_RAE (retinol activity equivalents) [2].

Mint has strongly mentholic, herbaceous, very aromatic and cooling aroma. Taste is spicy, minty cool, sweet, fragrant and slightly pungent. Aftertaste is herbaceous, minty and cooling. The presence of essential oils in the leaves and other parts of the plants gives it a very appealing aroma. It is the most widely used herb. Mint is a popular flavor found in desserts, beverages, baked goods, ice cream, liquors, sauces, confectionary, candies, and after dinner mints. The crushed leaves can be used in jellies, beverages, sherbets, soups, sauces, stew, meat fish and vegetables. The oil is used to flavor chewing gum, candy, and mints [2, 27]. The mint leaves can be used as an effective novel nutritional bio-agent up to 15 g/kg to improve the performance of broiler chicks, mainly due to its active component [28]. Replacement of 50% of nitrite with mint essential oil is a good approach in order to put down harmful effects of nitrite in sausage and to enhance functionality of the product [29]. Mint may be used to modify microbial fermentation of milk with the intention of producing dairy products with higher antioxidant and enhanced anti-ACE activities (angiotensin-1 converting enzyme) [30].

Addition of 5% dry mint powder increase antioxidant activity (DPPH method – 54.51 mg TEAC/g – TEAC Trolox equivalent antioxidant capacity), total polyphenol (258.20 mg GAE/g – GAE – gallic acid equivalent) and total ash content (0.8%) of Linz biscuits with compare to control variant without addition (DPPH – 3.10 mg TEAC/g; 86.01 mg GAE/g; 0.71%). These biscuits were also very good evaluated from sensory point of view, especially minty cool taste and aftertaste [12].

6. Lemon balm (*Melissa officinalis* L.)

Lemon balm, member of the family *Lamiaceae* is a perennial bushy plant and is upright, reaching a height of about 1 m with square stems. The soft, hairy leaves are 2 to 8 cm long and either heart-shaped. The leaf surface is coarse and deeply veined, and the leaf edge is scalloped or toothed. The flowers, white or yellowish are in loose; small bunches from the axils of the leaves and bloom from June to October. The flower consists of five fused sepals, five petals, two or four stamens, and four lobed ovaries. The seeds are very small, ovate, dark brown, or black in color. The plant dies down in winter, but the root is perennial [2, 31, 32]. The leaf of *Melissa officinalis* contains flavonoids (quercitrin, rhamnocitrin, luteolin), polyphenolic compounds (rosmarinic acid, caffeic acid and protocatechuic acid), monoterpenoid aldehyde, monoterpene glycosides, triterpenes (ursolic and oleanolic acids), sesquiterpenes, tannins, resin and essential oils (0.1 average, with citral-geraniol and neral, linalool, eugenol, citronellal, geraniol) [12].

Lemon balm has a sweet, lemon, fresh aroma, fresh lemony, sweet taste with a slightly mint hint. The oil has a very pleasant fresh sweet lemony aroma. The aromatic balm leaves are often used in beverages and as a seasoning in salads, dressings and sauces, as well as in cooked foods, in soups and stews. The leaves goes well with teas, vinegars, stewed fruits, jellies, puddings, and custards. It can be added to fish, poultry, eggs [2, 27]. Addition of 5% dry lemon balm powder increase antioxidant activity (DPPH method – 48.24 mg TEAC/g – TEAC Trolox equivalent antioxidant capacity), total polyphenol (227.39 mg GAE/g – GAE – gallic acid equivalent) and total ash content (1.16%) of Linz biscuits with compare to control variant without addition (DPPH – 3.10 mg TEAC/g; 86.01 mg GAE/g; 0.71%). These biscuits were also very good evaluated from sensory point of view, especially lemon taste, aroma and aftertaste [12]. Lemon balm powder (0.1, 0.5 and 1% addition) had positive effects on sensory evaluation of hamburger patties. The pH of all patties decreased with longer storage period. The 2-thiobarbituric acid value, volatile basic nitrogen content, and the total microbial counts of hamburger patties with 1% of lemon balm powder addition were lower, compared to those of the control group without addition of lemon balm powder. Lemon balm powder in hamburger patties had significantly delayed lipid peroxidation [33]. The beer enriched with lemon balm had a pleasant appealing and harmonious flavor and aroma [34]. The pig's diet with 100 ml of lemon balm per day for 10 days before slaughter had significant influence of lemon balm extract on drip loss 24 h post mortem in comparison with control pigs was observed. This extract also improved significantly lightness and yellowness of fresh pork (24 h). The extract improved significantly antioxidative stability in 5-days stored pork [35].

7. Rosemary (*Rosmarinus officinalis* L.)

Rosmarinus officinalis L. is a medicinal plant that belongs to the *Lamiaceae* family and is commonly known as rosemary. Besides the culinary uses due to the characteristic aroma, this plant is also widely employed by indigenous populations, where it grows wild. Rosemary is woody, evergreen perennial small shrub up to 2 m high. It has branched, and narrow leaves that are bright green above, with rolled-in margins and densely hairy below. The branches are rigid and the stem is square, woody, and brown. The flowers are small, pale purple or bluish and appear in cymose inflorescence. This is herb originates from Mediterrean region [2, 36]. The active constituents include essential oil up to 2.5%. Composition of oils is as follows: *alph*a-pinene 12%, *beta*-pinene, camphene 22%, mycrene 1.5%, *alpha*-phellandrene, limonene 0.5–1%, *alpha*- and *y*-terpinene, paracyme-ne 2%, *bet*a-caryophyllene 3%, linalool 0.5–1% terpine-1ol-4, a-terpineol 1.5%, borneol 3–5%, isoborneol, *cis*-thuy-anol-4, *trans*-thuyanol-4, *p*-cymene-8-ol, bornyl-actate, a-phenchyl-actate, 1,8-cineol 30%, caryophylline-ox-ide, humulene-epoxide I and II, 3-hexanon, methyl-heptenon, camphor 30%, verbenon, carvon 0.4%. The oil is clear, colorless to pale yellow mobile liquid. In leaves are phenolic acids (rosmarinic, chlorogenic and caffeic), bitter diterpenes (carnosol, carnosic acid, rosmanol), triterpens (oleanic and ursolic acid), triterpene alcohols (α-amyrin, β-amyrin, betulin), as well as several flavonoids and their glycosides (diosmetin, luteolin, genkwanin) [2, 37]. In 100 g of dried rosemary is possible to find 1280 mg of calcium, 61.2 mg of vitamin C, 1.74 mg of vitamin B_6 and 156 μg RAE (retinol activity equivalents) [2].

Rosemary has sweet and fresh, fragrant, slightly eucalyptus-like aroma and is slightly camphoraceous, minty, balsamic undertones and fresh, bittersweet flavor. The taste is somewhat peppery, spicy, warming and herbaceous with bitter and camphoraceous aftertaste. Rosemary is a popular flavoring for meat and meat products, baked goods and Mediterranean recipes. Fresh or dried leaves can be used for special accent with cream soups made of leafy greens, poultry, stew, and sauces. The leaves and flowering tops are used in lamb roast, mutton preparations, fish dishes, marinades, bouquet garni, with baked fish, rice, salads, occasionally with eggs preparations, dumplings, apples, summer wine cups, and fruit cordials, and in vinegar and oil. Dries leaves and extractives are used to season fried chicken, salad croutons, baked products, confections, and nonalcoholic beverages [2, 27]. Rosemary extract (350 ppm) was very effective antioxidant on quality and stability of ground chicken meat and comparable to the other commercial antioxidants, so can be a good substitution to many synthetic antioxidants used in meat industry [38]. Results showed that tri-methylamine-nitrogen value of rosemary extract and vitamin E treated samples of fried fillets of Nile tilapia were significantly lower than those of the control samples without rosemary extract [39]. Results revealed that rosemary extract retarded oxidative changes in chilling and frozen fried fillets of Nile tilapia whereas rosemary extract 0.1%, 0.2% and vitamin E 0.1% were not as effective as rosemary extract 0.3% on oxidative stability. The modeling results showed that soluble phenolic content in yogurt increased with increasing the concentration of rosemary extract mixed with skim milk and strongly correlated with antioxidant activity and decreased over the same time period. Apparent viscosity does not affect as concentration supplemented. The use of rosemary extract as a natural antioxidant could increase the shelf life of dairy products by inhibiting oxidation. A more thorough understanding of the mechanisms of lipid auto-oxidation in milk may lead to a better understanding of how added natural antioxidants, such as rosemary oleoresin, can help inhibit such oxidation and sensory changes in milk and dairy products. Rosemary antioxidants are in most applications more effective than vitamin E (synthetic), BHA (butylated hydroxyanisole), BHT (butylated hydroxytoluene), TBHQ (tertiary butylhydroquinone) and others. A new application for rosemary-derived antioxidant, extend the shelf life of milk powder and other dairy products [40, 41].

8. Conclusions

Medicinal herbs are most often defined as any part of a plant that is used in the diet for its aromatic properties. Recently, however, herbs have also been identified as sources of various phytochemicals, many of which possess important biological activity which is interesting for different kind of industry; nowadays very important and big interest of medicinal herbs can be visible in food technology. In this chapter are summarized selected kinds of medicinal herbs especially from Lamiaceae family (oregano, sage, lavender, mint, lemon balm and rosemary). Chapter described botanical characteristics, bioactive compounds, sensory properties (aroma, taste), using in gastronomy as well as food industry especially for producing food with added value. Development of food products enriched by medicinal herbs will continue to grow through the 21st century as consumer demand for healthful products.

Acknowledgements

This publication was supported by the project: The formulation of novel compositions and properties study of the polysaccharides based edible films and coatings with antimicrobial and antioxidant plant additives SK-BY-RD-19-0014.

Conflict of interest

The author declares no conflicts of interest.

Author details

Eva Ivanišová[1*], Miroslava Kačániová[2], Tatsiana A. Savitskaya[3] and Dmitry D. Grinshpan[4]

1 Faculty of Biotechnology and Food Sciences, Slovak University of Agriculture in Nitra, Nitra, Slovakia

2 Faculty of Horticulture and Landscape Engineering, Slovak University of Agriculture in Nitra, Nitra, Slovakia

3 Faculty of Chemistry, Belarusian State University, Minsk, Republic Belarus

4 Research Institute for Physical Chemical Problems, Belarusian State University, Minsk, Republic Belarus

*Address all correspondence to: eva.ivanisova@uniag.sk

References

[1] Awuchi ChG. Medicinal plants: The medical, food and nutritional biochemistry and uses. International Journal of Advanced Academic, Research, Science, Technology and Engineering. 2019;5;220-241.

[2] Charles DJ. Antioxidant properties of spices, herbs and other sources. New York: Springer;2013. 610 p.

[3] Opara EL, Chohan M. Culinary herbs and spices: their bioactive properties, the contribution of polyphenols and the challenges in deducing their true health benefits. International Journal of Molecular Science. 2014;15;19183-19202.

[4] Liberal Á, Fernandez Á, Polyzos N, Petropolus SA, Dias M, Pinela J, Petrović J, Soković M, Ferreira ICFR, Barros L. Bioactive properties and phenolic compound profiles of turnip-rooted, plain-leafed and curly-leafed parsley cultivars. Molecules, 2020;85;55-66. DOI: 10.3390/molecules25235606

[5] Zhao Ch, Liu Y, Lai S, Cao H, Guan Y, Cheang WS, Liu B, Zhao K, Miai S, Riviere C, Capanoglu E, Xiao J. Effects of domestic cooking process on the chemical and biological properties of dietary phytochemicals. Trends in Food Science and Technology.2019;85;55-66. DOI: org/10.1016/j.tifs.2019.01.004

[6] Senay TL. Systematic review on spices and herbs used in food industry. American Journal of Ethnomedicine. 2020;7;1-10. DOI: 10.36648/2348-9502.7.1.20

[7] Abdelkader M, Ahcen B, Rachid D, Hakim H. Phytochemical study and biological activity of sage (*Salvia officinalis* L.). International Journal of Bioengineering and Life Science. 2014;8;1253-1257.

[8] Ličina B, Stefaković OD, VasiĆ SM, Radojević ID, Dekić MS, Čomić LR. Biological activities of the extracts from wild growing *Origanum vulgare* L. Food Control. 2013;33;498-504. DOI: org/10.1016/j.foodcont.2013.03.020

[9] Peter KV. Handbook of herbs and spices. USA: CRC Press;2004. 376 p.

[10] Kintzios SE. Oregano. The genera *Origanum* and *Lippia*. London: CRC Press;2002. 296 p.

[11] Gutiérrez-Grijalva EP, Salapicos-Salas M, Leyva-López N, Criollo-Mendola M, Vazquez-Olivo G, Heredia JB. Flavonoids and phenolic acids from oregano: occurrence, biological activity and health benefits. Plants. 2018;7;1-10. DOI: 10.3390/plants7010002

[12] Chis MS, Muste S, Paucean A, Man S, Sturza A, Petrut GS, Muresan A. A comprehensive review about antimicrobial effects of herb and oil oregano (*Origanum vulgare* sp. *hirtum*). Hop and Medicinal Plants. 2017;25;17-27.

[13] Ivanišová E, Krajger E, Bojňanská T. Nutrition profile of biscuits with medicinal herbs. Materials of 4rd International Scientific Practical Conference Innovative Technologies in Bakery Production. 2020; 76-79.

[14] Jakovljević M, Jokić S, Molnar M, Jašić M, Babić J, Jukić H, Banjari I. Bioactive profile of various *Salvia officinalis* L. preparations. Plants. 2019;8;1-30. DOI: 10.3390/plants8030055.

[15] European Medicines Agency. Assessment report on *Salvia officinalis* L. folium and *Salvia officinalis* L. aetheroleum. [Internet]. 2010;39. Available: https://www.ema.europa.eu/en/documents/herbal-report/final-assessment-report-salvia-

officinalis-l-folium-salvia-officinalis-l-aetheroleum-revision-1_en.pdf

[16] Ghorbani A, Esmaeilizadeh M. Pharmacological properties of *Salvia officinalis* and its compounds. Journal of Traditional and Complementary Medicine. DOI: 2017;7;433-440. org/10.1016/j.jtcme.2016.12.014

[17] Sharifi-Rad M, Ozcelik B, Altin G, Daskaya-Dikmen C, Martorell M, Ramírec-Alarcón K, Alarcón-Zapata P, Morais-Braga MFB, Carneiro JNP, Leal ALAB, Countinho HDM, Gyawali R, Tahergorabi R, Ibrahim SA, Sahrifi-Rad R, Shropou F, Salehi B, Contreras MM, Sharifi-Rad J. *Salvia* spp. plants-from farm to food applications and phytopharmaco therapy. Trends in Food Science and Technology. 2018;80;242-263. DOI: org/10.1016/j.tifs.2018.08.008

[18] Javanmard M. Application of edible coatings incorporated sage (*Salvia officinalis*) alcoholic extract for inhibition of *Aspergillus flavus* growth in pistachio kernel. Iranian Journal of Food Science and Technology. 2012;9;85-90.

[19] Cegielka A, Syymanczuk H, Piwowarek K, Dasiewicz K, Slowinski M, Wronska K. The use of bioactive properties of sage preparations to improve the storage stability of low-pressure mechanically separed meat from chickens. Poultry Science. 2019;98;5045-5053. DOI: 10.3382/ps/pez242

[20] Prusinowska R, Śmigielski KB. Composition, biological properties and therapeutic effects of lavender (*Lavandula angustifolia* L.) a review. Herba Polonica. 2014;60;56-66. DOI: org/10.2478/hepo-2014-0010

[21] Adnan M, Hussain J, Tahir M, Shinwari Z. Proximate and nutrient composition of medicinal plants of humid and sub-humid regions in north-west. Pakistan Journal of Medicinal Plants Research. 2020;4;339-345. DOI: org/10.5897/JMPR09.505

[22] Kűcűkyilmar K, Kiyma Z, Akdag A, Cetinkaya M, Atalay H, Ates A, Gursel F.E, Bozkurt J. Effect of lavender (*Lavandula stoechas*) essential oil on growth performance, carcass characteristics, meat quality and antioxidant status of broilers South African Journal of Animal Science. 2017;42;178-185. DOI: org/10.4314/sajas.v47i2.9

[23] Taskaya L, Yapici HH, Metin C, Alparslan Y. The effect of lavender (*Lavandula stoldas*) on the shelf life of a traditional food: hamsi kaygana. Food Science and Technology. 2017;38;711-718. DOI: org/10.1590/1678-457x.12417

[24] Tafrihi M, Imran M, Tufail T, Gondal TA, Caruso G, Sharma S, Sharma R, Atanassola M, Atanassou L, Fokou PVT, Pezzani R. The wonderful activities of the genus *Mentha* not only antioxidant properties. Molecules. 2021;26;1-22. DOI: 10.3390/molecules26041118

[25] Rita P, Animesh DK. An updated overview on peppermint (*Mentha piperita* L.). International Research Journal of Pharmacy. 2011;2;1-10.

[26] Mainasara MM, Bakar MFA, Waziri AH, Musa AR. Comparison of phytochemical, proximate and mineral composition of fresh and dried peppermint (*Mentha piperita*) leaves. Journal of Science and Technology. 2018;10;85-91. DOI: 10.30880/jst.2018.10.02.014

[27] Padmini E, Valarmathi A, Usharani M. Comarative analysis of chemical composition and antibacteroaô activities of *Mentha spicata* and *Camellia sinensis*. Asian Journal of Experimental Biological Sciences. 2010;1;772-781.

[28] Trugo L, Finglas PM. Encyclopedia of Food Sciences and Nutrition. USA: Academia Press;2003;6000 p.

[29] Abdel-Wareth AA, Kehravs S, Sűdek KH. Peppermint and its respective active component in diets of broiler chickens: growth performance, viability, economics, meat physico chemical properties, and carcass characteristics. Poultry Science. 2019;98;3850-3859. DOI: org/10.3382/ps/pez099

[30] Barzegar MMM, Badi H. Production of functional cooled sausage by *Mentha piperita* essential oil as a natural antioxidant and antimicrobial material. Journal of Medicinal Plants. 2012;11;1-12.

[31] Amirdivani S, Baba SA. Changes in yogurt fermentation characteristics and antioxidant potential and *in vitro* inhibition of angiotensin converting enzyme upon the inclusion of peppermint, dill and basil. LWT-Food Science and Technology. 2011;44;1458-1464. DOI: org/10.1016/j.lwt.2011.01.019

[32] Moradkhani H, Sargsyan E, Bibak H, Naseri B, Sadat-Hosseini M, Fayazi-Barjin A, Meftahizade H. *Melissa officinalis* L. a valuable medicine plant: A review. Journal of Medicinal Plants Research. 2010;4;2753-2759.

[33] Miraj S, Kopaei R, Kiani S. *Melissa officinalis* L: A review study with and antioxidant prospective. Journal of Evidence-Based Complementary and Alternative Medicine. 2017;22;387-394. DOI: 10.1177/2156587216663433

[34] Hyun-Joo L, You-Jung Ch, Yang-LL Ch, Jae-Joon L. Effects of lemon balm on the oxidative stability and the quality properties of hamburger patties during refrigerates storage. Koreans Journal of Food Science and Animal Resource. 2014;34;533-542. DOI: 10.5851/kosfa.2014.34.4.533

[35] Dordević S, Popović D, Despotolić S, Veljović M, Atanacković M, Cvejič J, Nedović V. Extracts of medicinal plants as functional beer additives. Chemical Industry and Chemical Engineering Quarterly. 2016;22;301-308. DOI: 10.2298/CICEQ150501044D

[36] Bahelka L, Nűrnberg G, Kűchenmeister V, Nűrnberg K. Meat quality, sensory properties and oxidative stability of pork after dietary supplementation of sage, lemon balm and oregano extracts. [Internet]. Available: https://digicomst.ie/wp-content/uploads/2020/05/2011_23_05.pdf

[37] Akshay K, Swathi K, Saksmi V, Boggula N. *Rosmarinus officinalis* L: an update review of its phytochemistry and biological activity. Journal of Drug Delivery and Therapeutics. 2018;9;323-330. DOI: 10.4155/fsoa-2017-0124

[38] Begum A, Sandhya S, Ali SS, Vinod KR, Reddy S, Banji D. An in-depth review on the medicinal flora *Rosmarinus officinalis* (*Lamiaceae*). Acta Scientiarum Polonorum, Technologia Alimentaria. 2013;12;61-73.

[39] Al-Hijazeen M, Aô-Rawashdeh M. Preservative effects of rosemary extract (*Rosmarinus officinalis*) on quality and storage stability of chicken meat patties. Food Science and Technology. 2016;39;1-5. DOI: org/10.1590/1678-457x.24817

[40] Fovad I, Madi M, Lamlom S, Attitalla I. Effect of rosemary extract and vitamin E on lipid peroxidation and the quality during chilling and frozen storage of fried nile tilapia fillets (*Oreichromis niloticus*). Journal of Basic and Applied Research in Biomedicine. 2021;7;1-10.

[41] Gad AS, Sayd AF. Antioxidant propertirs of rosemary and its potential uses as natural antioxidant in dairy products: a review. Food and Nutrition Sciences. 2015;6;179-193. DOI: 10.4236/fns.2015.61019

Chapter 3

Structure: Activity and Emerging Applications of Spices and Herbs

Adeyemi Ojutalayo Adeeyo, Tshianeo Mellda Ndou, Mercy Adewumi Alabi, Hosana Dumisani Mkoyi, Erinfolami Motunrayo Enitan, Daniso Beswa, Rachel Makungo and John O. Odiyo

Abstract

Herbs and spices are plant parts (herbs from leaves and spices from other parts) that are conventionally used in their fresh or dried state for flavouring, natural condiments, preservatives and for medicinal purposes. Worldwide, most spices are classified on the basis of taste, season of growth, economic importance, growth habit and plant part used. Black pepper, chilies, small cardamom, ginger and turmeric are some of the widely used spices while common herbs include thyme, basil and bay leaves. These herbs are basically classified according to usage, active constituents and period of life. Secondary metabolites such as Eugenol, thymol, limonene, cuminaldehyde, curcumin, piperine, quercetin, luteolin in these plant parts have been found to be responsible for anticancer, antimicrobial, antiviral, antidiabetic, antioxidant, anti-inflammatory and hypocholesterolemic effects. Their application in water fortification, milk and cheese processing, production of beauty products and pesticides among others could not be underestimated. Finally, adulteration, toxicity and allergic reactions are some of the identified limitations and challenges often encountered in the use of herbs and spices.

Keywords: herbs, spices, water fortification, emerging applications, food preservation

1. Introduction

Herbs, spices and derived extracts have been used since ancient times to improve sensory characteristics of food, as preservatives as well as their nutritional and health properties [1]. Herb is derived from the Latin word '*herba*', meaning grass, green stalks or blades which refers to the leafy part of a plant used either in its fresh or dried state, altering the taste of the food with the aim of flavour enhancement. On the other hand, any other part of a plant; seed, bark, root, fruit, or flower, often used in the dried state is called a spice. Common examples of spices are cloves bud, turmeric rhizome, cinnamon bark, garlic bulb, ginger rhizome, peppercorn berries and cumin seeds (**Figure 1**) [2]. Each can be differentiated by their growing condition, taste, and part used [3]. Technically, herbs are usually grown in temperate or cooler climate, while spices are grown in the tropics [4]. Some plants can be

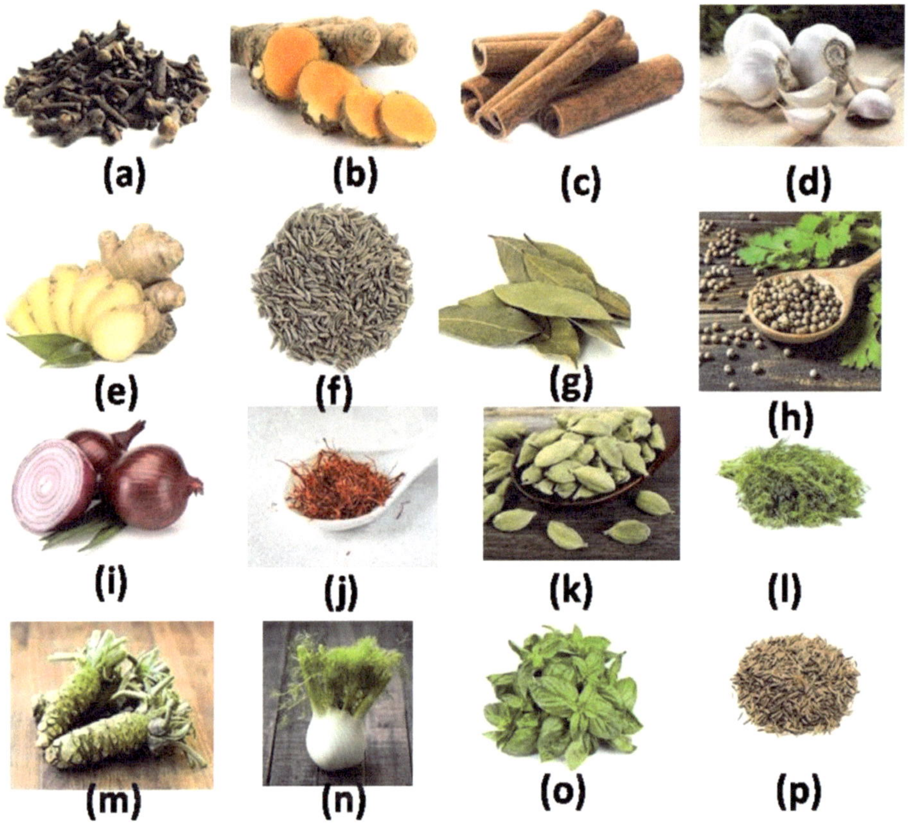

Figure 1.
Some common spices in use; (a) clove (b) turmeric (c) cinnamon (d) garlic (e) ginger (f) cumin (g) bay leaf (h) coriander (i) onion (j) saffron (k) cardamom (l) dill (m) wasabi (n) fennel (o) basil (p) caraway.

both herb and spice. For example, Coriander leaves and seeds are used for the production of both herb and spice, respectively [5]. For many centuries, herbs and spices have been used generally and basically in enhancing organoleptic properties of food like taste and flavour. However, newer applications have been reported in recent times. They have gained importance as potential sources of natural food preservatives due to the growing interest in the development of safe and effective natural preservatives which has been better alternatives to chemical additives [6, 7].

Furthermore, various compounds derived from herbs and spices have been reported for medicinal activities such as antimicrobial, antiviral, anti-inflammatory and antioxidant [8, 9]. Certain herbs and spices that have been reported for cancer prevention, cholesterol lowering effects and overall protection of human health [10]. In folk medicine, turmeric is used for gynaecological problems, stomach diseases, liver diseases, infectious diseases, and blood diseases and has been suggested for the treatment of proinflammatory diseases, cancer, diabetes, obesity, and atherosclerosis [11]. Turmeric, native to India and Southeast Asia, is commonly used as food colouring in Asian dishes, such as curries.

Herbs and spices have also been used in water enrichment. Herbs have been used in the production of functional beverages which are useful in boosting immune system, increase vitality, body weight control and fighting degenerative diseases. They are also used in the production of flavoured or enhanced water which also offer nutritional benefits [12]. More advanced application of herbs and spices is in dairy products, cosmetics and production of insecticides [13–15]. Herbal products have been researched and tested in skin care and reported for mildness, efficacy, biodegradability, low toxicity, cleansing ability, emulsification, moisturising, skin appearance, feel, fragrance, and lubrication [16, 17]. Clove buds' oils possess insecticidal properties [5]. To this end, the chapter therefore covers the recent application of herbs and spices as important natural products, in addition to information on the different types, classification, bioactivities and bioactive compositions, as well as the current limitations in optimization and disadvantages in the use of herbs and spices. A total of 102 articles were reviewed in the study, which deal directly with the subject having removed articles out of the scope of study. Articles used for the development covers the year 1990 to 2021.

2. Economic benefits of herbs and species

The use of herbs and spices were report as far back as 2000 to 1500 B.Cs in India and Egypt respectively which was later introduced to other countries of the world due to globalisation [18]. Economically, the main spice in the international trade is pepper and its price determine the value of spices in general. In 2012, the annual global trade in spices was 6–7 lakh tonnes valued at US$3–3.5 billion [19]. The European Union has the largest imports of spices in value terms, worth US$2.2 billion and consisting 44% retail sales to consumers, 41% sales to the food manufacturing sector and 15% to the catering sector. In South Africa, the annual spice trade is worth US$94 million with the potential of increase as consumers desire better taste in food [19].

3. Classification and examples of herbs and spices

The classifications of herbs and spices as described in literature Chhetri et al., 2019; [3, 20–24] are presented in **Tables 1–3**. **Table 1** shows the class, sub classes, super orders, orders and families of some spices. Spices can be conventionally classified on the basis of taste as hot, mild or aromatic. Spices can also be classified based on season of growth which can be annual, biennial or perennial, on the basis of growth habit which can be shrubs, trees, climbers or rhizomes or on the basis of plant part used (**Table 2**). Additionally, spices can be classified on the basis of their economic importance as either major spices or minor spices. Major spices are black pepper, chilies, small cardamom, ginger and turmeric. All other spices asides these are considered as minor spices [3, 22, 23].

Herbs are basically classified according to usage, active constituents and period of life (**Table 3**). When classified according to usage, herbs can be medicinal, culinary, aromatic and ornamental. Medicinal herbs as the name implies have therapeutic properties and are used in the treatment of illnesses. Culinary herbs are used majorly in cooking because of their strong flavours. Ornamental herbs are used for decoration owing to their bright colours [24]. When classified on the basis of active ingredient, herbs can be classified as aromatic (volatile oils), astringents (tannins), bitter (phenolics, saponins and alkaloids), mucilaginous (polysaccharides) and nutritive (food). Aromatics herbs have pleasant odours and are used medicinally as well as in flavouring. They are subdivided into stimulant herbs, used to increase energy and activity of the body. Astringent herbs help to tighten, contract or tone living tissues and this helps to halt discharges. Bitter herbs can be further divided into laxative bitter herbs, diuretic herbs or saponin-containing herbs. Mucilaginous herbs help to eliminate toxins from the intestinal systems and function as antibiotic, antacid, demulcent, emollient and detoxifier in nature [21].

Class	Subclass	Super order	Order	Family	Examples
Angiospermae	Dicotyledoneae	Sympetalae	Campalunatae	Solariaceae	Chilli, paprika, red pepper
				Pedahaceae	sesame
				Compositae	Camomile, chicory, tarragon
		Archichlamydaeae	Piperales	Piperaceae	Cubeba, long pepper, pepper
			Ranales	Myristicaceae	Mace, nutmeg
				Lauraceae	Bay leaf, cassia, cinnamon
				Magnoliaceae	Star-anise
			Rhoeadales	Cruciferae	Mustard, wasabi
			Myrtiflorae	Myrtaceae	allspice, clove
			Umbelliflorae	Umbelliferae	Anise, caraway, celery, chervil, coriander, cumin, dill, fennel, parsley
	Monocotyle-doneae		Liliiflorae	Liliaceae	Garlic, onion
				Irldaceae	Saffron
			Scitamineae	Zingiberaceae	Cardamom, ginger, turmeric
			Orchidales	Orchidaceae	Vanilla

Table 1.
Taxonomic classification of spices [21].

Category	Classes	Examples
Degree of taste	Hot spices	Capsicum (chillies), Cayenne pepper, black and white peppers, ginger, mustard
	Mild spices	Paprika, coriander
	Aromatic spices	Allspice (pimento), cardamom, cassia, cinnamon, clove, cumin, dill, fennel, fenugreek, mace and nutmeg
	Aromatic vegetables	Onion, garlic, shallot, celery
Growth habit	Shrubs	Rosemary, chillies, pomegranate
	Trees	Nutmeg, clove, cinnamon, tamarind, garcinia, Japanese pepper
	Climbers	Black pepper, tailed pepper, vanilla
	Rhizomes	Cardamom, ginger, turmeric, mango ginger, galangal, asafoetida
Season of growth	Annual	Coriander, cumin, fennel, fenugreek, ajowan, black cumin, aniseed, mustard, chilli
	Biennial	Onion, parsley
	Perennial	Cardamom, turmeric, ginger, black pepper, saffron, clove, nutmeg, asafoetida, cinnamon

Category	Classes	Examples
Part usage	Bark	Cinnamon, cassia, tejpat
	Rhizome	Ginger, turmeric, sweet flag, greater galangal
	Fruit	Pepper, cardamom, chilli, coriander, cumin, fennel, celery, aniseed, ajowan, caraway, dill, pepper long, star anise, allspice, tamarind
	Seed	Cardamom, fenugreek, mustard, pomegranate, nutmeg, poppy seed
	Rind	Kokam, camboge
	Bulb	Garlic
	Stem	Celery, lovage
	Pod	Vanilla
	Stigma	Saffron
	Root	Horse radish, angelica, lovage
	Flower bud	Caper
	Unopened flower bud	Clove
	Berry	Juniper berry
	Aril	Mace

Table 2.
Classification of spices based on taste, growth condition and plant part usage [3, 21–24].

Criteria	Class	Examples
Industrial Usage	Medicinal	Echinaceae, feverfew
	culinary	Basil, parsley, mint
	Ornamental	Lavender, chives
Seasonal Usage	Annual	Anice, basil, borage, calendula, chamomile, dill dukat, marjoram, parsley, shiso, saffron
	Biennial	Prime rose, caraway seeds, mullein, viper's bugloss
	Perennial	Alfalfa, aloe vera, arimony, asafetida, bee balm, bay leaves, thyme, dill, fennel, Echinacea, lavender, lemon balm, pepper mint, spear mint, mitsuba, oregano, rose mary, sage, salad burnet, yarrow, water cress.
Active ingredient	Aromatic	*Stimulant*: Fennel, ginger, garlic, lemon grass *Nervine*: Ginger, catnip
	Astringent	Pepper mint, raspberry
	Bitter	*Laxative*: Aloe, cascara, licorice, pumpkin, senna, yellow dock, yucca, barberry, gentian, safflower, golden seal *Diuretic*: Asparagus, Blessed thistle, burdock, butcher's broom, buchu, corn silk, dandelion, parsley *Saponin-containing*: Alfalfa, yucca, ginseng, gotu kola, schizandra
	Mucilaginous	Aloe, burdock, dandelion, glucomannan, Irish moss
	Nutritive	Apple, roseships, orange, wheat germ, spirulina, red clover, cauliflower, cabbage, broccoli, accerola, asparagus, oatstraw, carrot

Table 3.
Usage, seasonal and nutritional classification of herbs [3, 22–24].

4. Bioactive compounds in herbs and spices

Bioactive compounds are produced as secondary metabolites in plants other than the primary biosynthetic compounds such as amino acids, proteins, carbohydrates, and lipids. The types of bioactive components that can be found in herbs include glycosides (e.g., saponins and anthraquinine glycosides), resins and phenol compounds (e.g., flavonoids, tannins and quinones). Some of these compounds are listed in **Table 4** and their structures in **Table 5**. The post-harvesting process of medicinal herbs is crucial in industrial production which affects the quantity and quality of the bioactive components [28].

Name	Bioactive compounds
Turmeric herb	Primarily monoterpenes and phenolic compounds
Coriander (Spice)	Alcoholic monoterpene
Chilli (Spice)	Capsaicin
Cinnamon (spice)	Eugenol
Clove (herb)	Eugenol
Curry Leaf	Oxalic acid, resin, carbazole alkaloids and volatile oils
Fennel (herb)	Trans-anethole, p-coumaric acid and rosmarinic acid
Garlic (herb/ spice)	Allicin, alliin, diallyl sulfide, diallyl disulfide, diallyl trisulfide, ajoene, and S-allyl-cysteine
Ginger (herb)	Phenolic and terpene compounds
Musterd (spice)	Methallyl cyanide
Pepper (spice)	Ascorbic acid, carotenoids, and other antioxidants

Table 4.
Bioactive compounds in herbs and spices (source: [5, 25–27]).

Herbs/Spices	Compound name	Structure
Basil	Eugenol	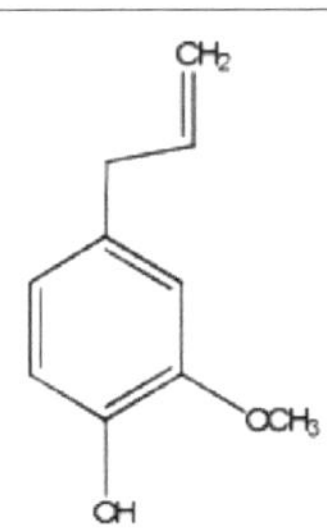
	Thymol	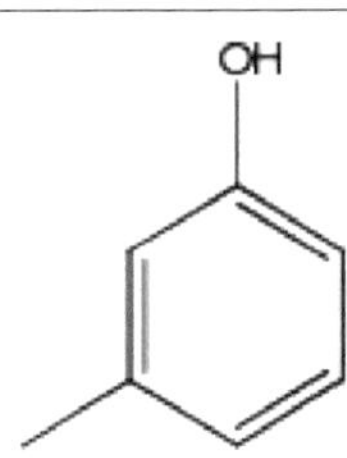

Herbs/Spices	Compound name	Structure
	Estragole	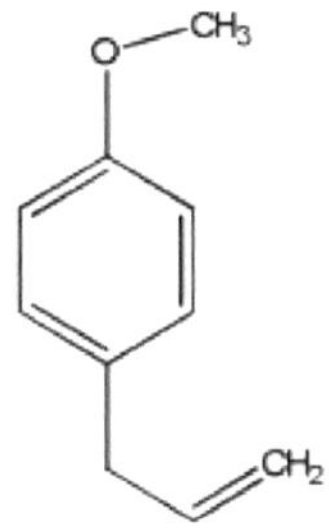
Celery leaves	Limonene	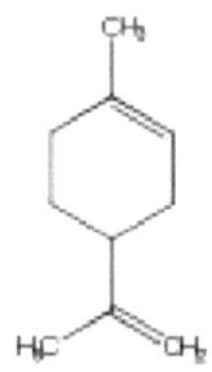
	b-selinene	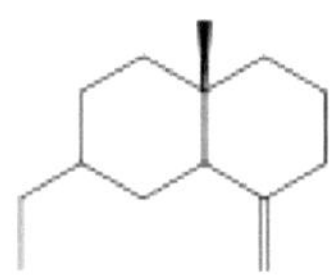
Clove oil	Eugenyl acetate	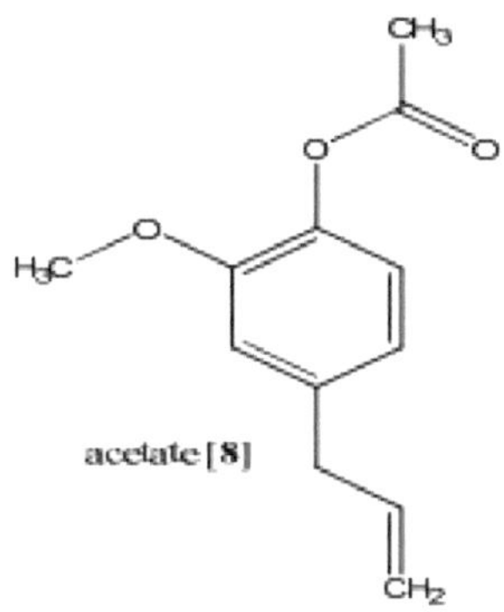
Cumin	Cuminaldehyde	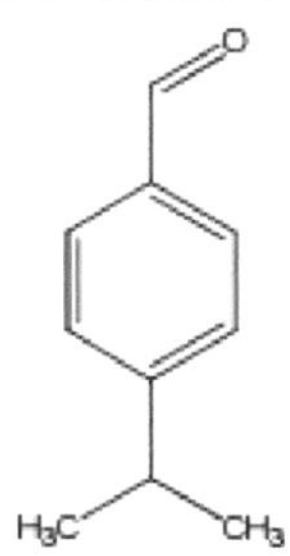
	b-pinene	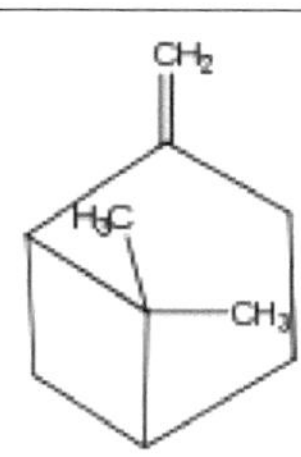
Curry leaf	Carbazole	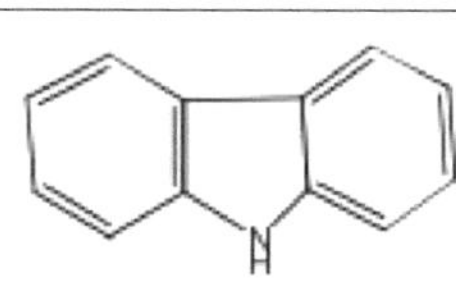

Herbs/Spices	Compound name	Structure
	a-pinene	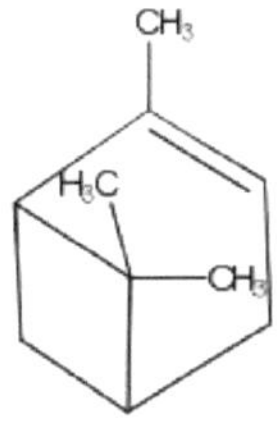
	d-terpenene	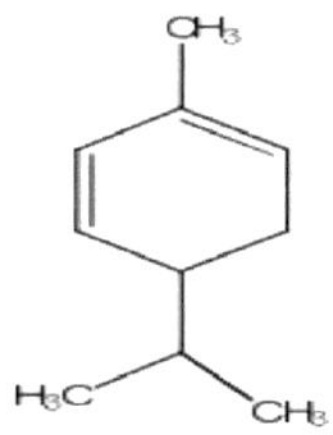
	b-phellandrene	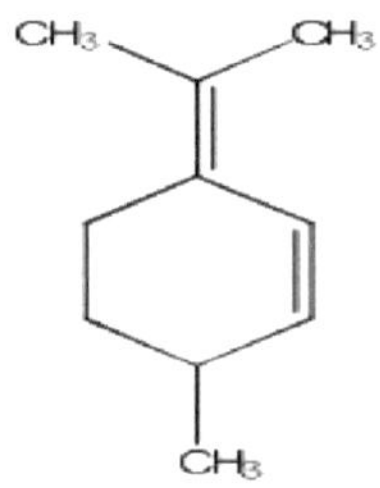
Ginger	Curcumin	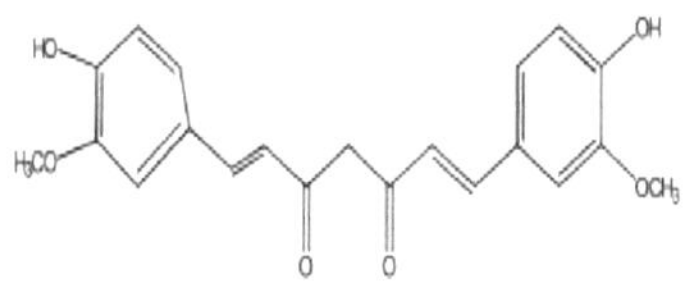
	Citral	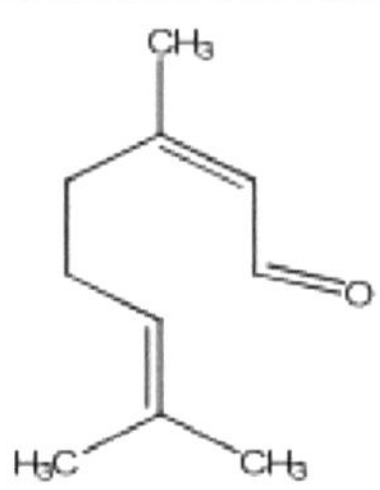
Nutmeg	Linalool	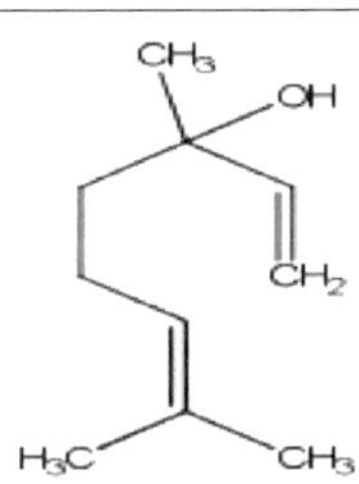
	Elemicin	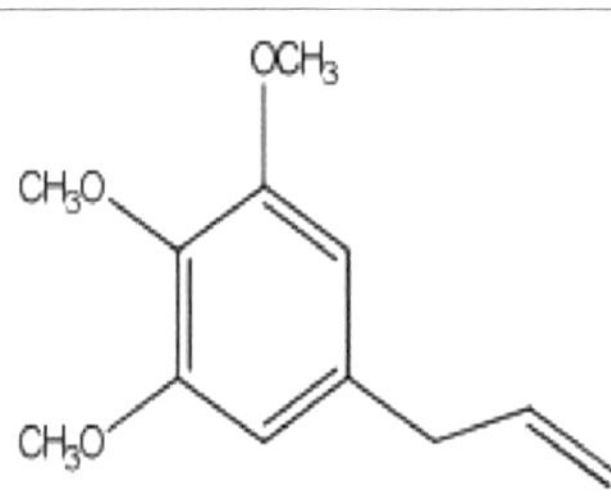

Herbs/Spices	Compound name	Structure
	a-sulphinyl-disulphide	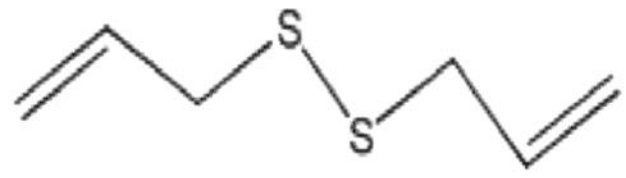
Black pepper	Piperine	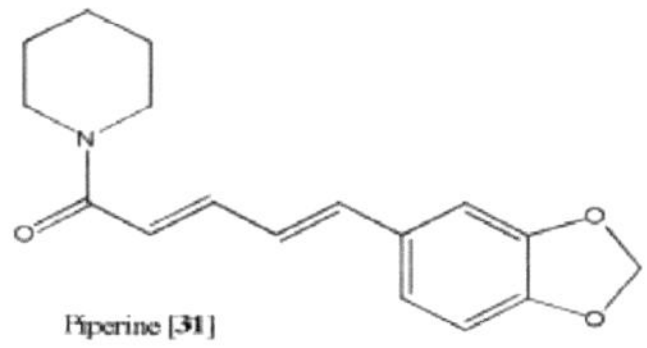 Piperine [31]
Star anise	Turmerone	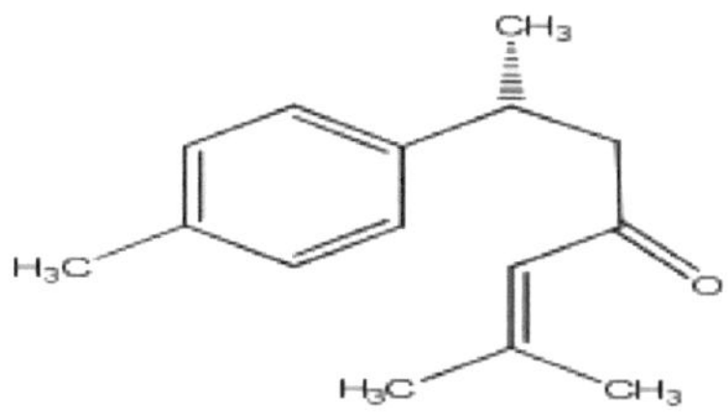
Onion	Quercetin	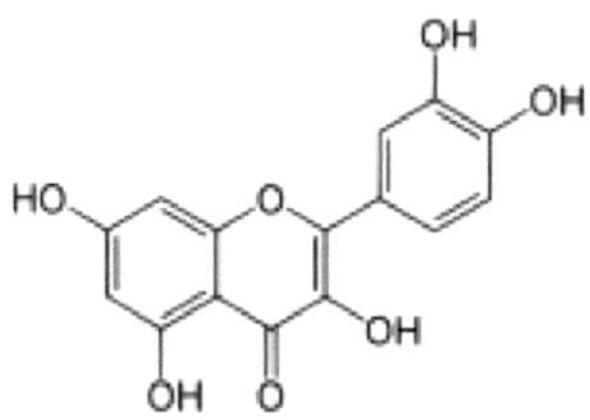
Fennelflower	Thymoquinone	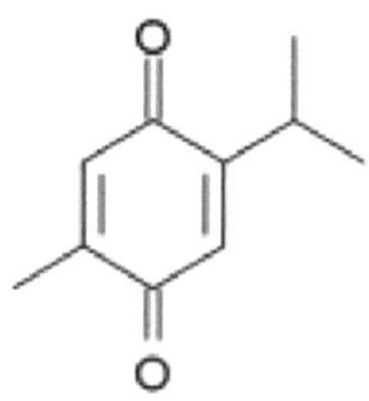
Red pepper	Capsaicin	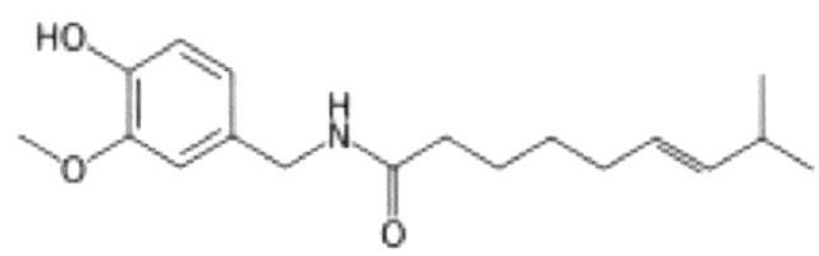
Parsley	Apigenin	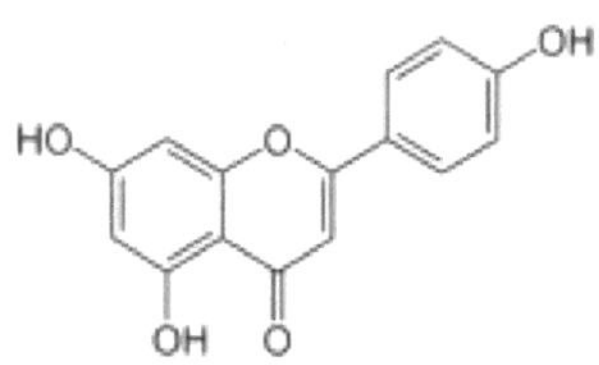
Oregano	Luteolin	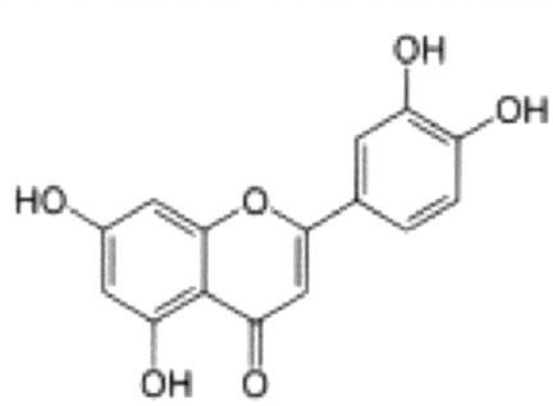
Saffron	Crocetin	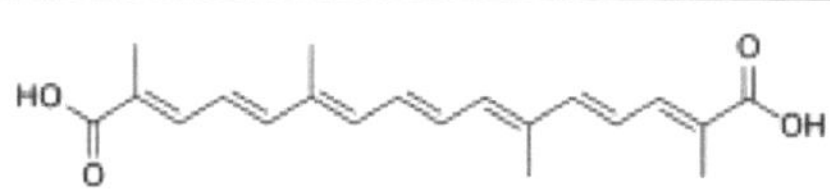

Herbs/Spices	Compound name	Structure
	Crocin	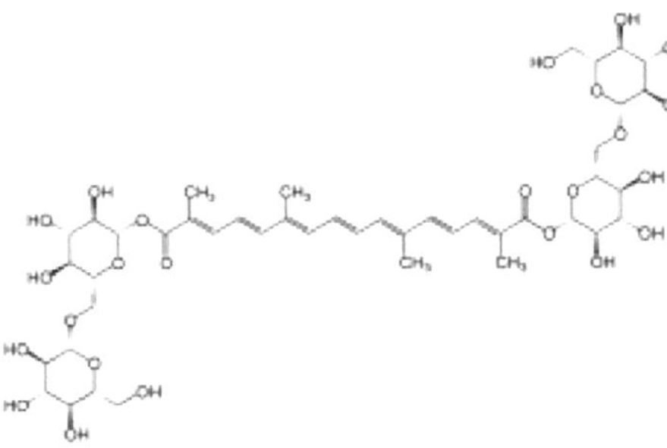

Table 5.
Structures of bioactive compounds in herbs and spices (source: [5, 27]).

5. Innovative functionality and medical application of herbs and spices

5.1 Antibacterial and antifungal activities

Phytochemicals such as phenolics, carotenoids and organosulphur compounds present in herbs and spices function for antimicrobial activity. Clove, oregano, thyme, cinnamon, cumin, rosemary, garlic, ginger, basil, fennel, coriander and galangal have been reported for antibacterial and antifungal activity [29]. Antimicrobial activity of clove bud oils possesses antibacterial and antifungal properties owing to the high level of eugenol present in the essential oil [30]. Curry leaves also exert antifungal activity [31]. Coriander and cinnamon were also reported for antifungal activity against *Aspergillus parasiticus, Cladosporium cladosporoides, Eurotium herboriorum, Penicillum chrysogenum* and *Aspergillus carbonarius* [32]. Galangal is a food additive used in Thailand and some other Asian countries and has been reported for antibacterial activity against *Staphylococcus aureus* and *Listeria monocytogenes.* The synergistic effect of galangal, rosemary and lemon iron bark was also reported [29]. Extracts of roselle, clove and rosemary were reported for antibacterial activity against *Escherichia coli, Vibrio parahaemolyticus, Pseudomonas aeruginosa, Salmonella enteritidis, Bacillus cereus, Candida albicans* and *S. aureus* [33].

5.2 Antiviral activity

A number of herbs and spices have been reported for antiviral activity [34]. Antiviral activity of turmeric was observed and documented in different viruses such as hepatitis virus, corona virus, influenza, Human Immunodeficiency virus (HIV) and others [34, 35]. Turmeric targets different cellular pathways, which further inhibiting the growth, and replication of viruses and this makes it an ideal candidate as an anti-viral drug. Antiviral activity of curcumin was observed against different viruses including hepatitis viruses, SARS coronavirus, influenza viruses, human immunodeficiency virus (HIV), herpes simplex virus, dengue virus and chikungunya virus [36]. Utomo et al. [37] reported that curcumin binds and inhibits the target receptors including SARS-CoV-2 protease, spike glycoprotein-RBD, and PD-ACE2, which are involved in virus infection.

Garlic produces an enzyme called alliinase and this enzyme has antiviral activities. Antiviral activity of garlic extract has been studied against influenza virusA/H1N1 in cell culture and it was found that it inhibits the virus penetration and proliferation in cell culture [38]. In another study conducted by Shojai et al. [39], garlic extract showed inhibitory activity on infectious bronchitis virus in chicken embryo. During the inception of COVID-19 pandemic, Ministry of AYUSH, India released an advisory of immunity and self-care of Ayurveda's spices [40]. This includes the use of spices such as turmeric, cumin, coriander, and garlic that are recommended in cooking. They have also advised taking herbal drinks, tea/decoction (kadha) made from basil, cinnamon, black pepper, ginger, and raisin once or twice in a day [40].

5.3 Anticancer activity

National Foundation for Cancer Research [41] mentions that herbs and spices are effective in the preventions and treatment of cancer. For decades, the National Cancer Institute and Memorial Sloan-Kettering Cancer Center in the United States have recognised the cancer preventive potential of herbs and spices from labiatae, zingiberaceae, and the unbelliferae family [10]. Some of the reported culinary herbs and spices for anticancer activities include basil, caraway, cardamom, clove, cumin, dill garlic, ginger, rosemary, saffron and thyme [42]. Likewise, Wigutow [43] reported turmeric, ginger, cayenne pepper, saffron, oregano and garlic to be one of the good cancer fighters. Epidemiological studies suggest that a high intake of raw and cooked garlic may provide a protective effect against stomach and colorectal cancers [44]. A commonly available spice, Saffron (*Crocus sativus* L.), used as a food flavouring spice has also been thoroughly reported for its cancer preventive and tumoricidal properties [45]. Research over the last 50 years indicated that curcumin, a polyphenolic ingredient in turmeric, can prevent cancer, and can be used to treat cancer [46]. Flaxseeds also known as linseeds, usually sprinkled on cereals, salads and desserts as nutritional booster is also a good source of lignans known as "phytoestrogens", which are studied for chemo-preventive properties. Various studies have shown that garlic and organosulfur compounds, especially diallyl disulfide, can slow the development of cancers of the skin, oesophagus, stomach, colon, liver, lung and the mammary glands [47].

5.4 Antidiabetic activity

In all cases of diabetes, development of one or more complicated chronic diseases such as neuropathy, retinopathy, nephropathy and cardiomyopathy are common. Culinary herbs and spices have been found useful in the treatment of diabetes [48]. Curcumin, an active component of turmeric, was reported to ameliorate diabetic nephropathy instreptozotocin-induced diabetic rats [49]. Supplementation of turmeric in patients with-ßovert type 2 diabetic nephropathy was also shown to attenuate proteinuria, IL-8 and can be administered as a safe adjuvant for these patients [50]. Cinnamon was also reported for its hypoglycaemic activity [51]. In addition, aniseed, bay leaf, cardamom, cinnamon, cumin, dill, ginger, hops, rosemary, saffron, sage have been examined in type 2 diabetes mellitus patients [52].

5.5 Antioxidant activity

Antioxidants can protect lipids and oils in food against oxidative degradation. When added to food, antioxidants control rancidity development, retard the formation of toxic oxidation products, maintain nutritional quality, and extend the shelf-life of products [27]. Natural antioxidants contained in spices help to reduce oxidative stress. Bakheit and Foda [53] determined the antioxidant activity of individual spices like black pepper, black cumin, and clove using (DPPH) free radical scavenging assay. Rosemary is one of the most effective spices widely used in food processing. It is the only spice commercially available for use as an antioxidant in

Europe and around the world [54]. Garlic has also been reported for antioxidant activity [55]. It has been documented by Wootton-Beard and Ryan [56] that natural antioxidant compounds are much effective than the synthetic compounds with regards to toxicity and carcinogenity. Antioxidants help to defend human bodies by deterring the formation of free radicals chain reaction. Moreover, antioxidant compounds are responsible for preventing diseases including cancer, cardiovascular disease, Alzheimer's disease, and muscular degeneration [56].

5.6 Hypocholesterolemic activity

Hypercholesterolemia, commonly known as high blood cholesterol, is a major risk factor for the development of atherosclerosis and occlusive vascular disorders [57]. Therapeutic lifestyles such as low saturated fat and cholesterol diet, weight management, and increased physical activity are vital for blood cholesterol regulation. Spices and herbs have also been reported for cholesterol-lowering activity [58]. Scientific evidence from several animal models revealed that curcumin from turmeric and capsaicin from red pepper are potent hypocholesterolaemic and hypolipidemic agents [59, 60]. Spices have been shown to possess good nutrient benefits with low calories, possess good inhibitory profiles on carbohydrate modulating enzymes, ACE and HMG-CoA reductase, which correlates to their total phenolic contents, phenolic profile and antioxidant properties. Ahmed et al. [61] reported that spices belonging to the Apiaceae family, for example, cumin, coriander, fennel and dill, are rich in monosaturated fatty acids and contain a good amount of polysaturated fatty acids and thus have great hypocholesterolemic effect.

5.7 Anti-inflammatory activity

Different studies have demonstrated an association between the typical Western diet rich in refined starches, sugars, saturated and transfatty acids but poor in fruit, vegetables, fibre, ω-omega-3 fatty acids and whole grains, which causes an increased tendency toward inflammatory disorders and related diseases, such as cardiovascular diseases, arthritis, or diabetes [62]. These signs can be prevented by eating or cooking food with herbs and spices that have medicinal properties to combat inflammation. Prevention is better than cure and healthy eating should be promoted to prevent inflammatory symptoms [63]. That is why turmeric is traditionally used in India in the treatment of rheumatic disorder because of its anti-inflammatory properties [64]. Ginger also has anti-inflammatory effect and has been researched to be effective in ameliorating arthritis pain [65]. Other herbs and spices reported for anti-inflammatory potential are cinnamon, garlic, black pepper and clove [63]. Herbs and spices have also been reported as anti-inflammatory food supplements against COVID-19 as excellent sources of vitamin C, for example, thyme, coriander, turmeric and cardamom [66].

6. Recent application of herbs and spices

6.1 Flavouring

Although herbs and spices are low-cost commodities, they have been valued as gold or jewels for many centuries being utilised as food additives all over the world. Herbs and spices are basically used in enhancing the flavour of food [13]. The addition of herbs and spices to vegetables, salad and fruits can help to improve the taste. Herbs and spices can be used as substitute for the less desirable taste promoters such as salt, sugar and fat. They generally add to appearance and smell of food [5]. African dishes such as jollof rice, soups and snacks as well as some drinks are flavoured using herbs and/or spices such as onion, chilli, turmeric, ginger, clove and tamarind [67]. Herbs such as basil, celery leaf, cumin, garlic also are important in African traditional snacks [5].

6.2 Preservatives

Green preservatives are becoming increasingly popular with new techniques of applications being developed [68]. Herbs and spices have been used to fortify foods throughout history not only as flavours but also as preservatives. Though used to enhance the organoleptic properties of food, they are also used in controlling natural spoilage by decreasing or eliminating foodborne pathogens thus increasing the shelf life [69]. Phenolic compounds present in herbs and spices are a major constituent responsible for their antimicrobial activity thus leading to preservation [1]. Chives, garlic, celery seed, tarragon, dill, black cumin, cinnamon, turmeric, cumin all have compounds functioning as preservatives in them [70]. Gallic acid, rutin and caffeic acid in black mustard, alicin and diallylsulfides in chives, garlic and eugenol in cinnamon prevent the growth of *E. coli* [71–73]. Capsicum in chilli pepper inhibits the growth of *Salmonella typhimurium* [74]. The antimicrobial efficacy of hydrosols of thyme, bay leaf, rosemary, sage and black cumin against *S. typhimurium* and *E. coli* has been reported [75]. Rosemary integration to rice cakes effectively inhibited *Bacillus cereus* and *S. aureus* [76]. The preserving function of herbs and spices can be linked to their antioxidant and antimicrobial activities [70, 77].

6.3 Dairy products

Antimicrobial properties of herbs and spices can be successfully used to control the growth of spoilage and pathogenic bacteria in dairy products. Phenolic compounds such as tea catechins, oleuropein, ferulic acid, ellagic acid and coumaric acid have been found to prevent the growth of some pathogenic bacteria (*S. aureus, S. enteritidis and L. monocytogenes*) and fungi [78]. Bakrm and Salihin [79] reported that addition of *Cinnamonum verum* and *Allium sativum* water extract in goat, cow and camel milk had no important effect on the acidification through fermentation. However, the presence of these two herbs in milk improved the proteolytic activity of the used cultures with the highest proteolytic activity gotten in cow milk yoghurt. Herbs and spices are also added to cheeses to impart unique flavours. These cheeses are regularly considered as specialty cheeses. Most spices impart specific flavours to cheeses, and some may affect the microbiological quality. Hamid and Abdelrahman [80] investigated the effect of adding 0.02% Cinnamon, Cardamom and Fenugreek powder to goat's milk curd after coagulation on the quality of the obtained white soft cheese. The additions of these spices enhanced the flavour and odour of goat's milk cheese. Herbs and spices also improved biological value and prolonged the shelf life of cottage cheese [80]. Black pepper, black cumin, and clove were also used to produce novel Mudaffara cheese [53]. Herbs and spices fortify dairy product acting as natural antioxidant, biopreservative, improvement of sensory qualities while also functioning for nutritional and medicinal purposes [13]. Herbs-fortified dairy products are a good source of antioxidant [81].

6.4 Essential in water and drink fortification

The production of flavoured and fortified water is another area in which herbs and spices have found application [82]. Asides the regular function of water for distribution of nutrient and maintenance of electrolyte balance, functional water (flavoured and fortified) has added medicinal functions of preventing illness and diseases. Herbs alongside vitamins, minerals, and amino acids are the main components of these beverages [12]. Beet root, ginger, and red ginseng have been used in fortification of quite a number of beverages and drinks [83, 84].

6.5 Herbal cosmetics

Exposure of human skin to sunlight and other atmospheric conditions causes production of reactive oxygen species, which can react with DNA, proteins, and fatty acids, causing oxidative damage and impairment of antioxidant system. Beauty products made from herbs are tested and preferred for low toxicity, mildness, moisturising, and cleaning activities. Herbal cosmetics have recently gained ground and natural ingredients such as herbs and spices have been incorporated into skin care formulation either directly or their essential oils [15]. Botanical extracts are multifunctional in nature because they possess various properties like photoprotection, antiaging, moisturising, antioxidant, astringent, anti-irritant, and antimicrobial activity, which are correlated with each other [85]. Turmeric is effective for the treatment as well as prevention of psoriasis and other skin conditions such as acne, eczema, sun damage, wounds and premature ageing since it inhibits the activity of phosphorylase kinase [86]. Garlic possess anti-inflammatory effect which reduces the inflammation of acne. Garlic oils are also useful in controlling sores, pimples and acne [87]. Eugenol present in clove is useful in keeping the skin dirt-free also reduces redness and inflammation of acne. Ginger possesses cleansing and antiseptic compounds in it and thus keep the skin smooth and without blemish and is used in many cosmetics for skin health [15].

6.6 Pest control

A number of herbs and spices have been reported for insecticidal potential and essential oil from Cinnamon is an example of such. Extracted oil from stem bark, leaves and fruits of *Cinnamomum camphora* were found to possess great fumigant toxicity against *Tribolium castaneum* and *Lasioderma serricone* [14]. Black pepper has also been reported for pest control. Scott et al. [88] reports that black pepper offers a unique biopesticide material that can be used in controlling small-scale insect outbreaks and also reduce the likelihood of development of resistance. Basil, sage and lemon thyme have all been researched for insecticidal activity [89].

7. Current challenges in the use of herbs and spices

Although several herbs and spices have been reported for great medicinal and flavouring benefits, there are a number of challenges confronting their use. The current challenges in the use of herbs and spices include toxicity, allergy as well as quality and adulteration.

7.1 Adulteration

The detection of adulteration in herbs and spices is important for value assessment in order to mitigate the health problems caused by undeclared constituents [90]. Adulteration can be direct and intentional which involves the practice of partially or fully substituted constituents with inferior ones. Adulteration can also be unintentional resulting mainly from the absence of a proper evaluation method and/or clerical errors [91]. Reported adulteration of herbs and spices include the addition of dried pawpaw seeds with black pepper, red beet pulp and tomato waste to pepper powder, exhausted clove added to good ones, grass seeds added to cumin seeds, exhausted ginger added to good ginger, capsicum added to ginger powder, wild *Curcuma* spp. added to turmeric powder and lots more [92].

Techniques have been developed to counter alteration including physical methods such as macroscopic and microscopic analysis [93] or analytical methods including chromatographic techniques, electrophoresis, spectroscopy, chemometrics and hyphenated techniques [94, 95]. Biotechnological [96] and hybridization methods, polymerase chain reaction, immunological and biosensors assays can all be used in adulterant detection [92].

7.2 Toxicity and allergy

Quite a number of studies have revealed the cytotoxicity, carcinogenicity, neurotoxicity, genotoxicity and teratogenicity of phytochemicals derived from herbs and spices [97]. Capsaicin has been reported to cause neural and retinal degeneration [98] and increase blood ATL level [99] in experimental animals. Chilli peppers was reported to cause hypertensive crisis in a 19 years old male [100]. Singh et al. [101] reported the cytotoxic effect of cinnamon extract on human and mouse cell lines. Eugenol at 0.06% concentration was also reported to have toxic effect on human skin cells [102]. Although herbs and spices have been reported for several health benefits, their use also has side effects just as possible in other medicinal plants [103]. Therefore, it is paramount that attention is paid to their dosage. Generally, herbs and spices should be consumed with the knowledge of their existing side effects [104]. As stated by Stiller [105], people's allergic reactions to spices and herbs can be either Type IV or Type I reactions. Occupational contact dermatitis is the most experienced Type IV allergy while rhinitis, bronchial asthma, gastrointestinal symptoms, oral allergy syndrome and anaphylactic shock are the Type I allergies most experienced.

8. Conclusion

Herbs and spices are products obtained from plants which have been used traditionally for their flavour enhancement properties and have also been scientifically proven to possess medicinal properties. Bioactive compounds present in these plants are responsible for their health benefits when they function for anti-oxidant, anti-inflammatory, anticancer, antimicrobial and antiviral activities. Besides the general use of herbs and spices in flavouring dishes, they have also found application in enrichment of water, other drinks and dairy products. They have been used for preservation of food, production of skin care product and pesticides. It was also established that bioactive compounds such as eugenol, curcumin and essential oils of a variety of herbs and spices are of great important, however, there is a need for more in-vivo studies for better evaluation and toxicological properties of herbs and spices.

Author details

Adeyemi Ojutalayo Adeeyo[1*], Tshianeo Mellda Ndou[2], Mercy Adewumi Alabi[3], Hosana Dumisani Mkoyi[4], Erinfolami Motunrayo Enitan[5], Daniso Beswa[6], Rachel Makungo[7] and John O. Odiyo[8]

1 Department of Ecology and Resource Management, Faculty of Sciences, Engineering and Agriculture, University of Venda, Thohoyandou, South Africa

2 School of Environmental Sciences, University of Venda, Thohoyandou, South Africa

3 Department of Microbiology, School of Sciences, Federal University of Technology, Akure, Nigeria

4 Department of Life and Consumer Sciences, College of Agriculture and Environmental Sciences, UNISA Science Campus, Florida, South Africa

5 Department of Biotechnology and Food Technology, Durban University of Technology, Durban, South Africa

6 Department of Biotechnology and Food Technology, University of Johannesburg, Johannesburg, South Africa

7 Department of Hydrology and Water Resources, Faculty of Sciences, Engineering and Agriculture, University of Venda, Thohoyandu, South Africa

8 Vaal University of Technology, South Africa

*Address all correspondence to: firstrebby@gmail.com

References

[1] Martinez-gracia C, Bermudez CAG, Cabellero-Volcarcel AM, Santaella M, Frontela C (2015). Use of herbs and spices for food preservation: Advantages and limitation. Current Opinion in Food Science, 6:38-43

[2] Davidson A (2010). The Oxford Companion to Food Oxford: Oxford University Press.

[3] Cengage (2018). Herbs and Spices. https://www.encyclopedia.com/plants-and-animals/botany/botany-general/herbs-and-spices Assessed 15th August 2021

[4] Agriculture and natural resources (2021). Using herbs and spices. University of Delaware. https://www.udel.edu/academics/colleges/canr/cooperative-extension/fact-sheets/using-herbs-and-spices/ Accessed 29th June, 2021

[5] Mann A. (2011). Biopotency role of culinary herbs and their chemical constituents in health and commonly used spices in Nigerian dish and snacks. Afr J Food Sci, 5(3):111-124

[6] Carocho M, Barreiro MF, Morales P, Ferreira ICFR (2014). Adding molecules to food, pros and cons: a review on synthetic and natural food additives. Comp Rev Food Sci Food Safety, 13: 377-399.

[7] Sanchez G, Aznar R (2015). Evaluation of natural compounds of plant origin for inactivation of enteric viruses. Food Environ Virol, 7:183-187.

[8] Carlsen MH, Halvorsen BL, Holte K, Bohn SK, Dragland S, Sampson L,Willey C, Senoo H, Umezono Y, Sanada C, Barikmo IE, Berhe N, Willett WC, Phillips KM, Jacobs DR Jr, Blomhoff R (2010). The total antioxidant content ofmore than 3100 foods, beverages, spices, herbs and supplements used worldwide. Nutr J, 9:3.

[9] Peters, K V (2001). Handbook of Herbs and Spices, CRC Press.

[10] Caragay A (1992). Cancer-preventive Foods and Ingredients. Food Technol, 46: 65.

[11] Gupta SC, Sung B, Kim JH, Prasad S, Li S, Aggarwal BB (2013). Multitargeting by turmeric, the golden spice: From kitchen to clinic. Mol. Nutr. Food Res, 57: 1510–1528.

[12] Mohammadi M, Khashayar P, Tabari M, Sohrabvandi S, Moghaddam AF (2016). Water fortified with minerals (Ca, Mg, Fe, Zn). Int J Med Res Health Sci, 5(11):107-115

[13] El-Sayed SM, Youssef AM (2019). Potential application of herbs and spices and their effect in functional dairy product. Heliyon, 5(6):e01989

[14] Guo S, Geng Z, Zhang W, Liang J, Wang C, Deng Z, Du S (2016). The chemical composition of essential oils from Cinnamomum camphara and their insecticidal activity against stored product pests. Int J Mol Sci, 17(11): 1836S

[15] Jahan F, Happy AA, Chowdhury MMH, Hossain MF (2019). Natural herbs and spices: A great resource for skin care cosmetics. Journal of Plant Sciences, 7(4):86-99

[16] Naik SR, Pilgaonkar VW, Panda VS (2006). Evaluation of antioxidant activity of Ginkgo biloba phytosomes in rat brain. Phytother Res, 11: 1013–1016.

[17] Xue J, Hao L, Peng F (2008). Residues of 18 organochlorine pesticides in 30 traditional Chinese medicines, Chemosphere 71:1051e1055.

[18] García-Casal MN, Pe˜na-Rosas JP, Gómez-Malavé (2016).Sauces, spices, and condiments: definitions, potential

benefits, consumption patterns, and global markets. Ann. N.Y. Acad. Sci. 1379 (2016) 3–16. doi: 10.1111/ nyas.13045

[19] Johnny's kitchen (2012). The trade in spices. https://www.johnnyskitchen.us/herbs-spices/the-trade-in-spices.h tml Accessed 23rd June, 2021

[20] Chhetri P, Vijayan AK, Bhat SK, Gudade BA, Bora SS (2018). An overview of grouping of spices. Indian Botanist, pp1-4

[21] Herbal Academy (2020). Herbal Terminology: Herbal Actions, Categories, Energetics, Flavors, and Properties. https://theherbalacademy.c om/herbal-terminology/ Accessed 24th June 2021

[22] Metre V, Ghorpade J (2013). An overview of the research on texture based plant leaf classification. Int J Comp Sci Net, 2:2271-5420

[23] Peter KV (2021). Conventional classification of spices. https://www.johnnyskitchen.us/herbs-spices/introduction.html Accessed 23rd June, 2021

[24] Rajak H (2020). Classification of herbs. https://hmhub.me/classification-of-herbs/ Accessed 24th June 2021

[25] Rubio L, Motilva M, Romero M (2013). Recent advances in biologically active compounds in herbs and spices: a review of the most effective antioxidant and anti-inflammatory active principles. Crit Rev Food Sci Nutr, 53(9):943-953

[26] Yashin A, Yashin Y, Xia X, Memzer B (2017). Antioxidant activity of spices and their impact on human health: A review. Antioxidants, 6(70): 1-18

[27] Khorshidi J, Mohammadi R, Fakhr TM, Nourbakhsh, H(2009). Influence of drying methods, extraction time, and organ type on essential oil content of rosemary (Rosmarinus officinalis L.) Nature and Science, 7(11): 42- 44.

[28] Juana F, Angel PJ, Manuel V (2012). Beneficial health effects of bioactive compounds present in spices and aromatic herbs. In studies in Natural Products. Chemistry 37:115-134

[29] Liu Q, Meng X, Li Y, Zhao C, Tang G, Li H (2017). Antibacterial and antifungal activities of spices International J Mol Sci, 18(6):1283

[30] Raghavenra H, Diwakr RT, Lokesh BR, Baidu KA (2006). Eugenol the active principle from cloves inhibit 5-lipoxygenase activity and leukotriene – C4 in human PMNL cells. Prostaglandins, Leukotrienes Essential Acids, 74:23-27

[31] Ray DP, Srivastava S (2006). Curry leaf (Murrayakoenigii): the aromatic biopesticide. J interacademicia, 10: 231-235

[32] Dimic G, Kocic-Tanackov S, Mojovic L, Pejin J (2015). Antifungal activity of lemon essential oil, coriander and cinnamon extracts on foodborne molds in direct contact and the vapour phase. J. Food Process Pres, 39:1778-1787

[33] Gonelimali FD, Lin J, Miao W, Xuan J, Charles F, Chen M, Hatab SR (2018). Antimicrobial properties and mechanisms of action of some plant extracts against food pathogens and spoilage microorganisms. Frontiers in Microbiology 9(1639):1-9

[34] Boukhatem MN, Setzer WN (2020). Aromatic Herbs, medicinal plant-derived essential oils, and phytochemical extracts as potential therapies for Coronaviruses: future perspectives plants. 9. 1-23. doi: 10.3390/plants9060800.

[35] Praditya D, Kirchhoff L, Brüning J, Rachmawati H, Steinmann J, Steinmann E (2019). Anti-infective Properties of the Golden Spice Curcumin. Front

Microbiol. 2019; 10: 912. doi: 10.3389/fmicb.2019.00912

[36] Johansen JS, Harris AK, Rychly DJ, Ergul A (2005). Oxidative stress and the use of antioxidants in diabetes: linking basic science to clinical practice. Cardiovasc Diabetol, 4(1):5-15.

[37] Utomo RY, Ikawati M, Meiyanto E (2020). Revealing the Potency of Citrus and Galangal Constituents to Halt SARS-CoV-2 Infection. Preprint article, doi:10.20944/preprints202003.0214.v1

[38] Mehrbod P, Amini E, Tavassoti-Kheiri M (2009). Antiviral activity of garlic extract on influenza virus. Iranian J Virol, 3(1): 19–23.

[39] Shojai TM, Langeroudi AG, Karimi V, Barin A, Sadri N (2016). The effect of Allium sativum (garlic) extract on infectious bronchitis virus in specific pathogen free embryonic egg. Avicenna J Phytomed, 6: 458–467.

[40] Ministry of Ayush (2020). Ayurveda Preventive Measures for self care during COVID-19 Pandemic https://www.ayush.gov.in/docs/Ayurveda%20Preventive%20Measures%20for%20self%20care%20during%20%20COVID-19%20Pandemic.pdf Accessed 30th June 2021

[41] National Foundation for Cancer Research (2020). Can herbs and spices treat cancer? http://www.nfcr.org/blog/can-herbs-and-spices-treat-cancer/ Accessed 19th July 2021

[42] Kaefer CM, Milner JA (2011). Herbs and spices in cancer prevention and treatment. In: Herbal medicine: Biomolecular and clinical aspects. 2nd edition Boca Raton (FL): CRC Press/Taylor & Francis

[43] Wigutow C (2016). Six cancer-fighting herbs and spices. https://www.mhs.net/news/2016/09/cancer-fighting-herbs-and-spices Accessed 19th July 2021

[44] Fleischauer AT, Poole C (2000). Garlic consumption and cancer prevention: meta-analyses of colorectal and stomach cancers Arab, L. Am J Clin. Nutr, 72(4): 1047.

[45] Abdullaev FI (2002). Cancer chemopreventive and tumoricidal properties of saffron (Crocus sativus L.). Exp Biol Med (Maywood). 227(1):20-25. doi: 10.1177/153537020222700104.

[46] Aggarwal, BB, Kumar A, Bharti AC (2003). Anticancer P otential of Curcumin: Preclinical and Clinical StudiesAnticancer Res, 23(1A): 363.

[47] Nouroz, F, Mehboob M, Noreen S, Zaidi F, Mobin T (2015). A review on anticancer activities of garlic (Allium sativum L.). Middle East J Sci Res, 23(6): 1145-1151

[48] Kaur KK (2020). Bioactive compounds within herbs and spices contributing to antidiabetic action in type 2 diabetis mellitus (T2DM) – A short communication. Acta Scientific Nutritional Health 4(1):88-92

[49] Lyantagaye SL (2011). Ethnopharmacological and Phytochemical review of Allium species (sweet garlic) and Tulbaghia species (wild garlic) from Southern Africa. Tanzanian Journal of Science, 37(1)

[50] Khajehdehi P, Pakfetrat M, Javidnia K, Azad F, Malekmakan L, Nasab MH, Dehghanzadeh G (2011). Oral supplementation of turmeric attenuates proteinuria, transforming growth factor-β and interleukin-8 levels in patients with overt type 2 diabetic nephropathy: a randomized, double-blind and placebo-controlled study. Scand J Urol Nephrol, 45(5):365-370

[51] Bandara T, Uluwaduge I, Jansz ER (2012). Bioactivity of cinnamon withspecial emphasis on diabetes mellitus: a review. Int. J. Food Sci. Nutr. 63(3): 380 -386.

[52] Adeniyi PO, Sanusi RA (2019). Antidiabetic herbs and spices. World Journal of Nutrition and Health., 7(1): 18-22

[53] Bakheit AM, Foda MI (2012). Sensory evaluation and antioxidant activity of new Mudaffara cheese with spices under different storage temperatures. J. Appl. Sci. Res. 8 (7): 3143–3150.

[54] Etter SC (2005). Rosmarius officinalis as an antioxidant. J Herbs Spices Med Plants, 11(1-2):121-159

[55] Alam K, Hoq O, Uddin S (2016). Medicinal plant Allium sativum-Areview. J Med Plants Stud, 4(6): 72–79.

[56] Wootton-Beard PC, Ryan I (2011). Improving public health?: the role of antioxidant-rich fruit and vegetable beverages. Food Res Int, 44: 3135-3148.

[57] Nelson RH (2013). Hyperlipidemia as a risk factor for cardiovascular disease. Prim Care 40(1):195-211

[58] Jinag A (2019). Health benefits of culinary herb and spices. Journal of AOAC International, 102(2):

[59] Kempaiah RK, Srinivasan K (2002). Integrity of erythrocytes ofhypercholesterolemic rats during spices treatment. Mol Cell Biochem, 236: 155-161.

[60] Srinivasan K, Sambaiah K, Chandrasekhara N (2004). Spices as beneficial hypolipidemic food adjuncts: A Review. Food Rev Int, 20:187-220.

[61] Sayed-Ahmad S, Talou T, Saad Z, Hijazi A, Merah O (2017). The Apiaceae: Ethnomedical family as source for industrial uses. Ind. Crops Prod, 109: 661-671

[62] Giugliano, D., Ceriello A, Esposito K (2006). The effects of diet on inflammation. Emphasis on the metabolic syndrome. J. Am. Coll. Cardiol. 48:677–685.

[63] Mueller M, Hobiger S, Jungbauer A (2010). Anti-inflammatory activity of extracts from fruits, herbs and spices. Food Chem, 12:987-996

[64] Krishnaswamy K (2008). Traditional Indian spices and their health significance. Asia Pacific J Clin Nutr, 17(S1): 265–268.

[65] Tapsell LC, Hemphill I, Cobiac L, Patch CS, Sullivan DR, Fenech M, RoodenrysKeogh JB, Clifton PM, Williams PG, Fazio VA, Inge KE (2006). Health benefits of herbs and spices: the past, the present, the future. Med J Aust, 85(4):S4-24.

[66] Mrityunjaya M, Pavithra V, Neelam R, Janhavi P, Prakash H, Ravindra PV (2020). Immune boosting, antioxidant and anti-inflammatory food supplements targeting pathogenesis of COVID-19. Frontiers in Microbiology, 11:2337

[67] Alabi MO (2007). Processing and utilization of selected food crops in Nigeria. Peace House Press, Gboko, Benue State, Nigeria, pp 138

[68] Tiwari BK, Valdramidis VP, O'Donnell CP, Muthukumarappan K, Bourke P, Cullen PJ (2009). Application of natural antimicrobials for food preservation. J Agric Food Chem, 57 (14): 5987–6000.

[69] Lai PK, Roy J (2004). Antimicrobial and chemopreventive properties of herbs and spices. Curr Med Chem, 11: 1451–1460.

[70] Gottardi D, Bukvicki D, Prasad S, Tyagi AK (2016). Beneficial effects of spices in food preservation and safety. Front Microbiol,7(1394):1-20

[71] Bhatia M, Sharma A (2012). Inhibitory activities of Brassica nigra,

Cinnamomum cassia (Blume) and Cuminum cymimum towards Esherichia coli and Staphylococcus aureus. Arch Appl Sci Res, 4: 1811-1815

[72] Rattanachaikunsopon P, Phumkhachorn P (2008). Diallysulfide content and antimicrobial activity against foodborne pathogenic bacteria of chives (Allium schoenoprasum). BiosciBiotechnolBiochem, 72:2987-2991

[73] Yadav AS, Singh R (2004). Natural preservatives in poultry meat. Indian J Nat Prod Resour 3:300-303

[74] Koffi-Nevry R, Kouassi C, Nanga YZ, Koussemon M, Loukou GY (2012). Antibacterial activity of two bell pepper extracts: Capsicum hydropiper (L.) Delarbre . J Evid Based Complement Altern Med, 2014:782830

[75] Tornuk F, Cankurt H, Ozturk I, Sagdic O, Bayram O, Yetim H (2011). Efficacy of various plant hydrosols as natural food sanitizers in reducing Escherichia coli O157:H7 and Salmonella typhimurium on fresh cut carrots and apples. Int J Food Microbiol. 48(1): 30–35.

[76] Lee SY, Gwon SY, Kim SJ. Moon (2009). Inhibitory effect of commercial green tea and rosemary leaf powders on the growth of foodborne pathogens in laboratory media and oriental-style rice cakes. J Food Prot. 72(5): 1107–1111.

[77] Tajkarimi MM, Sowmya HV, Swarnalatha SP, Negi PS (2014). Antifungal activity of essential oils and their combination in in-vitro and in-vivo conditions. Arch Phytopathol Plant Protect, 47:564-570

[78] Bin S, Yi-Zhong C, John DB, Harold C (2011). Potential application of spice and herb extracts as natural preservatives in cheese. J. Med. Food, 14: 284–290

[79] Bakrm, SA, Salihin BA (2013). Effects of inclusion of Allium sativum and Cinnamomumverum in milk on the growth and activity of lactic acid bacteria during yoghurt fermentation. Amer-Euras. J. Agric. Environ. Sci, 13: 1448–1457.

[80] Hamid OIA, Abdelrahman NAM (2012). Effect of adding Cardamom, cinnamon and Fenugreek to goat's milk curd on the quality of white cheese during storage. Int. J. Dairy Sci, 7: 43–50.

[81] Bandyopadhyay M, Chakraborty M, Raychaudhuri U (2007). A process for preparing a natural antioxidant enriched dairy product (Sandesh). LWT – Food Sci Technol, 40(5):842-851

[82] International Herbal Water Foundation (2008). Value Added Water Based Beverages Specification.https://www.academia.edu/9063800/Proposal_and_Draft_Standard_Flavored_Standard_Water_by_international_herbal_water_foundation_to_Food_Safety_and_Standards_Authority_of_India. Accessed 22-07-2021

[83] Park H, Lee M, Kim K, Park E, Paik H (2018). Antioxidant and antigenotoxic effect of dairy products supplemented with red ginseng extract. J Dairy Sci, 101:1-9

[84] Srivastava P, Prasad SGM, Mohd NA, Prasad M (2015). Analysis of antioxidant activity of herbal yoghurt prepared from different milk. Pharma Inno J 4:18-20

[85] Pal RS, Pal Y, Saraswat N, Wal P, Wal A (2019). Current review on herbs for derma care. The Open Dermatology Journal, 13:41-46

[86] Aburjai T, Natsheh FM (2003). Plants used in cosmetics. Phytotherapy Research, 17(9):987-1000

[87] Lyantagaye SL (2011). Ethnopharmacological and Phytochemical review of Allium species

(sweet garlic) and Tulbaghia species (wild garlic) from Southern Africa. Tanzanian Journal of Science, 37(1)

[88] Scott IM, Jensen HR, Philogene BJR, Arnason JT (2008). A review on Piper spp (Piperaceae) phytochemistry, insecticidal activity and mode of action. Phytochemistry review 7(1):65

[89] Kasrati A, Jamali CA, Bekkonche R, Wohlmuth H, Leach D, Abbad A (2015). Comparative evaluation of antioxidant and insecticidal properties of essential oils from five Moroccan aromatic herbs. J Food Sci Technol 52(4):2312-2319

[90] Asensio L, Gonzalez I, Garcya T, Martyn R (2008). Determination of food authenticity by enzyme linked immunosorbent assay (ELISA). Food Control, 19:1e8

[91] Zhao Z, Hu Y, Liang Z, Yuan JP, Jiang Z, Leung KS (2006). Authentication is fundamental for standardization of Chinese medicines. Planta Medica 72: 865e874.

[92] Sasikumar B, Swetha VP, Parvathy VA, Sheeja TE (2016). Advances in Adulteration and Authenticity Testing of Herbs and Spices . In: Advances in Food Authenticity Testing, pp 585-624

[93] Revathy SS, Rathinamala R, Murugeshan M (2012). Authentication methods for drugs used in Ayurvedha, Siddha and Unnani systems of medicine: an overview. Int J Pharm Sci Res 3: 2352e2361

[94] Meuren M (2010). Spectrophotometric techniques. In: Lees, M. (Ed.), Food Authentication and Traceability. Wood head publishing, Cambridge, pp. 184e185.

[95] Zhang Q, Thomas D, Acworth I (2013). Evaluation of Herb and Fruit Juice Adulteration and Authenticity by Colometric Array Detection and Pattern Recognition. Planta Medica 79:125.

[96] Yip PY, Chau CF, Mak CY, Kwan HS (2007). DNA methods for identification of Chinese medicinal materials. Chinese Med 2: 9.

[97] Guldikena B, Catalkayab G, Ozkanb G, Ceylanb FD, Capanoglub E (2021). Toxicological effects of commonly used herbs and spices. In: Toxicology pp 201 – 213

[98] Ritter S, Dinh TT (1990). Capsaicin-induced neuronal degeneration in the brain and retina of preweanling rats. J Comp Neurol, 296(3):447–461

[99] Chanda S, Mould A, Esmail A, Bley K (2005). Toxicity studies with pure trans-capsaicin delivered to dogs via intravenous administration. Regul Toxicol Pharmacol, 43(1):66–75.

[100] Patane S, Marte F, La Rosa FC, La Rocca R (2010). Capsaicin and arterial hypertensive crisis. Int J Cardiol, 144(2): e26–e27.

[101] Singh R, Koppikar SJ, Paul P, Gilda S, Paradkar AR, Kaul-Ghanekar R (2009). Comparative analysis of cytotoxic effect of aqueous cinnamon extract from Cinnamomum zeylanicum bark with commercial cinnamaldehyde on various cell lines. Pharm Biol, 47(12): 1174–1179

[102] Prashar A, Locke IC, Evans CS (2006). Cytotoxicity of clove (Syzygiumaromaticum) oil and its major components to human skin cells. Cell Prolif, 39(4):241–248

[103] Adeeyo AO, Edokpayi JN, Alabi MA, Msagati TAM, Odiyo JO (2021). Plant active products and emerging interventions in water potabilisation: disinfection and multidrug resistant pathogen treatment. Clin Phytosci, 7(1): 1-16

[104] Khanal A, Devkota HP, Kaundinnyayana S, Gyawali P, Ananda R, Adhikari R (2021). Culinary herbs

and spicesin Nepal: A review of their traditional uses, chemical constituents, and pharmacological activities. Ethnobot Res App, 21:1-18

[105] Stiller D (2011). Effects and side effects of spices. Allergologie, 34(8): 412-426

Chapter 4

Health Benefits and Functional and Medicinal Properties of Some Common Indian Spices

Vinod Kumar Paswan, Chandra Shekhar Singh, Garima Kukreja, Durga Shankar Bunkar and Basant Kumar Bhinchhar

Abstract

India is the largest producer and consumer of some important common spices. Major Indian spices include pepper, cardamom, ginger, turmeric and chilies. Commercial cultivation in India is undertaken on 27 spices besides the herbal spices. Spices and herbs are mostly used as seasonings to impart flavors, pungency, aroma and color in the food. In addition, spices enhances shelf life of the food by preventing and delaying the spoilage and by preserving the sensory attributes of food products. Spices contain several important phytochemicals like aromatic compounds, essential oils, phenolics and pigments which imparts characteristic flavor and aroma and gives a herbal appeal to the food and beverages and enhances their consumer acceptability. In addition the active components of these herbs and spices are endowed with tremendous functional properties and medicinal values providing several health benefits and immunity. The era of Covid-19 has seen spiked consumption of spices and herbs based health drinks and concoctions for providing these health benefits and immunity. The present chapter deals with the characteristics of some important Indian spices, their usages, active components present in them along with exploring their health benefits, functional and immunomodulant properties.

Keywords: Indian spices, herbal food products, functional foods, seasonings, phytochemicals, bioactive components

1. Introduction

India has been famous for varieties of spices since the ancient time for its exotic flavor, taste and medicinal values, therefore known as the home of Spices [1]. Spices means whole or ground form obtained from natural plants or vegetable products which has been used for imparting flavor, aroma and pungency to foods and also used for seasoning of foods. It also has non-food applications in dyeing, perfumery products and neutraceutical industries. It mask the spoiled flavor of meat that enhance the shelf life of foods [2]. Different parts of the plants or tree are used as spices such as fruits, stigma, bark, seeds, leaves, kernel, aril, bulbs, berries etc.

Around the world about more than 70 types of spices are grown, whereas pepper, cardamom, ginger, turmeric and chillies are the most common spices widely grown in India. However India is the largest producer as well as consumer of spices. Commercial cultivation in India is undertaken on 27 spices besides the herbal spices. The most famous spices of India is black pepper, which is known as the king of spices. Kerala got first position in the production of black pepper with contributing about 97% of the total production however cardamom known as the queen of spices which has been also used as essential commodity in the world. The leading spice producing states in India are the Andhra Pradesh, Karnataka, Kerala, Gujarat, Madhya Pradesh, Maharashtra, Orissa, Rajasthan, Tamil Nadu and West Bengal. Spices are mostly used as flavoring agent in a number of foodstuffs like curries, bakery products, pickles, processed meat, beverages, liqueurs etc. They enhance or change the flavors of the foods. These herbs and spices endowed with tremendous functional properties and medicinal values provide great health benefits and immunity [3, 4].

2. Classification of spices

Indian spices can be categorized based on its plant parts used, origin and flavor and economic importance. The classification is further given as hereunder.

2.1 Based on its plant parts

It is categorized based on its leaf, root, bulb, fruit, rhizome, bark, seed, pod, Kernel, bud, floral parts, latex, berry and aril. Classification is given as follows:

- Seed: Cumin, black cumin, fenugreek, coriander, fennel, ajwain, poppy, aniseed and mustard.
- Bulb: Onion, garlic, leek and shallot.
- Bark: Cinnamon and cassia
- Fruit: Chili, cardamom, allspice and kokum
- Leaf: Mint, curry-leaf, bay-leaf, chive, rosemary and savory
- Rhizome: Turmeric, ginger, and galangal
- Pod: Vanilla and tamarind
- Kernel: Nutmeg
- Floral part: Saffron, savory, caper and marjoram
- Bud: Clove and caper
- Latex: Asafoetida
- Aril: Mace and anardana
- Berry: Black pepper, juniper and allspice

2.2 Based on origin and flavor

Based on the origin and flavor spices can be classified as aromatic spices, pungent spices, phenolic spices and colored spices. Classification is given as follows:

- Pungent spices: Ginger, chili, black pepper and mustard

- Phenolic spices: Clove and allspice

- Aromatic spices: Cardamom, aniseed, celery, cumin, coriander, fenugreek and

- cinnamon.

- Colored spices: Turmeric, saffron and paprika

2.3 Based on economic importance

Based on economic importance Indian spices divided into two groups i.e. major and minor spices.

2.3.1 Major spices

Major spices are contributing a principle share in spice trade industry globally and contribute about 75–90% of the total imported exchange. Small cardamom, black pepper, chili, turmeric and ginger are comes under major spices.

2.3.2 Minor spices

Apart from five major spices, all other are known as minor spices. They are further divided into five sub groups. They are stated as follows:

- Bulbous spices: Garlic, onion, leek and shallot

- Seed spices: Coriander, cumin, black cumin, fennel, aniseed, celery, mustard, poppy and caraway.

- Aromatic spices: Clove, cinnamon, allspice, aniseed and nutmeg

- Leafy spices: Curry leaf, mint, rosemary, bay-leaf, and parsley.

- Acidulant tree spices: Tamarind, kokum and anardana

3. Common Indian spices

Common Indian spices, parts used and active compounds present in them are listed in **Table 1** and their usage and health benefits are presented in **Table 2** and discussed in this section.

3.1 Chilies (Mirch)

Red chili is the frequently used spice in our daily life which belongs of genus Capsicum, that is most famous consumed spices all around the world [5]. Chillies

Spices Name	Scientific Name	Plant part use as spice	Active compounds
Ginger	*Zingiber officinale* Rosc.	Rhizome	Gingerol and shogaol
Turmeric	*Curcuma longa* L.	Rhizome	Curcumin
Coriander	*Coriandrum sativum* L.	Leaf & Fruit	Geraniol
Cumin	*Cuminum cyminum* L.	Fruit	Aldehyde cumino
Cardamom (small)	*Elettaria cardamomum* Maton	Fruit,Seed	Cineole, pinene, sabinene and porneol
Cardamom (Large)	*Amomum subulatum* Roxb.	Fruit,Seed	Cineole, pinene, sabinene and porneol
Chili	*Capsicum annuum* L.	Fruit	Capsaicin
Fenugreek	*Trigonella foenum-graecum* L.	Seed	Rhaponticin and isovitexin
Aniseed	*Pimpinella anisum* L.	Fruit	Anethole
Ajwain	*Trachyspermum ammi* L.	Fruit	Thymol
Caraway	*Carum carvi* L.	Fruit	D-carvone and D-limonere
Cinnamon	*Cinnamomum zeylanicum Breyn*	Bark	Eugenol, cineole and cinnamaldehyde
Garlic	*Allium sativum* L.	Bulb	Allicin
Kokam	*Garcinia indica* Choisy	Rind	Anthocyanin
Saffron	*Crocus sativus* L.	Stigma	Crocin and crocerin
Pepper	*Piper longum* L.	Fruit Long	Peperine
Clove	*Syzygium aromaticum(L)* Merr.& Perry	Unopened Flower bud	Eugeniol
Asafoetida	*Ferula asafoetida* L	Root & Rhizome	Ferulic ester
Bay Leaf	*Laurus nobilis* L.	Leaf	Eugenol, methyl eugenol and elemicin
Nutmeg & Mace	*Myristica fragrans* Houtt.	Seed	Myristicin
Poppy seed	*Papaver somniferum* L.	Seed	Thiamin, folate,
Allspice	*Pimenta dioica* (L) Merr.	Fruit & Leaf	Eugenol
Rosemary	*Rosmarinus officinalis* L.	Leaf	Carnosic acid
Sage	*Salvia officinalis* L.	Leaf	Rosmarinic Acid
Oregano	*Origanum vulgare* L.	Leaf	Carvacrol and thymol
Tamarind	*Tamarindus indica* L.	Fruit	Limonene, geraniol, safrole and cinnamic acid
Rosemary	*Rosmarinus officinalis* L.	Leaf	Rosmarinic acid, carnosol, and carnosic acid
Capsicum	*Capsicum annuum* L.	Fruit	Capsaicin
Paprika	*Capsicum annuum* L.	Fruit	Capsaicin
Celery	*Apium graveolens* L.	Fruit & Stem	Umbelliferone and Alpha-linoleic acid
Dill	*Anethum graveolens* L.	Fruit	Limonene
Cassia	*Cinnamomum cassia.*Blume	Bark	Cinnamaldehyde
Mustard	*Brassica juncea* L.Czern	Seed	Allyl isothiocyanate
Parsley	*Petroselinum crispum* Mill.	Leaf	Myristicin & limonene

Spices Name	Scientific Name	Plant part use as spice	Active compounds
Star Anise	*Illicium verum* Hook.	Fruit	Shikimic acid
Sweet flag	*Acorus calamus* L.	Rhizome	Asarones
Greater Galanga	*Alpinia galanga* Willd.	Rhizome	1′-ace-toxychavicol acetate
Horse Radish	*Armoracia rusticana* Gaertn.	Root	Allyl isothiocyanate
Vanilla	*Vanilla planifolia* Andr.	Pod	Vanillin

Table 1.
List of common spices used in India, parts used and active compounds present in them.

are having differnet size, shapes and color. The red color of chillies is due to presence of capsanthin apart form a carotenoid pigment. The pungency of chillies is due to the presence of alkaloid capsaicin which is measured in terms of scoville value. Capsicum oleoresin of red chili is used for ointments, which are used to get relief from pain, swelling and inflammation [6, 7]. Generally smaller the size more is the pungency. Ground chili is used in most of the Indian gravies and vegetable dishes. It is also used in day to day preparation foods like chutney, sauses, pickles, dehydrated chili etc.

3.1.1 Uses and health benefits

- It is used as food seasoning agent.
- It is a stimulant of ptyalin present in saliva which helps in digestion.
- A green chili is rich in Vitamin C & vitamin A.
- It is carminative and antiflatulence agent.
- It stimulates blood circulation.
- It is good for sore throat.

3.2 Turmeric (Haldi)

Turmeric grown in India includes 60% of the overall area uses for spices and condiments belong to the Zingiberaceae family which is commonly cultivated in India and Southeast Asia. It is known by different names such as kunyit (Indonesian and Malay), besar (Nepali) and haldi or pasupu in some Asian nations. There are about 70 species of turmeric of which 30 species are found in India. Turmeric obtained from the rhizome of Curcuma longa plant which accounts 96% of the total turmeric obtained from this variety in India [8], however, *Curcuma aromatica* is another variety of turmeric which is accounts 4% of the area under cultivation. Turmeric rhizome contains 5% essential oil and the coloring substance present in it is known as curcumin which has been used as medicine since the many years ago because it having several pharmacological properties like anti-inflammatory, anti-neoplastic, and anti-angiogenic. It is “Generally Recognized as Safe.” By Food Drug Administration (FDA), and consumption of 12 g/day of curcumin was safe without any toxic effect [9]. It is used ground in curry powder, meat and egg dishes, in pickles and as a coloring substance in cakes and rice. It is also used in lemon rice,

Spices	Uses	Benefits	Picture of spices
Cardamom	It is commonly used in sweets and pharmaceutical sector as a flavor and smell enhancer.	It is widely used in stomach disorder and problems of respiratory system. Chewing of whole cardamom is also good for coping with diabetes.	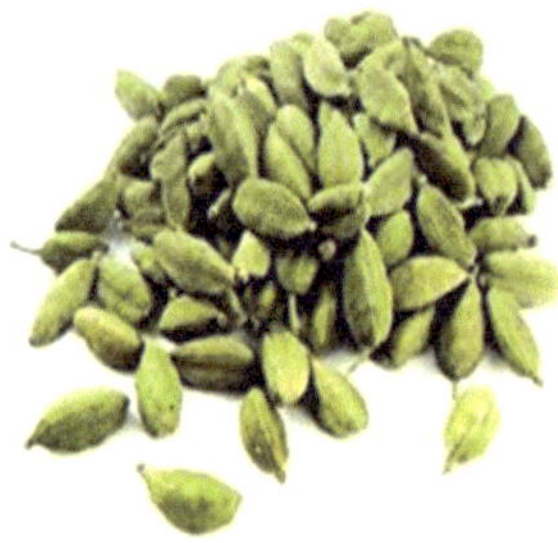
Chili	Chili is a principle ingredient adding to the food for hot flavor.	It reduces the cholesterol and also helps in burning calories. A green chili is rich in Vitamin C & vitamin A.	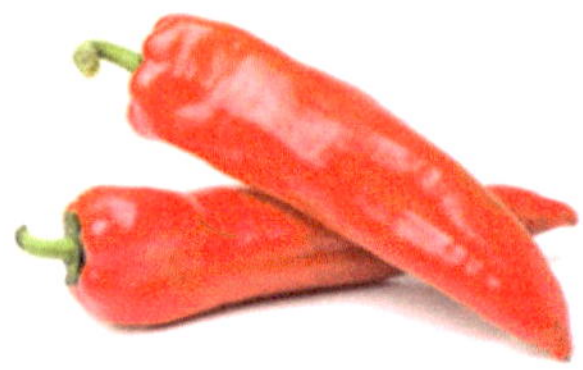
Cinnamon	It is used for mainly for preparing masalas and seasoning food.	It reduces blood cholesterol with natural production of insulin.	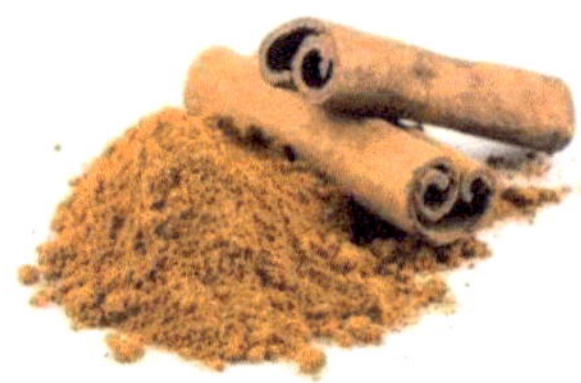
Coriander	Its leaves and seeds are used in cooking. The oil of coriander is used as antimicrobial property and as a natural fragrance in perfumery industry.	It is used in allergies, poor digestion, aching joints and rheumatism.	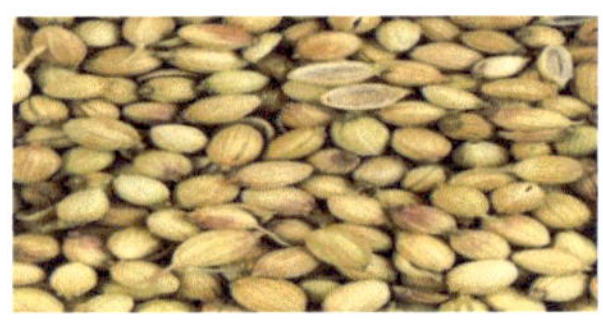
Clove	Clove is highly valued medicine for their carminative, stimulant, antiflatulent and antihelmenthic properties.	It is mostly used in many households as an aid to prevent the minor disorders like indigestion, flatulence, tooth ache etc.	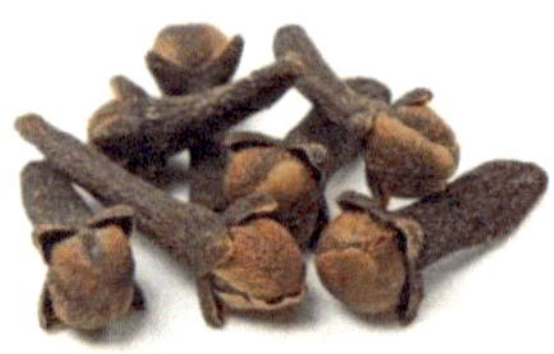
Fenugreek	It is mainly used as a green leafy vegetable and seeds are used for seasoning and preparing *Masalas*. It also has medicinal uses.	Fenugreek seed tea or sweet fudge is good for increasing breast milk. It also helpful for treating diabetes and lowering cholesterol	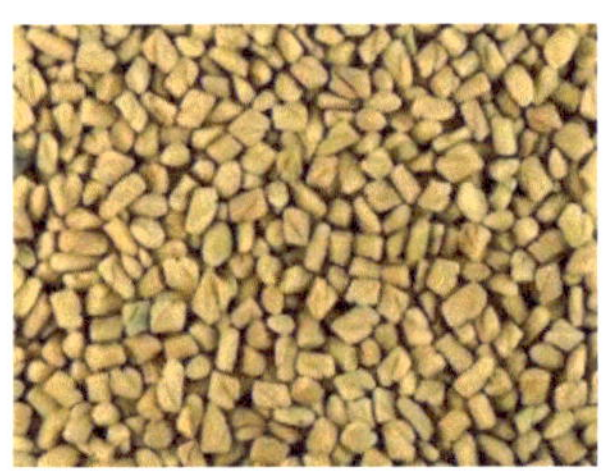
Garlic	It is use as condiment for flavoring of dishes.	It is used to treat various digestive disorders. Allicin uses intestinal synthesis of vitamin B.	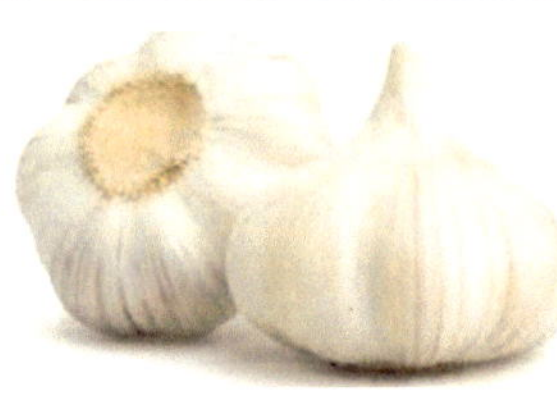

Spices	Uses	Benefits	Picture of spices
Ginger	Ginger oleoresin used for flavoring soft drinks and in medicine. Ginger Tea, ginger concoction effective in Cold & coughs.	It is used as carminative and gastro intestinal stimulant. It reduces opacity of cornea.	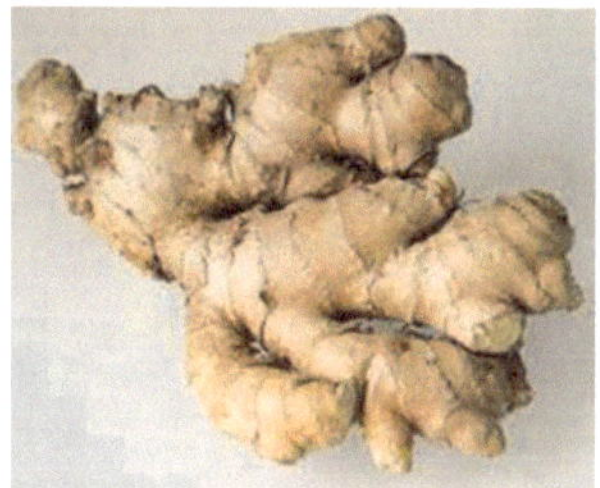
Turmeric	Used as blood purifier & antibiotics. It is also used in cooking and skin care products.	Turmeric powder can be used for healing cuts and wounds. It is used as anti-oxidant due to presence of phenolic bioactive compound of curcuminoids	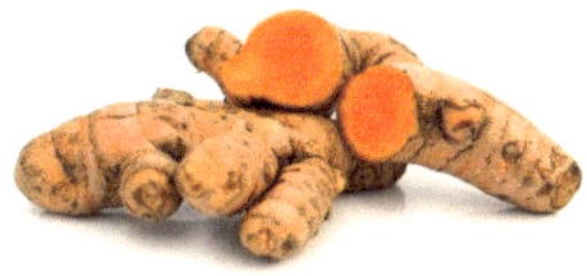
Black Pepper	It is mainly used in cooking, particularly for garnishing.	It is used effectively in the treatment of rheumatism and muscular pain, intestinal gas and headache.	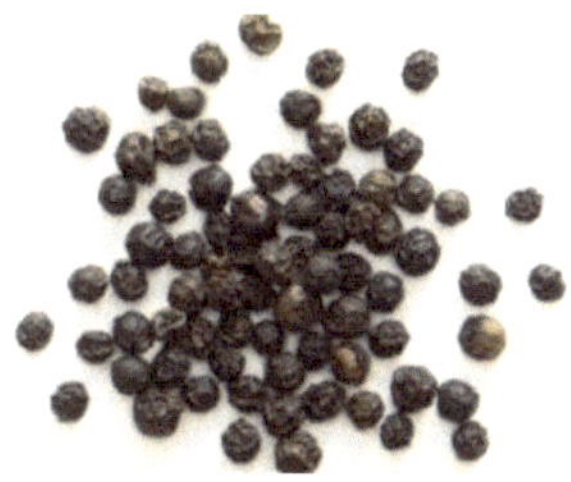
Cumin	It is used for cooking and it also possesses medicinal properties.	It is a good source or iron and keeps immune system healthy. Water boiled with cumin seeds is good for coping with dysentery.	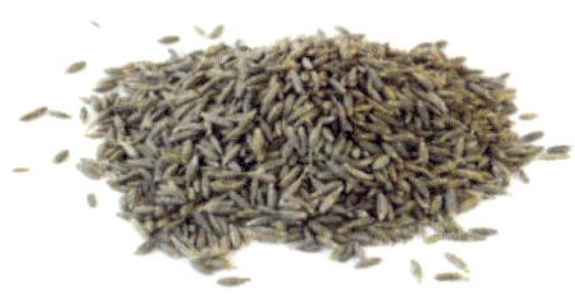
Ajwain	Even a small number of fruits tend to dominate the flavor of a dish.	Ajwain is used in traditional Ayurvedic medicine primarily for stomach disorders such as indigestion, flatulence diarrhea and colic	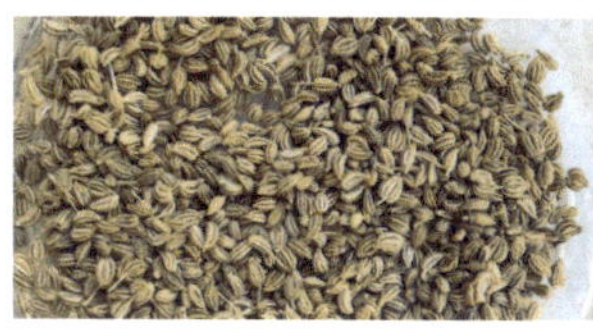
Aniseed	It is used a mouth refresher and used after the taking meals. It is also used in preparation of cakes, bread, cookies, and non-vegetarian dishes.	It is mildly carminative and used in treating colic pain.	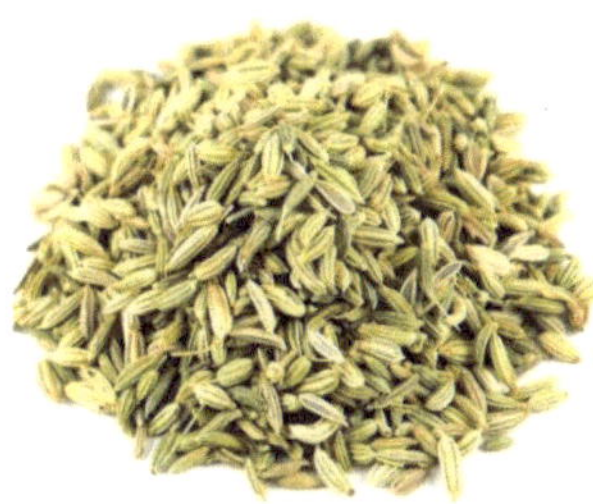
Caraway	Its seeds are used to flavor the cakes, biscuits, cheese, apple sause and cookies.	The combination of black cumin and caraway seeds oils have been used to killed parasites and worms, detoxify, ameliorate amoebic dysentery, shigellosis, abscesses, old tumors, ulcers of the mouth, and rhinitis.	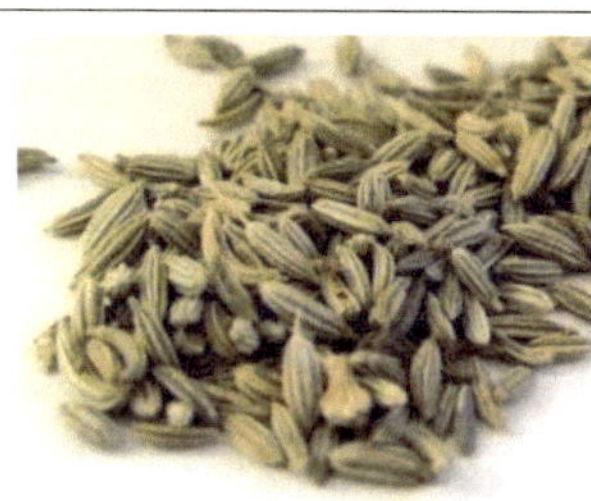

Spices	Uses	Benefits	Picture of spices
Kokum	Its colorful red juice is used for the manufacture of beverages	In traditional medicine, such as Ayurveda, kokum is prescribed for edema, rheumatism, delayed menstruation, constipation and other bowel complaints, and intestinal parasites	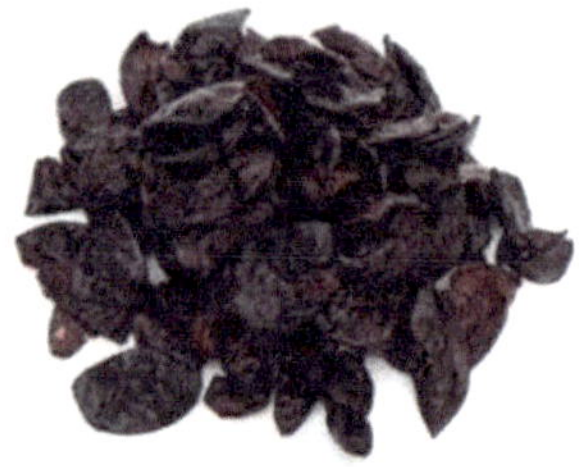
Saffron	It is used for cooking as well as in beauty products. It is mainly used in sweet dishes. It has good medicinal properties.	It helps to cope with skin diseases. It is a good remedy for cough, cold and asthma.	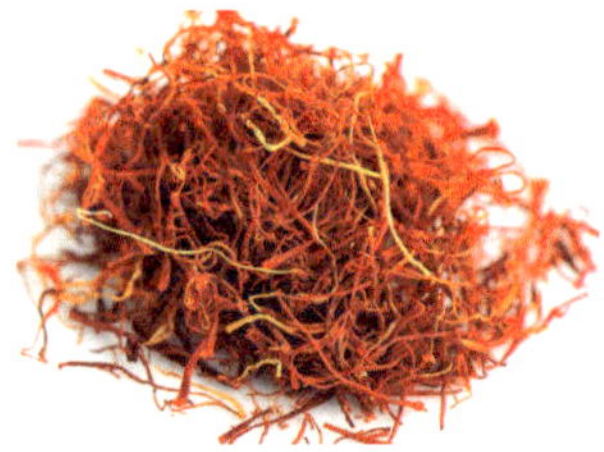
Asafoetida	It is used for seasoning food especially snacks and has medicinal uses.	A good medicine for whooping cough and stomach ache caused due to gas.	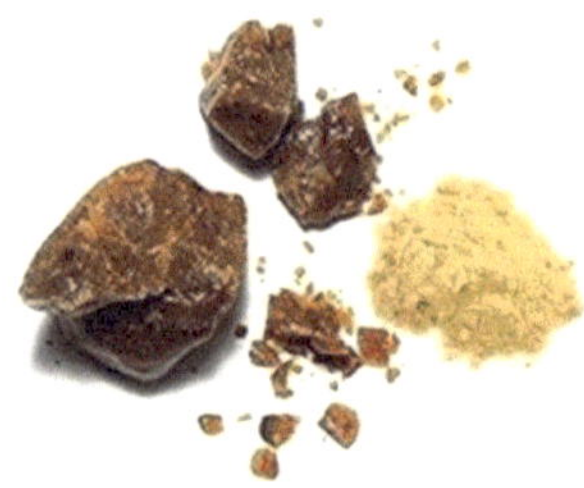
Bay leaf	It is used in cooking to add a specific flavor to food. It also has some medicinal properties.	Its oil possesses antifungal and anti bacterial.	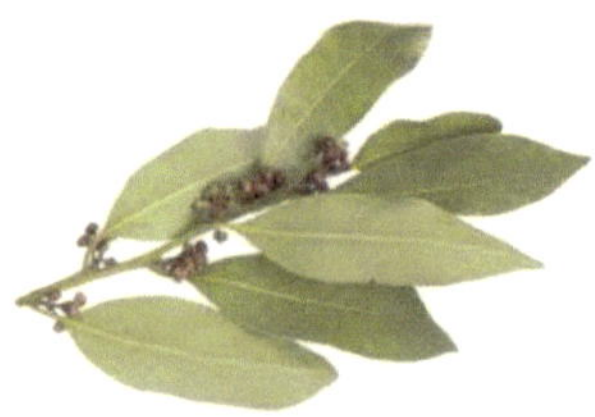
Nutmeg & Mace	It is used in powdered form for garnishing and also for masala preparation. It is used in soaps, perfumes and shampoos.	It is beneficial for the treatments of asthma, heart disorder and foul breath.	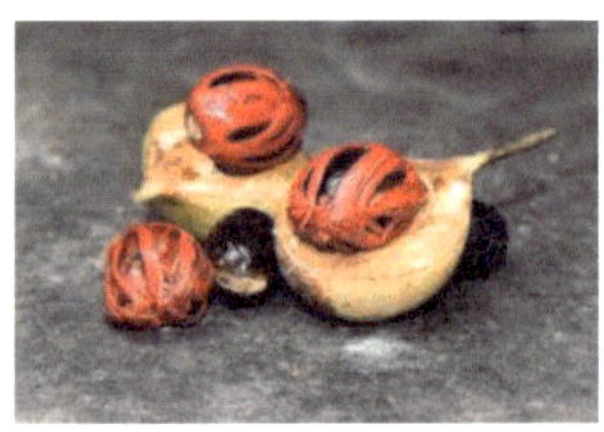
Poppy seed	Its seeds are good source of thiamin, folate, and important minerals like calcium, iron, magnesium, manganese, phosphorus and zinc.	It also effective in paralysis, facial palsy, migraine, amnesia related problem. Its powder if taken with water is effective in treating hemorrhoids	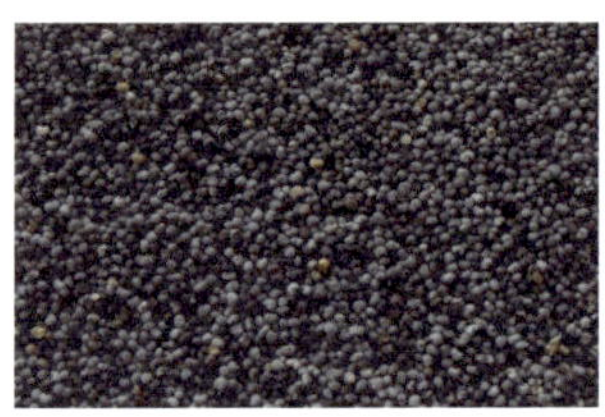

Table 2.
Uses and benefits of some common Indian spices.

sambar, dal, kadhi, and khichdi and in marinating meat. The most common adulteration in turmeric is metanil yellow or lead salts. India is the largest producer as well as exporter of Turmeric spice to the USA, U.K and Japan. Curcuminoids are responsible for yellow color and present 2–4% in turmeric.

3.2.1 Uses and health benefits

- It is used as anti-oxidant due to presence of phenolic bioactive compound of curcuminoids.
- Generally used for flavoring & coloring food.
- Principal using in manufacture of curry powders.
- Turmeric oleoresin is used instead of powder in pickles, gelatin, butter & cheese.
- Essential oil of turmeric is antimicrobial, antiseptic & antibacterial (due to sodium salts of curcumin & curcuminoids.
- Used as blood purifier & antibiotics.

3.3 Cardamom (Elaichi)

The common name of cardamom is Ellettaria cardamomum belong to the family Zingiberaceae and popularly known as the Queen of spice. The cardamom contains 2–10% volatile oil with the characteristic pleasant odor. The active compounds present in the oil cineole, terpinyl acetate, pinene, sabinene and porneol. It is used in coffee, sweet preparation, cookies, breads, cakes and preserves as flavoring substances. Cardamom is sometimes sold in the market after the extraction of essential oil. All species of cardamom are used as kitchen cooking spices. Besides the above uses it can be also helpful in flatulent indigestion and to stimulate the urge for food in humans with anorexia [10, 11].

3.3.1 Uses and health benefits

- Green cardamom is an essential ingredient in Indian sweets, puddings, yogurt and ice creams.
- Whole form important in chai masala, a special hot tea beverage.
- Aid in digestion, prevents nausea and vomiting.

3.4 Garlic (Lassan)

Garlic (Allium sativum L.) belongs to the family Liliaceae is native to Asia however it is also grown China, North Africa (Egypt), Europe, and Mexico. Its bulb growing to 25–70 cm height with flowers, which is used for flavoring of varieties of foods to enhance the taste, nutritive value and digestion. The principle compound present in the garlic is allin (inactive form) which is converted to allicin (active form) by the enzyme allinase which has been recognized for antifungal and antiviral activities. Allicin further converted in to allyl disulphide which is responsible for pleasant flavor [12]. It is used in recipe like rasam, chutney, pulav, sauses, and most of the non-vegetarian dishes. A numbers of pharmacological activities are found in garlic like anthelmintics, anti-inflammatory, antioxidant, and antifungal with low side effects. (Alam, Hoq, & Uddin, 2016).

3.4.1 Uses and health benefits

- It is used to treat various digestive disorders.
- It is possess platelet aggregation inhibitor factor.
- Use as condiment for flavoring of dishes.
- Garlic oil is used as an insecticide.
- Garlic has antibacterial property (allyl disulfide oxide) against gram positive and gram negative bacteria.
- Allicin uses intestinal synthesis of vitamin B.
- Extract of the garlic can lower the serum cholesterol levels and prevent heart diseases

3.5 Ginger (Adrak)

It is the root of the plant Zingiber officinale Roscoe. Bioactive compounds present in the ginger are gingerol and shogaol. It has the pungency like lemony or camphory note. The flavoring compound has sharp burning sensory stimulation [13]. The pungency of dried ginger is more and valuable for the taste. Whole root is used for curries, pickles, chutney, preserve and dried fruits. Ground ginger is used in masala, pulav, pongal, all non-vegetarian foods. It is also used different beverages such as tea, lime juice and butter milk. It is used as appetizer, laxative, Indigestion, Asthma, Bronchitis [14, 15].

3.5.1 Uses and health benefits

- It is used as carminative and gastro intestinal stimulant.
- Ginger oleoresin used for flavoring soft drinks and in medicine.
- Ginger provides relief in piles, Rheumatism and Head ache.
- It reduces opacity of cornea.
- Fresh ginger juice is useful for diabetics.
- Ginger Tea, ginger concoction effective in Cold & coughs.
- It’s improves the blood supply and heart muscles.

3.6 Coriander (Dhania)

Coriandrum sativum L. (Umbelliferae) is native of Meditarian region. It is mainly known for its fresh characteristic spring like aroma. The coriander seed contains 0.5 to 1.0% essential oil which possesses an active compound geraniol. Coriander leaves are rich in vitamin C (250 mg/100 g), and vitamin A (5,200 IU/100 g). The roasted and ground coriander is used in curry powder as an ingredient. It is used as thickening and flavoring agent in the cookery. Coriander is used to make pastries, synthetic syrup and drinks. It also acts as preservative in meat preparation. Previously coriander is used to effective in digestive problem, respiratory and urinary systems [16, 17].

3.6.1 Uses and health benefits

Seeds are chewed to correct the foul breath.

- An infusion of seeds is useful for flatulence, indigestion, vomiting & intestinal disorders eliminating symptoms related to female reproductive parts.
- Oleoresin (5%) used in flavoring beverages, pickles, sweets & other delicacies.
- Coriander is used for urethritis, cystitis, urinary tract infection, urticaria, rash, burns, sore throat, vomiting, indigestion, nosebleed, cough, allergies, hay fever, dizziness and amebic dysentery.
- The oil of coriander is used as antimicrobial property and as a natural fragrance in perfumery industry.

3.7 Clove (Laung)

It is the small reddish flower bud of the tree Syzygium aromaticum of the family Myrtaceae. Indonesia is the famous for cloves flower buds which is used around the world in cuisine [18]. In India it is grown in Nilgiris, Tembasi hills and Kanyakumari district in Tamilnadu state and Kottayam and Quilon districts in Kerala. The major component of the essential oil is Eugeniol and oil content about 15%. The oil of clove is frequently used in Ayurveda and Chinese medicine as a painkiller in dental problems [19]. Eugeniol present in the clove have antioxidant properties which retard the foods from get rancid. Eugenol esters are used as flavoring agent. Presence of strong and hot pungent taste, cloves is used as flavoring and dietary additives in meats and bakery products specially. We can blend the flavor of clove with both sweet and savory dishes. Due to its antioxidant properties it is act as preservative. It is popularly used in pan masala, betel nuts and chewing gums. A number of actions reported in clove such as analgesic property, anesthetic action, antibacterial property, antiparasitic action, antidotal property, antioxidant action, antiperspirant action, antiseptic property, carminative action, deodorant, digestive disorders, rubefacient action, stimulant property, stomachic action [20, 21].

3.7.1 Uses and health benefits

- It is mostly used in many households as an aid to prevent the minor disorders like indigestion, flatulence, tooth ache etc.
- Clove is highly valued medicine for their carminative, stimulant, antiflatulent and antihelmenthic properties.
- The dried buds are used as an analgestic and anesthetic.

- Among the spices, cloves are reported to have the highest antioxidant properties.
- It has aromatic and mild flavor.
- Used as a flavoring in bakery products & sweets, meat products pickles
- Clove bud oil is used in pharmaceuticals and dental formulation.

3.8 Black pepper (Kaali Mirch)

It is the fruits of plant black pepper and belongs to the family Piperaceae. Black pepper is used as both a spice and medicine. The native place of pepper is Kerala the Southern State of India. Kerala produces nearly 95% of the total pepper output. It is dried small round berry of a tropical vine with small white flower. Pepper possess its pleasant pungency and aroma due its oleoresin, which is present in the cells of pericarp. Peperine (4–10%) is the major constituent present in the pepper responsible for the biting taste of black pepper. Chavirine, peporidine and piperethine are the others alkaloids present in the small amount in pepper. The seeds of pepper also contain crude fiber range from 8 to 18%. Peppers are good source of Manganese, Iron, Calcium, Potassium, Vitamin A, C, K, Zinc, Chromium and other nutrients.

A numbers of medicinal benefits are found in peppers such as antihypertensive, anti-Alzheimer's, antidepressant, antiplatelets, anti-inflammatory, antioxidant, antipyretic, antitumor, antiasthmatic, analgesic, antimicrobial etc. It also stimulates the secretion of Hydrochloric acid in the stomach, resulting improves the digestion.

3.8.1 Uses and health benefits

- It is used with hot milk for throat infection.
- It is used effectively in the treatment of rheumatism and muscular pain, intestinal gas and headache.
- It is believed that peperine increase the bioavailability of other medicines by increasing their absorption and delaying their metabolism.
- Ancient Indian home remedies prescribe pepper as all antidote to cough and chest congestion.

3.9 Cinnamon (Dalchini)

Cinnamon (*Cinnamomum verum*) related to Lauraceae family is the most common spices used in the every household and commonly cultivated in the India, Sri Lanka, Bangladesh, and Nepal [20]. Cinnamon is obtained from the bark of the Cinnamon tree. The bark having 1% essential oil and the active compounds present in the oil are eugenol, cineole and cinnamaldehyde. It is used for making garam masala powder. It is also act as antioxidant due to presence of methyl hydroxyl chalcone polymer. Cinnamon having many important chemical constituents likes cinamaldehyde, cinnamic acid, and cinnamate that are providing many promising health benefits such as antioxidant, anti-inflammatory, antidiabetic, anti-microbial, immunity boosting, cancer and heart disease protecting abilities [22, 23]. The use of cinnamon with ginger stimulates the blood circulation and digestion [24].

3.9.1 Uses and health benefits

- It is use as antipyretic, lowering in body temperature, antiseptic, astringent, inflammatory problem, carminative, diaphoretic, fungicidal, stimulant, and stomachic.

- The powdered spice cinnamon bark in water is applied to overcome headaches and neuralgia.

- It regarded as a folk remedy for indurations (of spleen, breast, uterus, liver and stomach) and tumors (especially of the abdomen, liver and sinews).

3.10 Ajwain

It related to the Family Umbelliferae and originated in India. The leaves and seeds of the ajwain plant are edible in nature. Its seeds are resembles with the other seeds of Family Umbelliferae like caraway, cumin and fennel. The taste and flavor of the seeds are same as the aniseed and oregano. Bioactive compound present in the essential oil is thymol, which gives its bitingly hot and bitter taste that numbs the tongue when chewed. It is widely used as a spice in curries. In Ayurveda ajwain is prescribed as medicines for stomach disorder like indigestion, flatulence [25] diarrhea and colic [16].

3.10.1 Uses and health benefits

- It is a household remedy for indigestion.

- It is known for its antispasmodic, stimulant and carminative effect.

3.11 Fenugreek (Methi)

The common name of Fenugreek is maithray (Bangla, Gujarati), methi or mithi (Hindi, Nepali, Marathi, Urdu and Sanskrit). It is a kind of hard lentil seeds with dark fawn color and astringent aroma. It contains both soluble and insoluble fiber with 5% bitter fixed oil [26, 27]. Taste of this spice is bitter and thus used in small quantities in seasonings like sambar and kadhi. It improves the flavor and keeping quality of pickles.

3.11.1 Uses and health benefits

- Fenugreek seeds are having many medicinal properties such as digestive disorders, bronchitis, tuberculosis infection, skin irritations, ulcers and menopausal symptoms, diabetes.

- It is used to reduce blood sugar level.

- It is also used with butter milk in the treatment of dysentery.

3.12 Aniseed (Somfu)

It is small dried seed of an annual herb and native to the East Mediterranean region. It is cultivated in a small area in Rajasthan, Punjab, U.P and Orissa. The major compound is anethole which has the flavor of liquorice. It is used a mouth refresher and used after the taking meals [28]. It is also used in preparation of cakes, bread, cookies, and non-vegetarian dishes.

3.12.1 Uses and health benefits

- An infusion of fennel is used to counteract flatulence.
- It is mildly carminative and used in treating colic pain.
- It is used as natural chief raw material in the pharmaceutics, perfumery, food and cosmetic industries.
- Aniseed essential oil is used to treat the cold and flu in aromatherapy.

3.13 Caraway

It is black dried seed has pleasant aromatic flavor and contain about 5% essential oil. The chief flavoring compound is D-carvone and D-limonere. Its seeds are used to flavor the cakes, biscuits, cheese, apple sause and cookies. Its fine powder is effective in cataract when applied at the early stages. From the ancient times caraway oil has been used by the women as secret the beauty. The combination of black cumin and caraway seeds oils have been used to killed parasites and worms, detoxify, ameliorate amoebic dysentery, shigellosis, abscesses, old tumors, ulcers of the mouth, and rhinitis.

3.13.1 Uses and health benefits

- It is used as a food flavorent.
- It is a mild stomachic and carminative.
- Its seeds have carminative effect.

3.14 Bay leaf (Tez Patta)

Bay leaf (Laurus nobilis) belongs to the family Lauraoeac and it is native to the Mediterranean and Asia. They are the dried aromatic leaves of laurel tree and contain 1–3% aromatic oil. Its oil is used in the preparation of pickling spice and flavoring of vinegar. The dried leaves are mainly used for developing flavor in meat, pulav, soups, fish, tomato pickle and birinj sweet.

3.14.1 Uses and health benefits

- It is used as flavoring agent in curries dishes.
- The leaves and fruits of bay leaf possess stimulant and narcotic properties
- Bay leaf helps relieve pain in joints, chest, womb and stomach.
- It also helps in digestion by stimulating gastric functions.

3.15 Asafoetida (Hing)

Asafoetida is also commonly known as Food of the God and native to Iran and Afghanistan. Asafoetida is an oleo gum resin exuded from the rhizome or root of ferula asafoetida. The flavor of asafoetida comes from the presence of a ferulic ester and sulfur containing volatile oil. It is good sources of protein, fiber, carbohydrates, calcium, phosphorous, iron, niacin, carotene and riboflavin. Asafoetida is very common and easily available spice in every home and effectively used in the treatment of indigestion, menstrual, pain, ear ache, body pains and tooth ache. It is available in the market mixed with starch (compound hing) to dilute the strong flavor.

3.15.1 Uses and health benefits

- It is used as an antimicrobial agent.
- It is increases the levels of detoxification enzymes in the body.
- It is also used in the treatment of chronic bronchitis and whooping cough.

3.16 Cumin seeds (jeera)

Cumin is especially grown in India, Syria, Iran and Turkey and related to the family Apiacae. The largest producer of cumin is India (70% of world cumin production) while the second largest producer is the Syria. The major importers of the Indian cumin are U.A.E, Central America, China and Vietnam. It contains essential oil 2 to 4% and the active compound is aldehyde cumino. The seeds are mainly used in curry and seasoning. It is also used in curry powder, sambar powder and rasam powder.

3.16.1 Uses and health benefits

- Cumin warm water drinking rehydrate the human body and keep refresh.
- It help in digestive system by enhancing the saliva secretion
- It improves the breast feeding in the lactating mother.
- Cumin seeds are used to lowers the blood sugar levels.
- It increases the hemoglobin level in the blood.
- It is act as very good antioxidant spice due to presence of anticarcinogenic agents such as thymol and dithymoquinone.

3.17 Poppy seeds

It is tiny kidney-shaped oilseed found from the poppy (Papaver somniferum). Currently poppy seed is legally cultivated and used in many countries mainly in Central Europe [20]. Its seeds are good source of thiamin, folate, and important minerals like calcium, iron, magnesium, manganese, phosphorus and zinc.

3.17.1 Uses and health benefits

- The seeds are used, whole or ground, as an ingredient in many foods.
- Poppy seeds are used as thickening agent and also give added flavor to the recipe.
- Commonly used in the preparation of korma, ground poppy seeds, along with coconut.
- In Indian traditional medicine it is used as a skin moisturizer.
- Poppy seeds oil is valuable commercial oil that has multiple culinary, industrial, and medicinal uses.

3.18 Nutmeg and mace

Nutmeg is the dried and hard seed or pit of the nutmeg fruit; however mace is the orange red fleshy covering of the nutmeg. It contains 7–14% essential oil and this oil contains a highly toxic compound is called myristicin. Nutmeg and mace are used in small amounts to flavor the pudding and fruit pie. It is used as ground state in the cakes, cookies, pies, chocolate, garam masala etc.

3.18.1 Uses and health benefits

- It has antimicrobial properties.

3.19 Saffron (Kesar)

Saffron is known as crocus sativa and it is grown in the dry land of Kashmir valley. Name of this spice given saffron due to the fragrant stigma found in the flower of the saffron fruits. It has matchless aroma among the all spices therefore sold costly in the market. For making one ounce of pure saffron 75000 flowers are needed. Saffron is used mainly for its yellow color. It has a pleasant aroma and an essential oil crocin and the coloring principle is crocerin. It is widely used is soups, sauses, mainly in rice dishes to give them bright yellow color and distinctive flavor. It is also used in many famous sweets like sandesh, rasmalai, kesar milk, ice-cream, halwa and shrikhand.

3.19.1 Uses and health benefits

- It is used as a sedative and also used for eye infection.

3.20 Kokum

Kokum (Garcinia indica choipsy) is cultivated in the western ghats in the Konkan, Goa, South Karnataka and Kerela. The color of the ripe fruit is the dark purple due to the presence of anthocyanin and having sufficient amount of malic acid. Its colorful red juice is used for the manufacture of beverages.

3.20.1 Uses and health benefits

- It is used as soring agent in cookery.

4. Use of spices and herbs for health benefits during Covid-19 pandemic

Corona virus disease (COVID-19) has been declared as a pandemic by World Health Organization. The disease significantly affected all age groups of peoples, mainly old age patients that are suffering from diabetes, hypertension, cerebral infarction, chronic bronchitis, Parkinson's disease, chronic obstructive pulmonary disease, cardiovascular disease, and cancer [29, 30]. In the case of positivity with COVID-19 peoples lose their immunity mild to severely, therefore the demand of the natural immunity booster like spices and herbs are widely undertaken. Spices have been known for their high antioxidant and antimicrobial activity due to presence of many bioactive compounds such as flavonoids, phenolic compounds, sulfur-containing compounds, tannins, alkaloids, phenolic and diterpenes [31, 32]. After reviewing the role of spices as an immunity booster, even the Ministry of AYUSH, Gov. of India has issued the guidelines on heral use based immunity promoting methods for self-care during the COVID-19 pandemic. The guidelines emphasizes the uses of spices like turmeric, cumin, coriander, and garlic that are suggested in cooking. The guidelines further advocates use of drink of herbal tea or decoction (kadha) made by basil, cinnamon, black pepper, ginger, and raisin once or twice in a day. Similarly, 150 ml hot milk with half teaspoon turmeric powder can also be taken once or twice in a day. Several spices such as clove, cinnamon, ginger, black pepper, and turmeric are used as immunity boosters along with their antiviral property [33, 34].

5. Conclusion

Commonly used spices in different foodstuffs are having broad spectrum of bio-functions due to presence of bioactive compounds (curcumin, crocerin, D-carvone, D-limonere aldehyde cumino, eugenol, capsaicin, thymol, gingerol etc.) which may provide promising health benefits to our body from the many common disorders like cough, cold, fever, headache, stomach problems, cancer etc. Presence of strong flavor and aroma spices are used in small quantities that impart lower calories to food, however it enriched the foods with varieties of essential minerals, although some spices derived form seed contain high amount of fat, protein and carbohydrates. In the present pandemic situation of covid-19, spices such as turmeric, ginger, clove, pepper, cinnamon, cardamom are widely used in different foods formulation like kadha, herbal tea, masala tea etc., which play major role to arrest or reduce the effect of this virus. After reviewing this chapter we can be able to used right spices in the appropriate disorders and get benefited by its amazing functional, medicinal and nutritional properties.

Conflict of interest

The authors declare no conflict of interest.

Author details

Vinod Kumar Paswan*, Chandra Shekhar Singh, Garima Kukreja,
Durga Shankar Bunkar and Basant Kumar Bhinchhar
Department of Dairy Science and Food Technology, Banaras Hindu University,
Varanasi, India

*Address all correspondence to: vkpaswan.vet@gmail.com

References

[1] Manay N, Shadaskarswamy, M. Foods, facts and principles. New age international Pvt Ltd., New Delhi. 1999; 321-334.

[2] Khanum F, Krishna SKR, Semwal AD, Vishwanathan KR. Proximate compostion and mineral contents of spices. The Indian Journal of Nutrition and Diet. 2001; 38 (3): 93 - 96

[3] Sachan AK, Doli RD, Kumar M. Carum carvi-An important medicinal plant. Journal of Chemical and Pharmaceutical Research. 2016; 8(3): 529-533.

[4] Khajehdehi P. Turmeric: Reemerging of a neglected Asian traditional remedy. Journal of Nephropathology. 2012; 1(1): 17-22.

[5] Maqsood S, Singh P, Samoon MH, Munir K. Emerging role of immunostimulants in combating the disease outbreak in aquaculture. International Aquatic Research. 2011; 3: 147-163.

[6] Ravindran PN, Nirmal Babu K, Sivaraman K. The Golden Spice of Life. In: Turmeric. The Genus Curcuma. Boca Raton, FL, USA: CRC Press; 2007, 1-14.

[7] Szallasi A. Piperine: Researchers discover new flavor in an ancient spice. Trends in Pharmacology Science. 2005; 26(9): 437-439.

[8] Chattopadhyay I, Biswas K, Bandyopadhyay U, Banerjee RK. Turmeric and curcumin: Biological actions and medicinal applications. Current Science of India. 2004; 87:44-53.

[9] Gupta, S. C., Patchva, S., & Aggarwal, B. B. (2013). Therapeutic roles of curcumin: Lessons learned from clinical trials. The American Association of Pharmaceutical Scientists Journal, 15(1), 195–218.

[10] Jafri MA, Farah, Javed K, Singh S. Evaluation of the gastric antiulcerogenic effect of large cardamom (fruits of Amomum subulatum Roxb). Journal of Ethnopharmacology. 2001; 75(2–3): 89-94.

[11] Duke JA, Bogenschutz-Godwin MJ, deCellier J, Duke PK. Elettaria cardamomum Maton (Zingiberaceae) Cardamon, Malabar or Mysore cardamon, in CRC Handbook of Medicinal Spices. 2003; 120-138.

[12] Benavides GA, Squadrito GL, Mills RW, Patel HD, Isbell TS, Patel RP, Darley-Usmar VM, Doeller JE, Kraus DW. Hydrogen sulfide mediates the vasoactivity of garlic. 2007; PNAS. 104: 17977-17982.

[13] Agrawal M, Walia S, Dhingra S, Khambay BPS. Insect growth inhibition antifeedant and antifungal activity of compounds isolated derived from Zingiber officinale roscoe, ginger rhizome. Pest Management Science. 2001; 57: 289-300.

[14] Kikuzaki H, Kobayashi H, Nakatani N. Constituents of Zingiberaceae, diarylheptanoids from rhizomes of Zingiber officinale, Phytochemistry. 1991; 30: 3947-3952.

[15] Sachan AK, Doli RD, Senah LD, Shuaib, M. Asparagus racemosus (Shatavari): An overview. International journal of pharmaceutical and chemical sciences. 2012; 1(3) 588-592.

[16] Gilani AH, Bashir S, Khan AU. Pharmacological basis for the use of Borago officinalis in gastrointestinal, respiratory and cardiovascular disorders. Journal of Ethnopharmacology. 2007; 114:393- 399.

[17] British pharmacopoeia, Introduction General Notices Monographs, medicinal and Pharmaceutical, British pharmacopeia commission, London. 2003; Volume-1 (A-I); 542-543.

[18] Duke JA, Bogenschutz-Godwin MJ, deCellier J. Duke PK. Syzygium aromaticum (L.) Merr. and L. M. Perry (Myrtaceae) Clavos, Clove, Clovetree, in CRC Handbook of Medicinal Spices. CRC Press, Washington DC. 2003, 281.

[19] Daniel AN, Sartoretto SM, Schmidt G, Caparroz-Assef SM, Bersani-Amado CA, Cuman RKN. Anti- inflammatory and antinociceptive activities a of eugenol essential oil in experimental animalmodels. Revista Brasileira de Farmacognosia. 2009; 19: 212- 217.

[20] Bhat KS, Vivek K. Biocidal potential of clove oils against Aede albopictus – A comparative study. African Journal of Biotechnology. 2009; 8 (24):6933-6937, 15.

[21] Delaquis PJ, Stanich K, Girard B, Mazza G. Antimicrobial activity of individual and mixed fractions of dill, cilantro, coriander and eucalyptus essential oils. International Journal of Food Microbiology. 2002; 74(1–2): 101-109.

[22] Khan A, Safdar M, Khan AMM, Khattak KN, Anderson RA. Cinnamon improves glucose and lipids of people with type 2 diabetes. Diabetes Care. 2013; 26 (12): 215- 218.

[23] Bajpai M, Pande A, Tewari SK, Prakash D. Phenolic contents and antioxidant activity of some food and medicinal plants. International Journal of Food Science and Nutrition. 2005; 56 (4): 287-291.

[24] Doli RD, Sachan AK, Vishnoi G, Shuaib Mohd, Imtiyaz Mohd. A review on surveillance of herbal medicines. International Journal of Phytopharmacology. 2016; 7(2): 68-72.

[25] Al-Zuhair H, El-Sayeh B, Ameen HA, Al-Shoora H. Pharmacological studies of cardamom oil in animals. Pharmacological Research. 1996; 34(1–2): 79-82

[26] Basu SK, Acharya SN, Thomas JE. Appilcation of phosphate fertilizer and harvest management for important fenugreek (Trigonella foenum-graecum L.) seed and forage yield in a dark brown soil zone of Canada. KMITL Science and Technology Journal. 2008; 8(1): 1 –7.

[27] Hardman R, Fazli FRY. Methods of screening the genus Trigonella for steroidal sapogenins. Planta Medica. 1972; 21: 131–138.

[28] Cheung SC, Szeto YT, Benzie IF. Antioxidant protection of edible oils. Plant Foods Human Nutrition. 2007; 62 (1): 39-42.

[29] Deng SQ, Peng HJ. Characteristics of and public health responses to the coronavirus disease 2019 outbreak in China. Journal of Clinical Medicine. 2020; 9: 575.

[30] Huang C, Wang Y, Li X, Ren L, Zhao J, Hu Y, Gu X. Clinical features of patients infected with 2019 novel coronavirus in Wuhan, China. The Lancet. 2020; 395(10223): 497–506.

[31] Patra K, Jana K, Mandal DP, Bhattacharjee S. Evaluation of the antioxidant activity of extracts and active principles of commonly consumed Indian spices. Journal of Environmental Pathology. Toxicology and Oncology. 2016; 35: 299-315.

[32] Yashin A, Yashin Y, Xia X, Nemzer B. Antioxidant activity of spices and their impact on human health: A review. Antioxidants. 2017; 6:70.

[33] Shrivastava R. Immunity boosters: Solutions from nature-herbs and spices. Journal of Renal Nutrition Metabolism. 2020; 6: 35-37.

[34] Srivastava AK, Chaurasia JP, Khan R, Dhand C, Verma S. Role of medicinal plants of traditional use in recuperating devastating COVID-19 situation. Medicinal Aromatic Plants (Los Angeles). 2020; 9: 359.

Chapter 5

Important Medicinal Plants in Ethiopia: A Review in Years 2015–2020

Abebe Ayele Haile

Abstract

Many studies on medicinal plants have been taking place in different parts of Ethiopia and the people use them for the preparation of traditional herbal medicine. The purpose of the current study is to review the assessment of the medicinal plants used in Ethiopia, to compile the components used, the method of preparation, the medical uses, and the compilation of the number of medicinal plants in 2015–2020. This review paper took place in the years 2015 to 2020 from the published papers. Various databases, such as Science Direct, PubMed, and Google Scholar, have been searched. The data were analyzed using frequency, percentages, charts, and numbers using the Microsoft Excel spreadsheet 2010. In Ethiopia, a total of 4,007 medicinal plants were identified from different areas by different authors in the years 2015–2020. But, from this total number of identified medicinal plants, there was a similarity between types of plant species. Therefore, this total result has present similarities in plant species and types found in different areas. In 2015, a total of 1,062 medicinal plants were identified from different areas by different authors. Similarly, 315, 613, 944, 341, 732 medicinal plants were identified by different authors in different study areas in the years 2016, 2017, 2018, 2019, and 2020 respectively. The years 2015 and 2018 were the years many plants of medicinal value were documented. The growth forms of medicinal plants were analyzed from 2015 to 2020 in the different study areas with different authors but with the same year and valued for each year and put the average one. To calculate the 2015 growth form of medicinal plants for example to calculate herbs, add all herbs identified by different authors in the same year, and take the average one. This method applied to all growth forms of medicinal plants each year. In all years (2015–2020) the dominant growth forms were herbs. The highest average of growth form was herb in the year 2020 which is 44.2%. In all years the least growth form was a climber. In all growth forms, the parts used for medicine were identified. Add each medicinal plant's parts in the same year and then take the average for all years. In 2020 year, the traditional healers mostly used leaves (56.3%) for the preparation of remedy. In general, in all year leaves was dominant for the preparation of remedy. Oral and dermal ways of the route of administration were the most important in medicinal plants to treat directly different ailments. The route of administration was varying in percentage from year to year and also, a place to place according to the potential of traditional healers and type of diseases. But, different study areas and years showed that oral administration was the dominant one. In 2019, most of the prepared remedy was taken orally. Crushing was the most important and more cited in the preparation of remedy in the year 2015–2020. Also, powdering, boiling, chewing, concoction, grinding, direct and immediate, chopping, squeezing, decoction, boiling/unprocessed use, liquid form, Homogenizing in water, heating, cooking, smoking, and fumigation are common methods of preparation of remedy. In general, this review highlights the situation of Ethiopian traditional medicinal plants associated with their knowledge from years to years. In addition, this review paper plays an important role in the extraction of potential medicinal plants to discover new drugs through detailed researches in the future.

Keywords: Ethiopia, Medicinal plants, new drugs

1. Introduction

Ethiopia is the sixth major country in tropical Africa in terms of the diversity of flora [1]. The country is endowed with rich flora, having more than 6,500 species of vascular plants out of which an estimated 12% are endemic and many plant species are used as medicinal plants [2, 3]. In Ethiopia, 80% of people depend on traditional medicine for their health care, and more than 95% of traditional medicinal preparations are made from plant origin [4]. Ethiopia is also a home for many languages, cultures and beliefs that have in turn contributed to the high diversity of traditional knowledge and practice of the people, which, among others include the use of medicinal plants [5, 6]. Ethiopian traditional medicines are greatly complex because the country harbors much cultures and endogenous knowledge [7].

Medicinal plants are plants that are used to treat diseases of humans and animals [8]. Traditional healers practice on these plants using their indigenous knowledge and hence, they are called traditional medicines. Primitive peoples in all ages have had some knowledge of medicinal plants derived as the result of trial and error [9]. Medicinal plants were traditionally used for health care and serve as the bases for the emergence of modern medicine. About 6,000 medicinal plants are believed to be used in traditional medicine globally [10–12]. Most of the medicinal plants are directly used from the wild and some from home gardens. However, home gardens played important role in cultivating and retaining medicinal plants beyond other useful plants [13]. Ethnobotanical knowledge as part of living cultural knowledge and practice between communities and the environment is essential for biodiversity conservation [14–16]. Most traditional medical treatments put into performing in Ethiopia rely on an amplification of disease that draw on both the “mystical” and “natural” base of medical circumstance and put together use of a holistic approach to management [17]. The usage of herbal medicine in Ethiopian patients in the treatment of diseases like cancer, liver, neurological and hepatic diseases were reported by some authors [18, 19]. In general plants are very important in Ethiopia to treat various ailments.

The present review was conducted to gather information about the plants used by people of Ethiopia in traditional medicine in the years 2015 to 2020, such as to highlight the description of medicinal plants including local name, the parts used, the preparation methods, traditional uses, and to compile the number of medicinal plants in each year till 2015 to 2020. This is believed to show the importance of traditional knowledge on treating ailments and elucidate the degree of development of this knowledge to marketable business.

2. Methods and materials

This review paper took place in the years 2015 to 2020 from the published papers. Various databases, such as Science Direct, PubMed, and Google Scholar,

Medicinal plants studied by and year	Name of study area	Habit of medicinal plants in percent (%)				Parts utilized in percent (%)						Method of preparation	Principal RA (%)		Total Medicinal Plants
		H	Sh	T	C	L	R	F	Se	St	Ot		Or	De	
[20]	Abaya District (Guji Oromia tribes),	30.3	48.8	20.9	—	30.2	39.5	16.3	—	14	—	Powder, crushing pounding, chewing, concoction	60.46	23.2	43
[21]	Abeshige district, Gurage Zone, SNNP	37.1	29.2	22.5	12	41.6	23.6	7.86	5.6	3.37	17.97	Crushing and pounding	51.7	23.6	89
[22]	Ada'a District,East Shewa Zone, Oromia	37	39	17	7	33.68	38.34	6.22	—	3.63	18.13	Concoction, Powdering, Grinding, Chewing	49.4	38.4	131
[23]	Adwa District, Tigray	28	36	28	8	52	24	4	8	—	12	Crushed/grinded or powdered.	79	12	25
[24]	Yalo Woreda in Afar	28	44	21	7	52.9	17	3.27		3.27	23.5	crushing and pounding	68	—	106
[25]	Dire Sheikh Hussein heritage South-eastern Ethiopia	29	33	31	7	36	26	5	10	7	16	Crushing, pounding, chewing, powdering, grinding, cutting	59	24	87
[26]	Boricha district Southern Ethiopia	16.67	45.24	33.33	4.76	59.3	12.2	—	—	16.3	12.2	Crushing and chewing, boiling	73	18	42
[27]	Bule Hora District,West Guji Zone	42.86	21.42	35.71	—	64.28	—	14.28	—	21.42	13.28	—	—	—	70
[28]	Chilga District, Northwestern Ethiopia	36	30	24	11	45.3	44.6	—	—	—	10.2	Crushing, grinding, boiled	50	33	101
[29]	Chiro district, West Hararghe	36.67	31.67	26.66	5	46.96	24.24	4.55	7.58	4.55	12.03	pounding and grinding, Boiled, squeezing	63.2	26.32	60
[30]	Dale District, Sidama Zone, SNNP	—	49	51	—	41	12	12	—	—	35	Crushing, chewing	76	9	42
[31]	Dale Sedi district, oromia	29.8	40.4	29.8	—	36.2	21.3	—	14.9	—	27.6	Crushing, grinding	57.5	19.2	47
[32]	Debark district, North Gondar	36.56	33.33	19.51	10.6	40	18.57	—	12.86	8.57	20	Crushing, pounded	56.67	29.63	93
[33]	Dega Damot Woreda, Amhara	31.1	35.4	26.8	6.7	25	37.5	8.125	8.125	8.125	13.6	Chopping, pounding and crushing	69	14.8	54

Medicinal plants studied by and year	Name of study area	Habit of medicinal plants in percent (%)				Parts utilized in percent (%)						Method of preparation	Principal RA (%)		Total Medicinal Plants
		H	Sh	T	C	L	R	F	Se	St	Ot		Or	De	
[34]	Dega Damot district, Amhara	30	40	25	5	36.5	15.4	5.8	21.2	1.9	19.2	Decoctions, liquid	44	26.5	60
[35]	Jeldesa Cluster, Dire Dawa Administration, Eastern Ethiopia	38.5	42.8	15	3.7	34	33	5	9	—	19	Crushing, pounding, concoction, squeez	57.7	27.1	52
[36]	Dugda District, Oromia	38.2	32.5	22.8	3.3	41	29	—	11	—	19	Pounding, crushing and cooking/boiling	60.13	34.64	88
[37]	Enarj Enawga District, East Gojjam, Zone, Amhara	47.75	31.53	11.71	9.01	35.81	39.53	3.8	6.05	2.79	12.02	Crushing, boiled, squeezed	43.72	26.98	111
[38]	Local Communities of Gambella	12.3	37.03	32.1	18.5	27	23	10	10	9	21	Squeezing, chewing, boiled, crushing, burning	61.73	18.51	81
[39]	Ganta Afeshum District, Eastern Zone of Tigray	39.88	33.52	21.39	2.89	38.62	17.06	9.58	11.38	2.09	21.27	Direct and immediate/ unprocessed use, grinding, boiling, etc.	24.3	22.8	173
[40]	Gera district, Ethiopia	35.7	28.6	23.2	8.9	75	5.4	3.6	8.9	—	7.1	Crushing, exudation, squeezing, concoction	41.1	26.8	63
[41]	Gondar town, North Western Ethiopia	8.9	11.8	64.7	—	40	30	—	3.3	—	26.7	Powder, crushed, chewed, boiled,	64.3	26.2	30
[42]	Gozamin Wereda, East Gojjam Zone	45	31	16	8	41.9	17.2	4.3	14	4.6	18	Crushing, squeezing, powdering, juice, etc.	51.61	24.73	93
[43]	Robe district Bale zone, Oromia	38	33	26	—	33.3	21.4	—	19	—	26.3	Crushed, boiled, chewed, powdered	44.5	34.7	42
[44]	Gubalafto District, Northern Ethiopia	50.37	29.6	14.8	5.9	41.01	32.7	5.9	6.7	2.9	10.8	Crush, powder, chew, grind, and squeezed	61.4	35.4	135
[45]	halaba people, southern Ethiopia	53.06	18.37	22.45	—	52.92	13.46	—	—	25	8.62	Crush, squeezedchewed, pound powder	68.9	28.5	58

Medicinal plants studied by and year	Name of study area	Habit of medicinal plants in percent (%)				Parts utilized in percent (%)						Method of preparation	Principal RA (%)		Total Medicinal Plants
		H	Sh	T	C	L	R	F	Se	St	Ot		Or	De	
[46]	Harari regional State, East Ethiopia	42.6	35.2	14.8	5.6	48.15	20.37	9.26	—	7.41	14.81	Crushing, squeezing, chewing and cooking	53.7	24.1	54
[47]	Hawassa Zuria District, Sidama zone	34	28	32	6	56	12	15	4	4	9	Grinding, chewing, boiling, eating, liquid	74	20	105
[48]	Horro Gudurru Woreda, Western Ethiopia	46.4	28.6	25	—	51.8	19.6	10.7	10.7	—	7.2	Grinding, crushing, chopping, decoction	57.1	33.9	81
[7]	Jigjiga town, Somali region, Ethiopia	26	39	35	—	32.7	30.8	3.85	9.6	3.85	19.2	Homogenizing in water, crushing, decoction, chewing	55.6	27.8	46
[49]	Kembatta Tembaro (KT) Zone, Southern Ethiopia	54	25	13	—	41	26	3	15	—	15	Crushing, decoction, chewing, squeezing	69	22	145
[50]	Kilte Awulaelo District, Tigray	44	38	12	6	40.98	34.43	2.7	5.8	2.9	13.19	Crushing, chewing unprocessed,	25	29.69	50
[51]	Kunama ethnic group in Northern Ethiopia	37	13	43	13	21.74	35.5	8.9	9.5	2.6	21.76	pounding/crushing, smoking,	50.43	30.43	115
[52]	LaelayAdi-yabo District, Northern Ethiopia	29	29	29	10	34	24	2.7	6	13	20.3	Crushing, grind	48.65	48.65	37
[53]	Libo Kemkem District, northwest Ethiopia	41.1	38	14.7	6.1	31.2	30.9	7.2	2	1.7	27	Crushing, grinding, concoction, boiling	44.9	37.7	163
[54]	Menz Gera Midir District, North Shewa Zone, Amhara	43.87	30.32	18.45	6.45	43.9	31	8	3	4	10.1	Pounding, powdering, squeezing	47.96	28.57	155
[55]	Minjar-Shenkora District, North Shewa Zone of Amhara	38.98	40.67	13.55	6.48	45.7	18.5	13.5			22.3	liquid forms, exudates, powder, smash	54.21	41.78	118
[56]	Misha Woreda, Hadiya Zone, southern Ethiopia	43	27	21	9	41	26				33	Crushing, powdering, Boiling, chewing	47	31	126

Medicinal plants studied by and year	Name of study area	Habit of medicinal plants in percent (%)				Parts utilized in percent (%)						Method of preparation	Principal RA (%)		Total Medicinal Plants
		H	Sh	T	C	L	R	F	Se	St	Ot		Or	De	
[57]	Raya Kobo District of Amhara Region	46.2	31.8	22	—	53.1	21.8	6.45	6.45	9.8	2.4	Grinding/pounding, Crushing, Boiling, Chewing, Squeezing	53.7	28.9	91
[58]	Sayo and Hawa Gelan Districts of Kelem Wollega Zone, Oromia	15.1	45.5	39.4	—	57.47	17.24	5.45	6.45	—	13.39	Concoction, squeezing, boiling, smoking, chewing	55	32	66
[59]	Seharti Samre District, Southern Tigray	39	42.2	14.4	4.4	44	16	4	8	3	25	Crushing, pounding, Chewing, Squeezing	64.6	35.4	90
[60]	Sheka Zone of SNNP State, Ethiopia	53	23.7	12.4	10.9	42	16	6	3	3	30	Liquid form, chewed.	47	33	266
[61]	Boricha District, Sidama Zone, South Region	30	39	16	15	59	10	—	7		24	Grinding, Decoction, homogenization, concoction	97.4	2.4	42
[62]	Abergelle, Sekota and Lalibela districts of Amhara region	15.69	19.6	60.13	4.57	32.08	32.08	—	11.32	—	24.52	Crushing, grinding, squeeze, fumigation	35.85	33.96	53
[63]	Tepi Town, Southwest Ethiopia	33.3	24.24	24.24	15.15	36.36	12.12	—	—	3.03	49.49	Crushing and grinding	75.75	9.09	33
[52]	Cheha district	49	19	29.41	2	65	14	5	10	3	3	Cooking, smoking, heating and boiling	69	24	102

N.B. H = herb, Sh = shrub, T = tree, mpts = medicinal plants, C = climber, L = leaf, R = root, F = fruit, Se = seed, St = stem, Or = oral, Ot = other, De = dermal, RA = Route of administration, SNNP = South nation and nationality of people.

Table 1.
List of medicinal plants studied by and year, study area, habit, parts utilized, mode of preparation in Ethiopia (2015–2020 years).

have been searched. The data were analyzed using frequency, percentages, charts, and numbers using the Microsoft Excel spreadsheet 2010.

3. Medicinal plants in Ethiopia

In Ethiopia many medicinal plants are useful for treatment of different health problems. As indicated in **Table 1**, (review of recent literature: 2015–2020 years) medicinal plants in Ethiopian pharmacopeia are studied in different parts of the country by different authors. The review was restricted to the years 2015–2020 because the study made so far is bulky. This review showed that the total number of medicinal plants documented varied from year to year. In 2015, a total of 1,062 medicinal plants were identified from different areas by different authors. Similarly, 315, 613, 944, 341, 732 medicinal plants were identified by different authors in different study area in years 2016, 2017, 2018, 2019 and 2020 respectively.

4. Identified medicinal plants in Ethiopian in the years 2015–2020

The pattern of number of identified medicinal plants per year in Ethiopia in the years 2015–2020 was different (**Figure 1**). In 2015, 1,062 of medicinal plants were identified. When compared to the year 2016, it was greater by 747. Years 2015 and 2018 were the years many plants of medicinal value were documented (**Figure 1**).

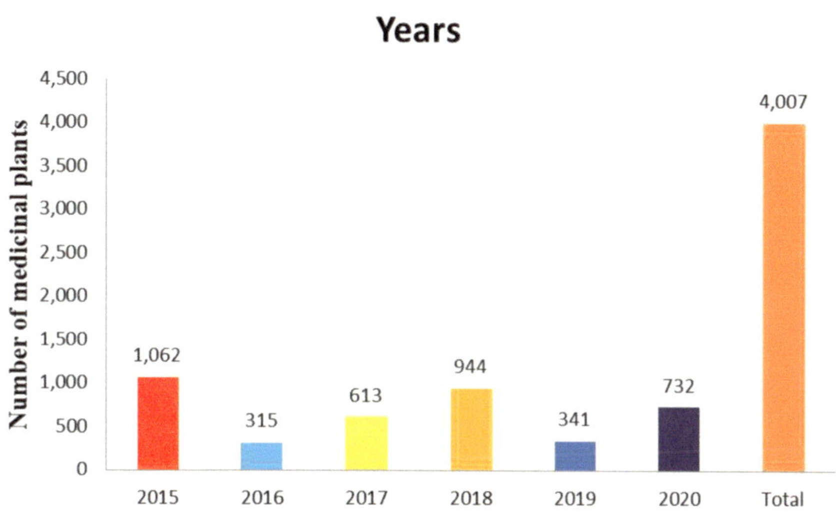

Figure 1.
Pattern of number of identified medicinal plants in Ethiopia years 2015–2020.

5. Growth forms (habits) of medicinal plants

The growth forms (habits) of medicinal plants was analyzed from 2015 to 2020 in different study area with different authors but with the same year and valued for each year and put the average one. To calculate the 2015 growth form of medicinal plants for example to calculate herbs, add all herbs identified by different authors in the same year and taken the average one. This method applied for all growth form

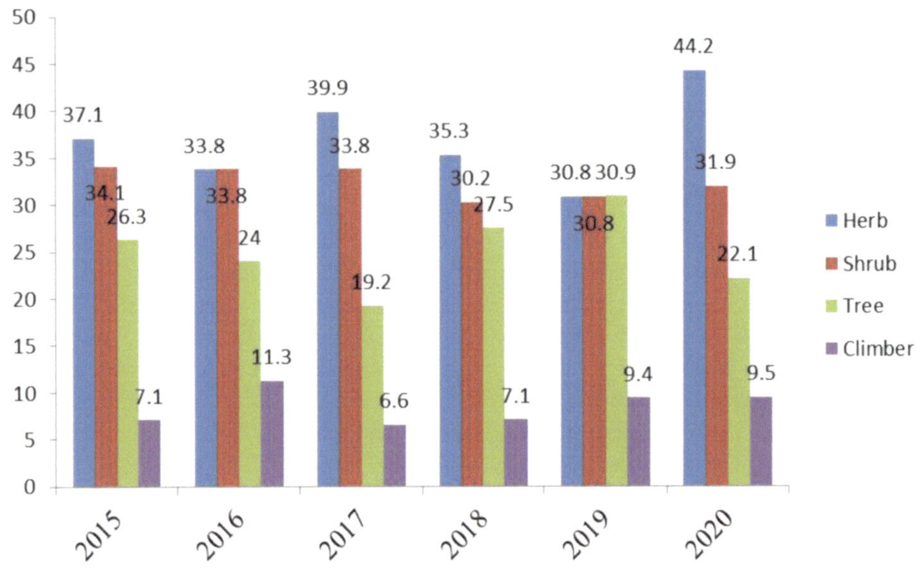

Figure 2.
Growth forms (habits) of medicinal plants years 2015–2020.

of medicinal plants to each year (**Figure 2**). In all years (2015–2020) the dominant growth forms were herbs. The highest average of growth form was herb in year 2020 which is 44.2% (**Figure 2**). In all years the least growth form was climber (**Figure 2**).

6. Parts of medicinal plants

In all growth forms, the parts used for medicine were identified. Add each medicinal plants parts in the same year and then taken the average for all years (**Figure 3**). In 2020 year the traditional healers mostly used leaves (56.3%) for the

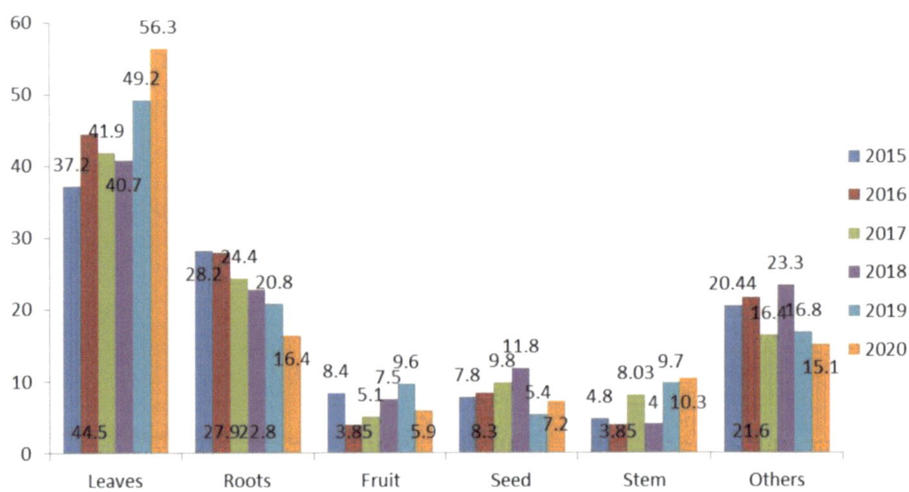

Figure 3.
Average of plant parts used in preparation of remedies 2015–2020.

preparation of remedy. In general, in all year leaves was the dominant for the preparation of remedy (**Figure 3**).

7. Route of administrations

Oral and dermal ways of route of administration were the most important in medicinal plants to treat directly different ailments. The route of administration was varying in percentage from year to year and also, place to place according to the potential of traditional healers and type of diseases. But, in different study areas and years showed that oral administration was dominant one (**Figure 4**). In 2019, most of the prepared remedy was taken orally.

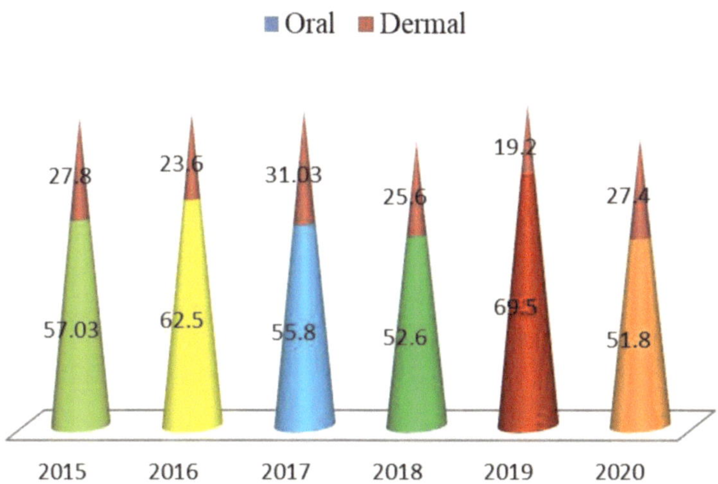

Figure 4.
Route of administration of remedies years 2015–2020.

8. Methods of preparation of medicinal plants

Crushing was the most important and more cited in the preparation of remedy in the year 2015–2020 (**Table 2**). Also, powdering, boiling, chewing, concoction, grinding, direct and immediate, chopping, squeezing, decoction, boiling/ unprocessed use, liquid form, Homogenizing in water, heating, cooking, smoking and fumigation are almost common for many traditional healers were shared methods to preparation of remedy.

9. Conclusion

All the medicinal plants reported in the current review work have been used in traditional medicine for the treatment of different human ailments in Ethiopia. But, the studied plants in the present review need further investigation for detailed extraction of natural products, pharmacological and biological activities as well as a safety control. Therefore, today's review is a gateway for a new researcher to

Plant family	Scientific Name	local name	Habit	used parts	Medicinal uses	Methods of preparation	References
Asteraceae	*Vemonia adoensis* Sch.Bep. ex Walp.	feres zeng	Herb	root	Menstrual disorder	Root is chewed with honey, then drunk the fluid	[32]
	Echinops hispidus Fresen	Kebericho	Shrub	Stem/root	Cough	Smoke the nasal cavity of the patient with dried stem or root	[64]
	Carthamus tinctorius L	Suf	Herb	Seed	Cough	—	[54]
	Tagetes minuta L	Gimie	Herb	Leaf	Black leg	Take the prepared remedy through orally.	[54]
	Echinops macrochaetus Fresen	kosorruu(or) koshshle	Herb	Stem	Ringworm	Fresh stem of this plant is chopped and fumigated to affected area.	[36]
	Helichrysum sp.	Nechilo	Shrub	Leaf	Impotency	—	[54]
	Artemisia abyssinica Sch.Bip.	Chikugn	Herb	Root/leaf	Common cold, evil eye, typhus	Nasal for common cold Neck hang for the evil eye	[54]
	Carduus leptacanthus Fresen.	guccino(or Amharic-	Herb	stem	Hemorrhoid	Crushed dry stem concocted with *Vernonia amygdalina* leaves mixed with water is taken orally	[20]
	Vernonia amygdalina Del.	Girawa	Shrub	leaf	Bloating	Crush and give with water	[53]
	Acmella caulirhizea Del.	yemider berbrie	Herb	leaf	Tonsillitis	Smashed and rubbed, take the juice	[64]
	Kleinia odora (Forssk.)	Wushie	Herb	leaf,stem	heart disease	—	[46]
Fabaceae	*Senna singueana* L	hambaha mbo (tig) key inchet	Shrub	Root	helmints, abdominal pain	Grind and mix with water, then drinking	[23]
	Tephrosia bracteolata' Guill. and Perr.	gerengerie	Herb	leaf	Body lice	—	[54]
	Lupinus albus L	gbto	Herb	seed	Hypertension	The prepared GB to will be eaten	[54]
	Senna septemtrionalis (Viv.) H.S. Irwin & Barneby.	hamashaka (sd)	Herb	leaf	Snake bite	Rubbing	[47]
	Crotalaria karagwensis Taub.	yeayt ater	Herb	leaf	Itchiness	Crush and powder, thencream with butter	[53]
	Pterolobium stellatum (Forssk.)Brenan	harengeemmaa/ kontir/kentafa	Shrub	Root	Rhumantic pain	Root boiled in a cooking dish and fumigating the leg with vapor.	[22]

DOI: http://dx.doi.org/10.5772/intechopen.97937

Plant family	Scientific Name	local name	Habit	used parts	Medicinal uses	Methods of preparation	References
	Albizia schimperiana Oliv.	Sesa/shimoro	Tree	Root	evil eye swelling	—	[47]
	Cicer arietinum L.	shimbra		seed	Malaria	Powdered, boiled and drunk	[55]
	Calpurnia aurea Benth	Digita	Shrub	leaf	eye disease, snake bite	—	[55]
	Vicia faba L.	Baaqelaa/or oral	Herb	seed	tapeworm	Fresh seeds are soaked in water overnight and eaten for five days	[36]
Lamiaceae	*Clerodendrummyricoides* (Hochst.) Vatke	Misrch	Shrub	leaf/root	evil eye & evil sprit	Crush, powder, then tie on the neck or take with tooth	[54]
	Satureja punctate Benth. Briq	lomishet	Herb	leaf	liver	Cooked fresh and drink the juice	[53]
	Ocimum lamifolium Hochst	demakese	Shrub	leaf	vaginal bleeding	Crush and Smearing in the vaginal part	[23]
	*Thymus schimperi*Ronniger	Tosign	Herb	Leaf	Lung tuberculosis	—	[54]
	Salvia schimperi Benth	Dibreq	Herb	Seed	Diarrhea	—	[54]
	Otostegia integrifolia Benth	Tunjut	Shrub	Whole plant	evil eye	Chopped and fumigate home using local stoves; chopped and used to take a smoke bath; people chew the leaves and spit into the mouth	[34]
	*Salvia nilotica*L	cheguri habesha(tig) hulegeb	Herb	Root	snake bite	Crushing, homogenize with water and drink a cup of the solution	[51]
Solanaceae	*Datura stramonium* L.	Astenagir/ etsefaris	Herb	Leaf	Ring worm	Rubbing and painting	[28]
	Solanum incanum L.	Enbuay/yekola	Herb	Root	Abdominal pain	Drinking Crushed and mixing with Water	[23]
	Nicotina tabaccum L.	Tinbaho	Herb	Leaf	Cough	Powdered and smoked	[55]

Plant family	Scientific Name	local name	Habit	used parts	Medicinal uses	Methods of preparation	References
	Solanum anguivi Lam.	zerch enboy	Shrub	Leaf	Mastitis	Dried and crushed leaves mixed with butter	[46]
	*Lycopersicon esculentum*Mill.	Timatim	Herb	Leaf	Spider poison	Leaf Chewed and put on the affected area	[33]
	Capsicum annuum L	Karia	Herb	Fruit	Malaria	—	[54]
	Solanum marginatum L	Geber embouy	Shrub	Leaf	Tapeworm	Take the prepared remedy through orally	[54]
	Solanum nigrum L.	Xunaye(sd)/ tkurawut	Herb	Leaf	Snake bite	Fresh leaf immediately after bit chewed and swallowing	[26]
	Withania somnifera (L.) Dunal.	bula(sd)/ girawa	Shrub	Root	Pneumonia	Fresh root is crushed andboiled then infusion is filtered and drunk in the morning for human until recovery and for four days for livestock.	[55]
Euphorbiaceae	*Euphorbia abyssinica* J. F. Gmel. T	Kulkual	Tree	Root/leaf	Jaundice	Crush, immerse in water, then drink or bake bread then eat	[54]
	Bridelia micrantha (Hochst.) Brain.	yenebr tifir	Tree	Bark	Expel placenta	Crush is then given with water	[55]
	Clutia lanceolata Forssk.	Fiyelefej	Shrub	Root	Diarrhea	Crush then tie on neck region	[53]
	Euphorbia tirucalli L.	Kinchib	Shrub	Sap	Swelling	Painting	[28]
	Croton macrostachyus Del.	Bisana	Tree	Leaf/root	Evil eye, Jaundice, Eye disease	—	[54]
	Ricinus communis L.	Qobboo (or) Gulo	Shrub	Seed	Impotency	The dried seeds are pounded, mixed with small quantity of latex from Aloe spp. And drunk two coffee cups before bedtime for two days	[23]
	Tragia cinerea (Pax) Gilbert & Radcl. Smith	alebelabit	Herb	Root	Kintarot	Fine powder of plant part mixed with butter /honey and drink before sexual intercourse with his partner.	[20]
	Phyllanthus ovalifolius A. Radclife-Smith	gurbi adi/ qechemo	Shrub	leaf	Scabies	Leaves squeezed by hand and applied on the skin	[24]

Plant family	Scientific Name	local name	Habit	used parts	Medicinal uses	Methods of preparation	References
Malvaceae	*Sida ovate* L	umer kope (or)	Herb	leaf	Swelling	Fresh leaves pounded tied on the swelling.	[54]
	*Gossypium barbadense*L.	Tit	Shrub	Root	Snake bite	Tie on neck or chew, absorb the Juice	[53]
	Malva parviflora Hojer	nacha	Shrub	leaf	Wound	Chew and cream with cotton	[54]
	Sida schimperiana ochst. exA. Rich.	harmellaa (or)/ chfrg	Shrub	Root/leaf	Evil eye, intestinal parasite	—	[46]
	Malva verticillata L	Lut	Shrub	Root	Headache	Crush the root and mix with water and wash the head	[47]
Rutaceae	*Citrus limon* (L.) Burm.f	betre lomi/ yeferenji lomi	Tree	fruit	Liver disease	—	[54]
	Clausena anisata(Willd.) Benth.	limich	Shrub	Root	Evil eye	Sniff, drink and fumigate with the concoction	[53]
	Citrus aurantium L.	Komtatie/bahre lomi	Shrub	leaf	Hypertension	Drink the juice leaf	
	Ruta chalepensis L.	Tenadam	Shrub	leaf	Evil eye	Crushed, powdered and sniffed	[41]
			Herb	leaf	Cough	Leaves boiled in milk are taken orally and take medicine orally for three days	[41]
				leaf	Malaria	Crushed the leaves of the plant with bulb of *A. sativumin* by adding ginger then drunk.	[24]
			Herb	leaf	flue	Leaf of *R. chalepensisis* pounded with bulb of *A. Sativum*, mixed with soup and used as a drink	[65]
Alliaceae	*Allium sativum* L.	nech shinkurt	Herb	bulb	Evil eye, malaria, virus. Asthma,	Sniff, drink and fumigate With concoction	[53]
Poaceae	*Cymbopogon martini*L	tejesar	Herb	Root	Evil eye	—	[54]
				leaf	Boost immunity of breastfeeding infants	The grassy leaf is boiled, macerated, cooled, and given to infants orally (esp. drenching).	[65]
	Arundinaria alpina K.Schum	qerqeha	Herb	Root	Shotelay	The root of *Arundinaria Alpina* is tied on the neck part of the body	[55]

Plant family	Scientific Name	local name	Habit	used parts	Medicinal uses	Methods of preparation	References
Amaranthaceae	*Achyranthes aspera* L.	telenj	Herb	Root/leaf	wound	Rubbing the leaf or root and applying for the wounded part	[28]
Acanthaceae	*Hypoestes forskaoli* (vahl) R.Br	gerbya	Shrub	Root	bone fracture	Tie Cut the root parts and tie the damaged part	[23]
	Justicia schimperiana (Hochst. Ex Nees)	Sensel/ Ciikkicho (sd)	Shrub	leaf	Helminthiases	The leaf is pounded, macerated, and drunk	[65]
Celastraceae	*Maytenus arbutifolia* (A. Rich.) Wilczek	atat	Shrub	Root	Kidney problem	—	[54]
Asclepiadaceae	*Calotropis procera* L.	Tobia/ginda/ qinba	Shrub	leaf	swelling	Warming the leaf and rubbing the swelled part.	
Simarobaceae	*Brucea antidysenterica* J.F. Mill.	abalo/ Waginos	Tree	leaf	wart	The leaf is crashed with *Clematis simensis*, *Brucea antidysenterica*, and *Oenanthe Palustris*, and the powder is applied on the affected part.	[28]
Cucurbitaceae	*Cucumis dipsaceus* Ehrenb.	Yeamora msa/ hafafelo (tig)	climber	Root	belly ache, snake bite, insect bite,	Grind and mix with water drinking	[62]
	Cucumis ficifolius A. Rich	yemdir embway	Herb	Root	Stomach ache, Gonorrhea, Rabies	—	[54]
Rubiaceae	*Coffee arabica* L.	buna	Tree	fruit	wound,	Apply the powder on affected part	[28]
Moraceae	*Dorstenia barnimiana* Schwienf.	work bemeda	Herb	Root	rabies	Grinding the roots of *Malva verticillata*, *Croton macrostachyus*, and *Cucumis ficifolius* separately and mixing them, then drinking with Skimmed milk, after that drinking coffee.	[28]
	Ficus vasta' Forssk	warka	Tree	Root	Eye disease	—	[54]
Rhamnaceae	*Rhamnus prinoides* L'Herit	gesho	Shrub	Shoot	tonsillitis	Crush and drink with water	[53]
Oleaceae	*Jasminum abyssinicum* Hochest. ex DC.	tenbelel	Tree	leaf	toothache	Take with teeth	[53]

Plant family	Scientific Name	local name	Habit	used parts	Medicinal uses	Methods of preparation	References
Polygalaceae	*Polygala abyssinica* Fres.	etse libona	Herb	Root	evil eye	Grinding the roots of *Polygala abyssinica, Carisa spinarum, Phytolacca dodecandra, Capparis tomentosa, Securidaca longepedunculata., Boscia angustifolia, Ruta halepensis,Sida schimperiana,* and *Croton macrostachyus,* then inhaling; additionally bandage	[28]
Convolvulaceae	*Dichondra repens* J.R.&G. Forst.	afer kocher	Herb	leaf	febrile illness	Rub, squeeze, then cream except the heart	[53]
Boraginaceae	*Cordia africana* Lam.	wanza	Tree	leaf	eye problem	Burn, then insert ash with butter	[53]
Capparidaceae	*Capparis cartilaginea* Decne	qelemberur	Tree	fruit	gastritis	Fruit coat is crushed and mixed with ½ glass water and 3 spoon sugar and taken orally	[62]
				Root	Ascaris	Dried roots crushed and boiled and consumed empty stomach	
				leaf	diarrhea	Fresh leaves crushed and mixed with water and sugar is added and consumed	
Loganiaceae	*Buddleja polystachya* Fresen.	anfar	Shrub	shoot	tonsillitis	Tie and cream concoction	[44]
Cuppressaceae	*Juniperus procera* Hochst ex. Engl.	Yehebesha tid	Tree	shoot	(painful swelling	The shoot is pounded, decocted, and drunk	[65]
				fruit	urine retention	Boil with TEJ then drink	[53]
Myrtaceae	*Eucalyptus globulus* (Labill.)	nechbahirzaf	Tree	leaf	Nasalinfluenza	Chopped, boiled and inhale the vapor	[55]
Rosaceae	*Rosa abyssinica* L	kega	Shrub	fruit	hypertension	Powdered, mixed with water and drunk	[53]
anunculaceae	*Clematis hirsuta* Perr.	yazohareg	climber	Leaf/stem	Swellings/ Wart, Eczema	Powdered and tied on affected part	[54]
Urticaceae	*Urera Philodendron* (A. Rich.) Wedd.	lankusso	Shrub	leaf	retained placenta	Chopped Leaves and mixed with water	[46]

Plant family	Scientific Name	local name	Habit	used parts	Medicinal uses	Methods of preparation	References
Ranunculaceae	*Thalictrum rhynchocarpum* Dill. and A. Rich	sire-bizu	Herb	Root	scrotum swelling	Crush and drink with Tella	[53]
Apocynaceae	*Carissa spirarum* L	agam	Shrub	apex	insect poison	For any poisoning by insects or animal bite, seven apexes from seven different places are collected and crushed.	[33]
Sapindaceae	*Dodonea angestifolia* L	kitkita	Shrub	shoot apex	chife	The apex is charred on an open fire and the powder is mixed with butter and applied on the affected area	[33]
Ebenaceae	*Eucleadivinorum* Hiern.	Dedho/kuliew (tig)	Shrub	Root	scorpion bite	Roots are chewed to relieve pain	[59]
Meliaceae	*Ekebergia capensis* Sparrm	Lol/sembo/ Olonchoo	Tree	bark	weight loss in children	—	[30]
Plantaginaceae	*Plantago lanceolata* L	gorteb	Herb	leaf	wound & bleeding	Crush leaf powder, then cream	[53]
Phytolacaceae	*Phytolacca dodecandra* L Herit	Endod/shebti	Shrub	Root	rabies	The dried root of the plant is powdered and mixed with local alcohol and a cup of solution drunk daily for twelve days. Vomiting is its side effect and, therefore, restricted to children and pregnant women	[30]
				leaf	gonorrhea	Leaves of *P. dodecandraand* roots of C. *Macrostachyus* are ground, powdered mixed with water and solution drunk with one to two cups of coffee	
				leaf	jaundice	Leaves are crushed, squeezed and one cup of juice taken daily for 21 days	
Brassicaceae	*Lepidium sativum* L	Feto/shenfa	Herb	seed	Amoebiasis, diarrhea	Seeds are ground into powder, mixed with honey and then taken for three day	[54]
Asparagaceae	*Asparagus africanus* L	yesiet kest	Shrub	aboveground	swelling	Above ground is crushed and homogenized in water for washing the swelling.	[66]
Caricaceae	*Carica papaya* L	Papaye/ papaayee	Shrub	seed	diarrhea	Seeds ground and boiled with coffee and taken with hone	[24]

Plant family	Scientific Name	local name	Habit	used parts	Medicinal uses	Methods of preparation	References
Vitaceae	*Cyphostemma adenocaula* (A.Rich.)	asserkush	climber	Root	rabies	Root boiled with milk, filtered and filtrate taken in empty stomach	[41]
Crassulaceae	*Kalancheo petitiana* A. Rich,	endahula	Herb	Root	ascaris	For ascaris, the root is cut with a knife of horn and chopped on unmovable stone, and mixed with water, it is squeezed between palms, applied in the left nose, then moved the stomach	[33]
Dipsacaceae	*Dipsacus Pinnatifidus* Steud. ex A. Rich.	Kelem/galam	Herb	leaf	rabies	Pound and give with water	[53]
Myrsinaceae	*Embelia schimperi* Vatke .	enkoko	Shrub	fruit	Tape worm	Row eaten; crushed, is drunk mixed with 'tela difdif'	[54]
Verbenacae	*Lippia adoensis* Hochst. exWalp	Koseret/kusaye	Shrub	leaves	fibril illness	The leaves squeezed and the filter is given through the nose and drink	[41]
plumbaginaceae	*Plumbago zeylanica* L.	Amera	Herb	Root/leaf	Wound	The crushed form of its root and leaf of *Dodonaea angustifolia*, with latex of *Calotropis proceraare* mixed together then creamed on the wound	[44]
Melianthaceae	*Bersama abyssinica* Fresen	azamir	Shrub	Leaf	Ascaris/ Hypertension,	The twig part of the leaf is crushed and powdered then boiled with tea and drunk	S [54]
Aloaceae	Aloe pulcherrima Tod.	eret	Herb	Root	Impotency	Crush and powder, then cream with butter	[53]
Linaceae	*Linum usitatissimum* L	telba	Herb	seed	Gastric	Pound, mix with honey, then drink	[54]
Anacardiaceae	*Rhus vulgaris* Oliv	Embis/yeregna qolo	Tree	Root	Evil eye	—	[54]
Tiliaceae	*Rewia ferruginea* Hochst. ex A. Rich.	lenquata	Shrub	bark	Expel placenta	Pilled the insider part and chopped emilizifyed then given to cattle, goat and sheep	[53]

N.B.Tig = Tigrigna, Sd = Sidamgna, Or = Oromigna.

Table 2.
List of most common medicinal plants used in Ethiopia with their local name, scientific name, family, parts utilized method of preparation, ailment treated and route of administration.

discover new drugs and screening chemicals resulting from these plants for against different health problems.

Conflict of interest

The authors declare that there is no any conflict of interests.

Author details

Abebe Ayele Haile
Department of Biology, Debre Berhan University, Debre Berhan, Ethiopia

*Address all correspondence to: abebeayele230@gmail.com

References

[1] Tizita E. The role of indigenous people in the biodiversity conservation in Gamo area of Gamo Gofa zone, Southern Ethiopia. *International Journal of Biodiversity and Conservation*. 2016; 8 (10):244-250. doi:10.5897/ijbc2015. 0893.

[2] Lulekal E, Kelbessa E, Bekele T, Yineger H. An ethnobotanical study of medicinal plants in Mana Angetu District, southeastern Ethiopia. *J Ethnobiol Ethnomed*. 2008; 4(1). doi: 10.1186/1746-4269-4-10.

[3] Unschuld P. Traditional Chinese medicine: Some historical and epistemological reflections. *Soc Sci Med*. 1987; 24(12):1023-1029. doi:10.1016/ 0277-9536(87)90018-9.

[4] Fassil H. Beyond Plants Professionals & Parchments: The role of home-based medicinal plant use and traditional health knowledge in primary health care in Ethiopia. *Ethnobotany Research and Applications*. 2005; 3:037. doi:10.17348/ era.3.0.37-50.

[5] Garedew B, Bizuayehu B. A Review on Ethnobotanical Study of Traditional Medicinal Plants Used for Treatment of Liver Problems in Ethiopia. *European J Med Plants*. 2018; 26(1):1-18. doi: 10.9734/ejmp/2018/38153.

[6] Teklehaymanot T, Giday M, Medhin G, Mekonnen Y. Knowledge and use of medicinal plants by people around Debre Libanos monastery in Ethiopia. *J Ethnopharmacol*. 2007; 111(2):271-283.

[7] Getachew Alebie and Abas Mehamed. An ethno-botanical study of medicinal plants in Jigjiga town, capital city of Somali regional state of Ethiopia. *International Journal of Herbal Medicine*. 2015; 4(6): 168-175.

[8] WHO. Traditional medicine fact sheet World Health Organization. 2008; 34.

[9] Hill AF. Economic Botany: a Text Book of Useful Plants and Plant products, second ed. Mc Graw Hill Book Company, Inc., New York. 1989; 560.

[10] Dawit Abebe., Debella A, Urga K. *Illustrated Checklist, Medicinal Plants And Other Useful Plants Of Ethiopia*. Addis Ababa, Ethiopia: Ethiopian Health and Nutrition Research Institute; 2003.

[11] Jima T, Megersa M. Ethnobotanical Study of Medicinal Plants Used to Treat Human Diseases in Berbere District, Bale Zone of Oromia Regional State, South East Ethiopia. *Evidence-Based Complementary and Alternative Medicine*. 2018; 2018:1-16. doi:10.1155/ 2018/8602945.

[12] Takele Bassa. Ethnobotanical Study of Medicinal Plants in WolaitaZone, Southern Ethiopia. *Journal of Health, Medicine and Nursing*. 2018; 48.

[13] Wolde Tenssay Z. Medicinal Plants:- Traditional Knowledge and Practices in Some Communities of Ethiopia. *International Journal of Ecotoxicology and Ecobiology*. 2017; 2(2):56. doi:10.11648/j. ijee.20170202.11.

[14] Girmay T. Assessment of Traditional Medicinal Plants used to treat human and livestock ailments and their threatening factors in Gulomekeda District, Northern Ethiopia. *International journal of Emerging Trends in Science and Technology*. 2017; 04(04): 5061-5070. doi:10.18535/ijetst/v4i4.03.

[15] Martin GJ. Ethnobotany a people and plants conservation manual. Chapman and Hall. London, UK. 1995.

[16] Behailu B, Temesgen A. Ethnobotanical value of medicinal plant diversity in Cheha district, Guraghe zone, Southern Nations, Nationalities and Peoples (SNNPR) of Ethiopia. *Journal of Medicinal Plants Research*.

2017;11(28):445-454. doi:10.5897/jmpr2017.6356.

[17] Pankhurst R. The History and Traditional Treatment of Rabies in Ethiopia. *Med Hist*. 1970;14(4):378-389. doi:10.1017/s0025727300015829.

[18] Girmay T. Assessment of Traditional Medicinal Plants used to treat human and livestock ailments and their threatening factors in Gulomekeda District, Northern Ethiopia. *International journal of Emerging Trends in Science and Technology*. 2017; 04(04): 5061-5070. doi:10.18535/ijetst/v4i4.03.

[19] Lulekal E, Rondevaldova J, Bernaskova E et al. Antimicrobial activity of traditional medicinal plants from Ankober District, North Shewa Zone, Amhara Region, Ethiopia. *Pharm Biol*. 2014; 52(5):614-620. doi:10.3109/13880209.2013.858362.

[20] Bekele G, Reddy P. Ethnobotanical Study of Medicinal Plants Used to Treat Human Ailments by Guji Oromo Tribes in Abaya District, Borana, Oromia, Ethiopia. *Universal Journal of Plant Science*. 2015; 3(1):1-8. doi:10.13189/ujps.2015.030101.

[21] Dagne Abebe and Belachew Garedew. Utilization of Traditional Medicinal Plants and Management in Darge-Walga Town, Abeshige District, Gurage Zone, Ethiopia. *Research Journal of Biological Sciences*. 2020; 15(4), 112-123.

[22] Kefalew A, Asfaw Z, Kelbessa E. Ethnobotany of medicinal plants in Ada'a District, East Shewa Zone of Oromia Regional State, Ethiopia. *J Ethnobiol Ethnomed*. 2015; 11(1). doi:10.1186/s13002-015-0014-6.

[23] Assefa T, Nigussie N, Mullualem D, Sinshaw G, Adimasu Y. The Role of Medicinal Plants in Traditional Medicine in Adwa District, Tigray, Northern Ethiopia. *Asian Plant Research Journal*. 2020:1-11. doi:10.9734/aprj/2019/v3i3-430067.

[24] Teklehaymanot T. An ethnobotanical survey of medicinal and edible plants of Yalo Woreda in Afar regional state, Ethiopia. *J Ethnobiol Ethnomed*. 2017; 13(1). doi:10.1186/s13002-017-0166-7.

[25] Demie G, Negash M, Awas T. Ethnobotanical study of medicinal plants used by indigenous people in and around Dirre Sheikh Hussein heritage site of South-eastern Ethiopia. *J Ethnopharmacol*. 2018; 220:87-93. doi:10.1016/j.jep.2018.03.033.

[26] Tamene S, Addisu D, Debela E. Ethno-medicinal study of plants in Boricha district: Use, preparation and application by traditional healers, Southern Ethiopia. Journal of Medicinal Plants Research. 2020; 14(7): 343-353. https://doi.org/10.5897/JMPR2020.6906.

[27] Yirefu T, Adugna B, Behailu B. Homegarden Plant use and their Traditional Management Practice in Bule Hora District, West Guji Zone, Southern Ethiopia. Agri Res& Tech: Open Access J. 2019; 21(4): 556168. DOI: 10.19080/ARTOAJ.2019.21.556168.

[28] Mekuanent T, Zebene A, Solomon Z. Ethnobotanical Study of Medicinal Plants in Chilga District, Northwestern Ethiopia. *Journal of Natural Remedies*. 2015; 15(2):88. doi:10.18311/jnr/2015/476.

[29] Amare F, Getachew G. An ethnobotanical study of medicinal plants in chiro district, West Hararghe, Ethiopia. *African Journal of Plant Science*. 2019;13(11):309-323. doi:10.5897/ajps2019.1911.

[30] Kewessa G, Abebe T, Demissie A. Indigenous Knowledge on the Use and Management of Medicinal Trees and Shrubs in Dale District, Sidama Zone, Southern Ethiopia. *Ethnobotany Research*

and Applications. 2015; 14:171-182. doi: 10.17348/era.14.0.171-182.

[31] Firaol Bekele, Bayecha Darge, Lulu Hordofa, Desta Goshu, Nurfeta Reta and Addisu Abebe. Survey of Ethno-Veterinary Medicinal Plants at Dale Sadi Districts of Oromia Regional State, Western Ethiopia. *Journal of Natural Sciences Research*. 2018; 8(19).

[32] Asmera Amde, Getinet Masresha, Hamer Hansha, Obsa Asafa. Ethnobotanical Study of Traditional Medicinal Plants in Debark District, North Gondar, Ethiopia. *International Journal of Scientific Research in Multidisciplinary Studies*. 2020; 6(11): 16-23.

[33] Messay Wolde-Mariam, Yayesh Limenih and Shemsu Umer. Ethnobotanical Study on Traditional Medicinal Plants in Dega Damot Woreda, Amhara Region, North Ethiopia. *International Journal of Research in Pharmacy and Chemistry*. 2015; 5(2): 258-273.

[34] Wubetu M, Abula T, Dejenu G. Ethnopharmacologic survey of medicinal plants used to treat human diseases by traditional medical practitioners in Dega Damot district, Amhara, Northwestern Ethiopia. *BMC Res Notes*. 2017; 10(1). doi:10.1186/s13104-017-2482-3.

[35] Shimels A, Atinafu K, Akalu M, Getachew M. Ethnobotanical study of medicinal plants used by agro pastoralist Somali people for the management of human ailments in Jeldesa Cluster, Dire Dawa Administration, Eastern Ethiopia. *Journal of Medicinal Plants Research*. 2017; 11(9):171-187. doi:10.5897/jmpr2016.6292.

[36] Wolditsadik Beyi M. Ethnobotanical Investigation of Traditional Medicinal Plants in Dugda District, Oromia Regio. *SM Journal of Medicinal Plant Studies*. 2018; 2(1):1-19. doi:10.36876/smjmps.1007.

[37] Simegniew Birhan Y, Leshe Kitaw S, Abebe Alemayehu Y, Minuye Mengesha N. Ethnobotanical Study of Medicinal Plants used to treat Human Diseases in Enarj Enawga District, East Gojjam Zone, Amhara Region, Ethiopia. *SM Journal of Medicinal Plant Studies*. 2017; 1(1):1-20.

[38] Megenase J, Tilahun Gelaye K, Kumar Dara P. Indigenous Knowledge and Practices on Medicinal Plants Used by Local Communities of Gambella Region, South West Ethiopia. *Int J Trop Dis Health*. 2019:1-14. doi:10.9734/ijtdh/2019/v39i230203.

[39] Kidane L, Gebremedhin G, Beyene T. Ethnobotanical study of medicinal plants in Ganta Afeshum District, Eastern Zone of Tigray, Northern Ethiopia. *J Ethnobiol Ethnomed*. 2018; 14 (1). doi:10.1186/s13002-018-0266-z.

[40] Gonfa N, Tulu D, Hundera K, Raga D. Ethnobotanical study of medicinal plants, its utilization, and conservation by indigenous people of Gera district, Ethiopia. *Cogent Food Agric*. 2020; 6(1): 1852716. doi:10.1080/23311932.2020.1852716.

[41] Zewdu Birhanu, Abyot Endale, Zewdineh Shewamene. An ethnomedicinal investigation of plants used by traditional healers of Gondar town, North-Western Ethiopia. *Journal of Medicinal Plants Studies*. 2015; *3*(2): 36-43.

[42] Amsalu N, Bezie Y, Fentahun M, Alemayehu A, Amsalu G. Use and Conservation of Medicinal Plants by Indigenous People of Gozamin Wereda, East Gojjam Zone of Amhara Region, Ethiopia: An Ethnobotanical Approach. *Evidence-Based Complementary and Alternative Medicine*. 2018; 2018:1-23. doi:10.1155/2018/2973513.

[43] Abadi B, Shimels A. Indigenous knowledge on medicinal plants used in and around Robe Town, Bale Zone,

Oromia Region, Southeast Ethiopia. Journal of Medicinal Plants Research. 2018; 12(16):194-202. doi:10.5897/jmpr2017.6445

[44] Chekole G. Ethnobotanical study of medicinal plants used against human ailments in Gubalafto District, Northern Ethiopia. *J Ethnobiol Ethnomed*. 2017; 13 (1). doi:10.1186/s13002-017-0182-7.

[45] Reta Regassa, Tesfaye Bekele, Moa Megersa. Ethnobotonical study oftraditional medicinal plants used to treat human ailments by halaba people, southern Ethiopia. *Journal of Medicinal Plants Studies*. 2017; 5(4): 36-47.

[46] Yeneayehu Fenetahun, Girma Eshetu, Abebe Worku and Taher Abdella. A survey on medicinal plants used by traditional healers in Harari regional State, East Ethiopia. *Journal of medicinal plants studies*. 2017; 5(1): 85-90.

[47] Tefera B, Kim Y. Ethnobotanical study of medicinal plants in the fDistrict, Sidama zone, Southern Ethiopia. *J Ethnobiol Ethnomed*. 2019; 15 (1). doi:10.1186/s13002-019-0302-7.

[48] Tadesse B, Dereje A. Survey of ethno-veterinary medicinal plants at selected Horro Gudurru Districts, Western Ethiopia. *African Journal of Plant Science*. 2015; 9(3):185-192. doi: 10.5897/ajps2014.1229.

[49] Ayenew A. An Ethnobotanical Study of Enset (<i>Ensete ventricosum</i> (Welw) Cheesman) in Angacha Woreda, Kembata-Tembaro Zone, South Region, Ethiopia. *American Journal of Life Sciences*. 2016; 4(6):195. doi:10.11648/j.ajls.20160406.18.

[50] Abraha Teklay. Traditional Medicinal Plants for Ethnoveterinary Medicine Used in Kilte Awulaelo District, Tigray Region, NorthernEthiopia. *Journal of Biology, Agriculture and Healthcare*. 2015; 5(19): 120-130.

[51] Meaza G, Tadesse B, Maria A, Piero B, Gidey Y. Traditional medicinal plants used by Kunama ethnic group in Northern Ethiopia. *Journal of Medicinal Plants Research*. 2015; 9(15):494-509. doi:10.5897/jmpr2014.5681.

[52] Fitsumbirhan Tewelde, Mebrahtom Mesfin, Semere Tsewene. Ethnobotanical Survey of Traditional Medicinal Practices in LaelayAdi-yabo District, Northern Ethiopia. International Journal of Ophthalmology & Visual Science. 2017; 2 (4): 80-87. doi: 10.11648/j.ijovs.20170204.11.

[53] Chekole G, Asfaw Z, Kelbessa E. Ethnobotanical study of medicinal plants in the environs of Tara-gedam and Amba remnant forests of Libo Kemkem District, northwest Ethiopia. *J Ethnobiol Ethnomed*. 2015; 11(1):4. doi: 10.1186/1746-4269-11-4.

[54] Seble W, Zemede A, Ensermu K. Ethnobotanical study of medicinal plants used by local people in Menz Gera Midir District, North Shewa Zone, Amhara Regional State, Ethiopia. *Journal of Medicinal Plants Research*. 2018; 12(21):296-314. doi:10.5897/jmpr2018.6616.

[55] Getu Alemayehu, Zemede Asfaw and Ensermu Kelbessa. Ethnobotanical study of medicinal plants used by local communities of Minjar-Shenkora District, North Shewa Zone of Amhara Region, Ethiopia. *Journal of Medicinal Plants Studies*. 2015; *3* (6): 01–11.

[56] Gebreyes T, Melesse M. Determination of informant consensus factor and fidelity level of ethnomedicinal plants used in Misha Woreda, Hadiya Zone, Southern Ethiopia. *International Journal of Biodiversity and Conservation*. 2016; 8 (12):351-364. doi:10.5897/ijbc2016.1020.

[57] Osman A, Sbhatu D, Giday M. Medicinal Plants Used to Manage Human and Livestock Ailments in Raya Kobo District of Amhara Regional State, Ethiopia. *Evidence-Based Complementary and Alternative Medicine*. 2020; 2020:1-19. doi:10.1155/2020/1329170.

[58] Abdeta D. Survey on Ethno Botany and Medicinal Animals at Sayo and Hawa Gelan Districts of Kelem Wollega Zone, Western Ethiopia. *Biomed J Sci Tech Res*. 2020; 28(2). doi:10.26717/bjstr.2020.28.004620.

[59] Araya S, Abera B, Giday M. Study of plants traditionally used in public and animal health management in Seharti Samre District, Southern Tigray, Ethiopia. *J Ethnobiol Ethnomed*. 2015; 11 (1). doi:10.1186/s13002-015-0015-5.

[60] Kassa Z, Asfaw Z, Demissew S. An ethnobotanical study of medicinal plants in Sheka Zone of Southern Nations Nationalities and Peoples Regional State, Ethiopia. *J Ethnobiol Ethnomed*. 2020; 16(1). doi:10.1186/s13002-020-0358-4.

[61] Asnake S, Teklehaymanot T, Hymete A, Erko B, Giday M. Survey of Medicinal Plants Used to Treat Malaria by Sidama People of Boricha District, Sidama Zone, South Region of Ethiopia. *Evidence-Based Complementary and Alternative Medicine*. 2016; 2016:1-9. doi:10.1155/2016/9690164.

[62] Assefa A, Bahiru A. Ethnoveterinary botanical survey of medicinal plants in Abergelle, Sekota and Lalibela districts of Amhara region, Northern Ethiopia. *J Ethnopharmacol*. 2018; 213:340-349. doi:10.1016/j.jep.2017.11.024.

[63] Garedew B, Abebe D. Ethnobotanical Study of Medicinal Plants Used for Treatment of Liver Diseases in Tepi Town, Southwest Ethiopia. *Asian Journal of Biological Sciences*. 2019; 12(4):648-655. doi:10.3923/ajbs.2019.648.655.

[64] Feto Haji A. Ethnobotanical Study of Medicinal Plants Used for the Treatment of Human and Livestock Ailments in Dawe Kachen District of Bale Zone, Southeast Ethiopia. *International journal of Emerging Trends in Science and Technology*. 2017; 04(04): 5043-5055. doi:10.18535/ijetst/v4i4.01.

[65] Tuasha N, Petros B, Asfaw Z. Medicinal plants used by traditional healers to treat malignancies and other human ailments in Dalle District, Sidama Zone, Ethiopia. *J Ethnobiol Ethnomed*. 2018;14(1). doi:10.1186/s13002-018-0213-z.

[66] Meragiaw M, Asfaw Z, Argaw M. The Status of Ethnobotanical Knowledge of Medicinal Plants and the Impacts of Resettlement in Delanta, Northwestern Wello, Northern Ethiopia. *Evidence-Based Complementary and Alternative Medicine*. 2016; 2016:1-24. doi:10.1155/2016/5060247.

Section 3

Medicinal Herbs

Chapter 6

Curcuminoids: The Novel Molecules of Nature

Sitabja Mukherjee and Santosh K. Kar

Abstract

Curcuminoids inactivate Nuclear Factor-Kappa B (NF-κB), a key pro-inflammatory transcription factor which is involved in inflammation and immune response in diseases like cancer. NF-κB activation is necessary to determine tumor microenvironment which controls migration and metastatis of cancer cells through chemokines and their receptors and involvement of some cell adhesion molecules. Therefore inhibition of NF-κB by curcuminoids could be a new approach in treatment of cancer by immune modulation. Curcuminoids are not bioavailable and therefore there were problems in efficacy. Now by using bioavailable curcuminoid formulations the problem has been resolved to a great extent. Out of 49 placebo controlled double blind clinical trials using curcuminoids, 17 have been found to be successful. Therefore curcuminoids could be developed as an adjunct therapy for diseases like cancer to save human life.

Keywords: Curcuminoids, Inflammation, Immunomodulation, Human clinical trial

1. Introduction

Curcuminoids are natural polyphenolic compounds present in the rhizome of *Curcuma longa* plant which are responsible for the yellow color of turmeric and it's medicinal properties [1]. Turmeric has been used for centuries not only to make Indian curry spicy but also for healing wounds, reducing pain and as antibacterial agent in our traditional system of medicine [2]. No one knew what component of turmeric was responsible for these medicinal properties till Vogel Peletier isolated the pigment from it in 1815 [3]. No structural studies could be done as the isolated pigment was found to be a mixture of oleoresin and oil. Finally Vogel A Jr. isolated the pure pigment in 1842 but he did not determine its structure [4]. After unsuccessful attempts by many chemists, Milobedzka J and Lampe V determined the chemical structure of curcumin to be diferuloylmethane and named it as curcumin in 1910 almost hundred years after it was first isolated in 1815 [5]. Later the same group synthesized the molecule in 1913 which established its structure firmly [6]. Subsequently K R Srinivasan developed chromatographic methods to separate curcumin and showed it to have three components [7, 8].

Using diverse extraction techniques and chromatographic methods which are coupled with sensitive mass spectrometric detection system to identify the extracted molecules we now know that turmeric contains atleast 235 specialized secondary metabolites which include 109 sesquiterpene and 68 monoterpene molecules besides the three Curcuminoid molecules which are the subject of discussion here [9]. The three molecules viz. Curcumin (which is the major Curcuminoid), demethoxycurcumin (DMC) and bisdemethoxycurcumin (BDMC) which are

IntechOpen

Name of compound	Structure & molecular weight (g/mol)	IUPAC name	Physical appearance	Molecular formula	Physical & chemical properties
Curcumin	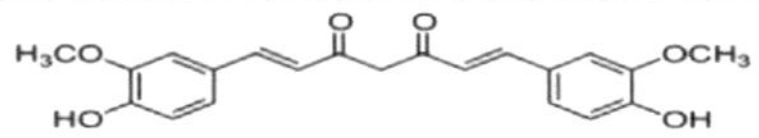 M.W : 368.38	1E,6E-1,7-bis(4-hydroxy-3-methoxyphenyl)-1,6-heptadiene-3,5-dione	Bright orange yellow powder	$C_{21}H_{20}O_6$	Melting Point: 183°C Boiling Point: 591.4°C at 760 mmHg Density: 1.3 ± 0.1 g/cm^3
Demethoxy Curcumin	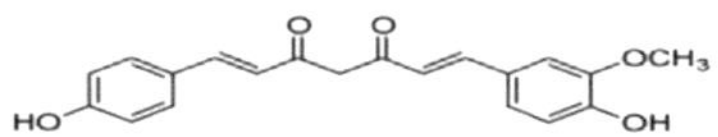 M.W : 338.37	1E,6E-1-(4Hydroxy-3-methoxyphenyl)-7-(4-hydroxyphenyl) hepta-1-6-diene-3,5-dione	Orange colored powder	$C_{20}H_{18}O_5$	Melting Point: 178°C-180°C Boiling Point: 573.4 ± 50.0 °C at 760 mmHg Density: 1.3 ± 0.1 g/cm^3
Bisdemethoxy Curcumin	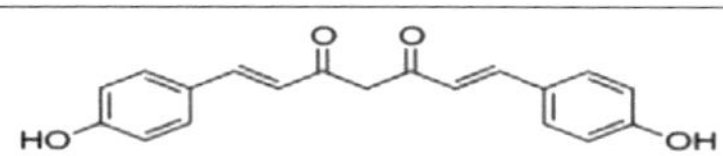 M.W : 308.33	(1E,6E)-1,7-Bis(4-hydroxyphenyl) hepta-1,6-diene-3,5-dione	Yellow colored powder	$C_{19}H_{16}O_4$	Melting Point: 226°C-231°C Boiling Point: 551.3 ± 45.0°C at 760 mmHg Density: 1.3 ± 0.1 g/cm^3

Name of compound	Structure & molecular weight (g/mol)	IUPAC name	Physical appearance	Molecular formula	Physical & chemical properties
Cyclocurcumin	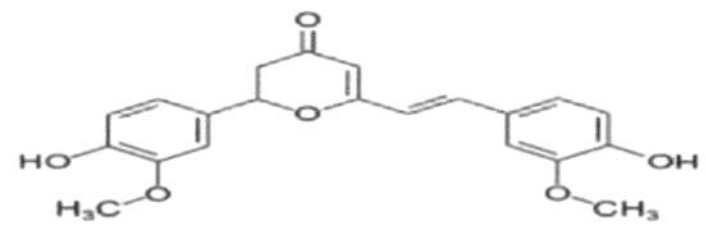 M.W : 368.38	2-(4-hydroxy-3-methoxyphenyl-6-[(E)-2-(4-hydroxy-3- methoxyphenyl) ethenyl]-2,3H-dihydropyran-4-one	Yellow colored powder	$C_{21}H_{20}O_6$	Melting Point: 179°C-226°C Boiling Point: 571.9 ± 50.0°C at 760 mmHg Density: 1.4 ± 0.1 g/cm^3

Table 1.
Structure and properties of curcuminoids present in turmeric.

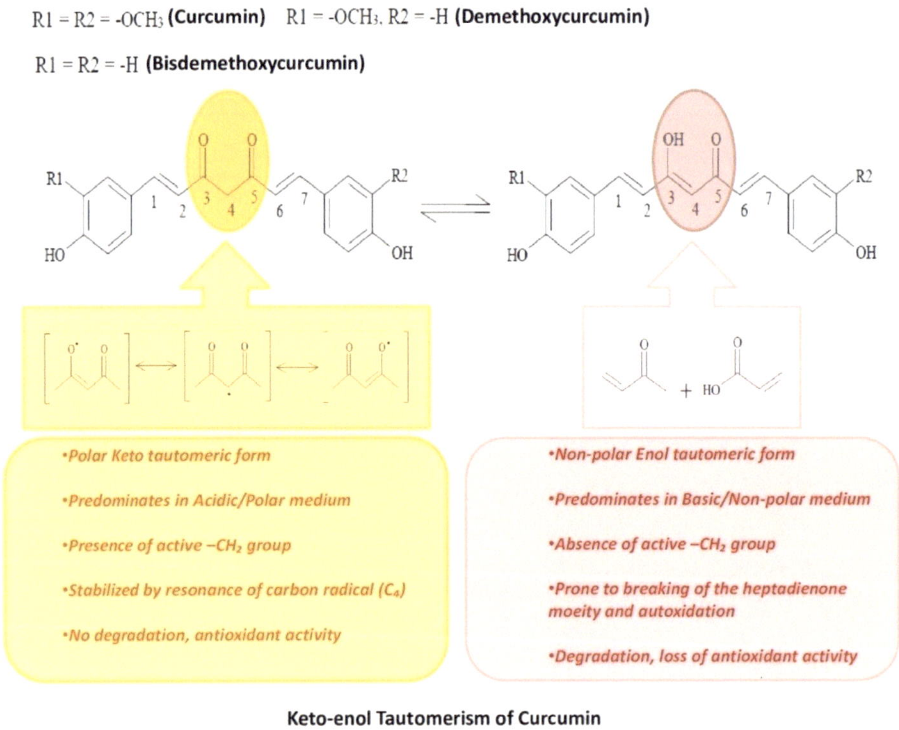

Figure 1.
Tautomeric forms of curcumin.

minor components of turmeric appear to have many medicinal properties. A fourth molecule called Cyclocurcumin which in the absence of α, β-unsaturated β-diketone motif is not considered as a Curcuminoid but an analog of Curcumin, has recently been identified to be present in the rhizome in much less concentration but with some interesting medicinal properties (**Table 1**) [10]. **Table 1** gives the structure of the four molecules and summarizes the chemical properties of the three curcuminoids and cyclocurcumin for comparison.

Each of the three curcuminoid molecules contains two aromatic o-methoxy phenolic groups, except BDMC which has only phenolic groups joined linearly through a seven carbon chain linker contain**ing** α, β-unsaturated β-diketone groups. The presence of this linker chain with the α, β-unsaturated β-diketone groups, a unique feature of curcuminoid molecules, allows the curcuminoids to remain either in the keto or enol form depending upon the ambient pH and exhibit biological activities (**Figure 1**) [11].

Every year more than 10 thousand papers are published worldwide describing the biological activity and therapeutic potential of Curcumin. Here we will discuss some of the properties of curcumin and will introduce the *Curcuma longa* plant. *Curcuma longa* has been cultivated in India and other south eastern countries with suitable weather and soil conditions for centuries [12]. Significant efforts have been made to understand the biosynthesis of these molecules in the rhizome and purify them from turmeric to study their chemistry. Efforts have been made to synthesize them in heterologous systems like E.coli and so that novel curcuminoids could be made and tested for their activities. We will also discuss how there has been concerted efforts to discredit curcumin as a lead molecule due to it's poor ADMET (absorption, distribution, metabolism, excretion, and toxicology) properties inspite of credibility of successful traditional usage to emerge as new neutraceutical drugs against diseases [13].

2. The *Curcuma longa* plant

Curcuma longa belongs to Zingiberaceae family which includes *Zingiber officinalis*, the source of ginger another very useful herb [14]. *Curcuma longa* grows to a height of 1 m as an upright, perennial plant displaying bright foliage and colored flowers. The plant is sterile as it produces seeds which are not viable but *Curcuma longa* can be vigorously propagated by using the rhizomes of the plant [15]. It does not grow in the wild and is thought to have arisen by selection and vegetative propagation of a hybrid between wild plant *Curcuma aromatica* which is, native to India and some other closely related species [16]. It is estimated that the genus *Curcuma* contains between 80 and 117 species, the majority of which are found in Southeast Asia, but some of which can also be found in the Himalayas, Southern China, Australia, and the Pacific Islands [16, 17]. Carolus Linnaeus, the famous Swedish taxonomist, coined the name Curcuma for the genus and included it in his book Species Plantarum, which was published in the year 1753. The plant derives its name "curcuma" from the Arabic word Kurkum, in reference to the yellowish color of its root [17].

To thrive, *Curcuma longa* requires temperatures ranging from 20^0Celsius to 35^0 Celsius, and significant rainfall during the monsoon season when it is cultivated [18]. Turmeric is best known for its culinary applications as a major component of curry powder, for which it has been dubbed "Indian saffron" as a cheaper alternative to the far more expensive saffron spice. Turmeric is also used in cosmetics and toiletries. Its active ingredient has a distinct earthy, slightly bitter, slightly hot peppery flavor and a mustardy smell. The genus *Curcuma* also contains a number of economically important species, such as *C. angustifolia* (short-leaved turmeric), *C. zedoaria* (also known as zedoary) and *C. amada* which is a slang term for "amazing" (mango ginger). Curcuma plants such as *C ornata*, which has beautiful green leaves and pinecone-like flowers of light pink color that lasts for a month, *C elata,* which can withstand cold climate conditions and produces extremely brilliant yellow flowers, and *C petiolata* 'Emperor' from Thailand, which produces pink colored flowers, are few examples which can be grown as house plants.

Erode, a city in the Indian state of Tamil Nadu, with suitable weather conditions and rainfall is the world's largest producer of turmeric and the world's most important trading center for the spice, earning it the nickname "Turmeric City" in addition to Sangli, a town in the Indian state of Maharashtra, which too is another significant trading center for turmeric throughout Asia. In a year, India produces 600,000 tons of turmeric, which accounts for 75% of the world's total annual production of 800,000 tons. The rhizomes, which are underground stems that look like roots and have a brown surface with bright orange or yellow interior flesh, are processed to produce a lemon yellow powder known as turmeric.

3. Extraction of curcuminoids from turmeric and it's synthesis in the laboratory

The extraction of curcumin from turmeric has become of immense commercial interest due to health benefitting medicinal properties of curcumin. For the process to be commercially viable it should be efficient, simple and the end product should be suitable for human consumption. Since India is one of the largest producers of turmeric, quite naturally there are a lot of activities with respect to extraction of curcuminoids from turmeric on a commercial scale. Typically, the content of curcuminoids in turmeric ranges from 2%-9% of the total dry weight depending upon origin of the plant and the conditions of the soil where it is grown. Even though Curcumin was first isolated as a pigment in the impure form by Vogel in the year 1815, the methods of curcuminoids extraction are being standardized till very recently. The most commonly used method for extracting curcumin from turmeric has been the employment of solvent extraction followed by column chromatography for separating curcuminoids from other molecules that are extracted. Soxhlet extraction, ultrasonic extraction, microwave, zone-refining and dipping methods have been tried, and among these the Soxhlet, ultrasonic and microwave extractions are the most commonly employed methods [19]. Recently, it has been reported that pulse ultrasonic and microwave-assisted extraction methods are superior to continuous extraction methods. As there is an increase in the use of curcumin in dietary supplements, researchers are continually developing newer extraction methods in order to increase the yield and quality of the end product. Green bio based methods which do not use surfactants or solvent are also being developed. When compared with the conventional ethanol/water based extraction methods, the surfactant free microemulsion (SFME) methods have been found to be more efficient in extracting curcuminoids [20]. Some of the newer methods use food grade molecules like triacylglycerol which can solubilize curcumin in the presence of water for achieving higher yield and use of supercritical carbon dioxide makes it a method free of any organic solvents [21]. Pilot plants based on supercritical carbon dioxide have been established in several countries for the extraction of curcumin from turmeric with the purpose of making the extraction process of curcumin a commercially viable one.

Column chromatography can separate curcumin from curcumin mix (a mixture of curcumin, demethoxycurcumin, and bisdemethoxycurcumin) by adsorbing the mixture on silica gel and then eluting with solvent mixtures such as dichloromethane/acetic acid or methanol/chloroform to yield three different fractions. The curcumin fraction is then purified further on silica gel using eluents such as chloroform/dichloromethane and ethanol/methanol mixtures. The high performance liquid chromatography (HPLC) technique has been used extensively in the detection and estimation of curcumin in different fractions. In general, reverse phase C18 columns are used as the stationary phase, with various gradients of solvents containing acetonitrile/water or chloroform/methanol used as the mobile phase [22]. Curcumin detection is simple and can be done by using absorption detectors in the visible range of 350 to 450 nm or in the UV region using a common detection wavelength in the range of 250 to 270 nm. Several researchers have also used HPLC-diode array and fluorescence detection methods. Another versatile tool for detecting curcumin is liquid chromatography-coupled mass spectrometry [23].

Lampe published the first paper on the synthesis of curcumin in 1918, a century after its isolation from turmeric. The procedure consisted of five steps, beginning with carbomethoxyferuloyl chloride and ending with ethyl acetoacetate. Later, Pabon reported a simpler method for the synthesis of curcumin in high yields using acetyl acetone and substituted aromatic aldehydes in the presence of boron trioxide (B2O3), trialkyl borate, and n-butylamine (**Figure 2**). This method was adopted by several research groups for all subsequent synthesis of curcumin with minor modifications. The primary step in all of these methods is the reaction of 2,4-diketones with appropriately substituted aromatic aldehydes. To prevent the participation of diketone in Knoevenagel condensations, it is complexed with boron. These reactions are best performed in anhydrous conditions and polar aprotic solvents, where curcumin can be easily separated from reaction mixtures. Primary and secondary amines are used as catalysts to provide the basicity required to deprotonate the diketone's alkyl groups. Scavengers such as alkyl borates are used to remove the water produced during the condensation reaction. Water, if not removed, can react with the diketone complex, reducing the curcumin yield. Under slightly acidic

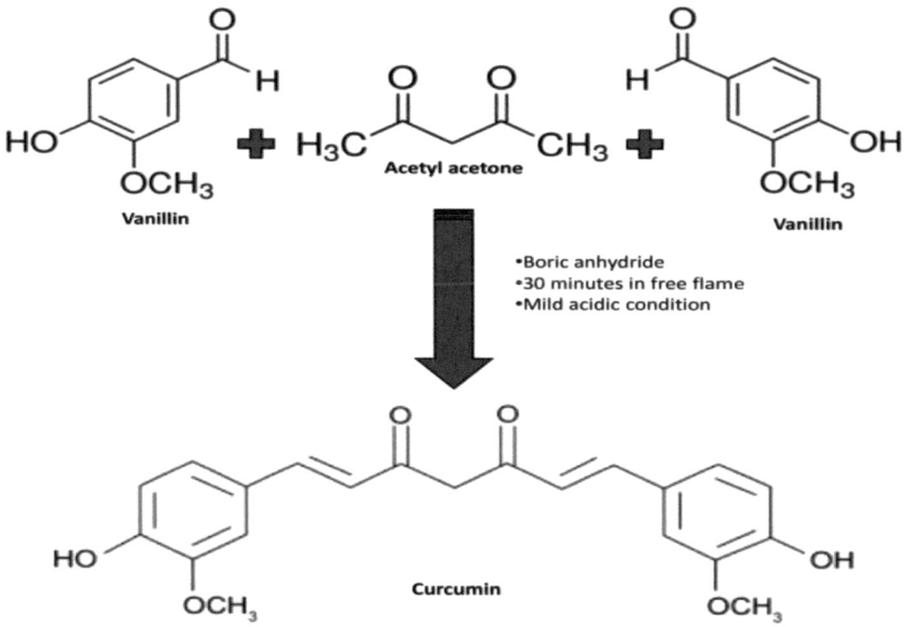

Figure 2.
Laboratory synthesis of curcumin.

conditions, the boron complex dissociates into curcumin. Washing and repeated precipitation followed by column chromatography can then be used to separate curcumin from this reaction mixture [24].

4. Chemistry of curcuminoids

The relative concentrations of the three curcuminoids in the turmeric vary depending upon the source of the rhizome used for propagation and the climatic conditions as well as fertility of the soil in which it is grown. Typically it varies between the following ranges: curcumin (70-80%), demethoxy curcumin (10-20%), and bisdemethoxy curcumin (3-6%) [25]. Because curcumin is the primary curcuminoid found in turmeric, it could be playing a significant role in the control of the medicinal properties of the mixture. It is equally important that we should investigate how the other two molecules contribute to curcuminoids' health benefitting effects like anti-inflammatory, anti-oxidant, and immunomodulatory properties [24].

Because the methylene group in curcumin contains two active hydrogen atoms and is flanked by two keto groups, the hydrogen atom attached to the carbon atom can migrate to the oxygen atom of the keto group, resulting in the keto-enol tautomeric forms (**Figure 1**) Extensive research over the last few decades have established the role of these distinct functional domains in curcumin's observed biological activities.

When the pH is between 3 and 7, it is the keto form that is predominantly found embedded in the lipid bilayer of membranes, while the enol form is found around pH 8. Curcumin's physicochemical and antioxidant properties are determined by this keto-enol-enol equilibrium. It is worth noting that when curcumin is present in the enol form, both aromatic rings at either end of the molecule can interact through extensive electron delocalization via the pi orbitals of the C=C bonds in the heptadiene linker. Due to these structural constraints, the aromatic rings at either end of the molecule must be in the same plane, transforming the whole molecule into a planar structure.

The two aromatic rings with hydroxyl and O-methyl groups can exist in separate planes and interact with other molecules independently. The keto form exhibits distinct physiological properties, whereas the enol form, which must be planar, degrades rapidly [26]. When curcumin is administered orally or via intraperitoneal injection, it is rapidly eliminated through the feces due to its low solubility, which results in decreased absorption and extensive systemic clearance due to its degradation or metabolic conversion to more water-soluble forms that are rapidly secreted out. In the gut, curcumin is converted enzymatically to more soluble forms such as glucuronide and sulphate conjugates or reduced to tetrahydrocurcumin and hexahydrocurcuminglucuronides [27].

Curcumin's fundamental antioxidant activity is entirely dependent on the presence of hydrogen on the phenolic or central methylene groups. By losing a proton, a phenoxy-radical can be generated from the curcumin molecule's phenolic groups, and similar reactions can generate a carbon radical from the central methylene group. Although the phenoxy radical is more stable than the carbon radical, experimental data from study of curcumin indicate that both phenoxy and carbon radicals contribute to curcumin's biological activity. The phenoxy or carbon radicals produced by curcumin molecules are resonance stabilized by extensive conjugation via the heptadiene linker. As a result, curcumin acts as a potent scavenger of various reactive oxygen species (ROS), including hydroxyl radicals, hydrogen peroxide, singlet oxygen, and superoxide anion, thereby preventing damage to macromolecules in circulation or present in tissue. As a result, the phenolic groups or active methylene groups are a critical component of the curcumin molecule which contribute to its bioactivity [28].

As with curcumin, the other two curcuminoids (demethoxycurcumin and bisdemethoxycurcumin) also contain phenolic hydroxyl groups, a heptadiene chain, and a diketone moiety, which contribute to their diverse therapeutic properties, including antioxidant, anti-inflammatory, and anticancer properties. Curcumin has the highest antioxidant capacity, followed by demethoxycurcumin and bisdemethoxycurcumin. This observation holds true only when curcuminoids are not degraded, as is the case when an acidic or polar medium is used. On the other hand, under basic or non-polar conditions, bisdemethoxycurcumin is more stable than demethoxycurcumin, which in turn is more stable than curcumin. Apart from pH or the nature of the medium the structure of the phenolic compounds has an effect on the stability of curcuminoids. The electron donating group like OH or OMe groups on the benzene rings has a preference for the enol tautomer. Thus, among the three curcuminoids, the equilibrium shifting toward formation of the enol tautomer is greatest for curcumin and least for bisdemethoxycurcumin due to the presence of two methoxy groups. Bisdemethoxycurcumin, on the other hand, is less susceptible to degradation than demethoxycurcumin, which is less susceptible to degradation than curcumin. In basic or non-polar solvents, the rate of degradation is as follows: curcumin >demethoxycurcumin> bisdemethoxycurcumin (**Figure 3**).

The activity of Curcuminoids is strongly influenced by the methoxy group. The antioxidant activity of curcuminoids is primarily due to the active methylene group; however, the presence of an electron-donating methoxy groups ortho to the phenolic hydroxyl group also contributes to the molecule's antioxidant activity via an inductive effect on the hydroxyl group. Curcumin has the highest antioxidant activity of the three curcuminoids due to the presence of two methoxy groups.

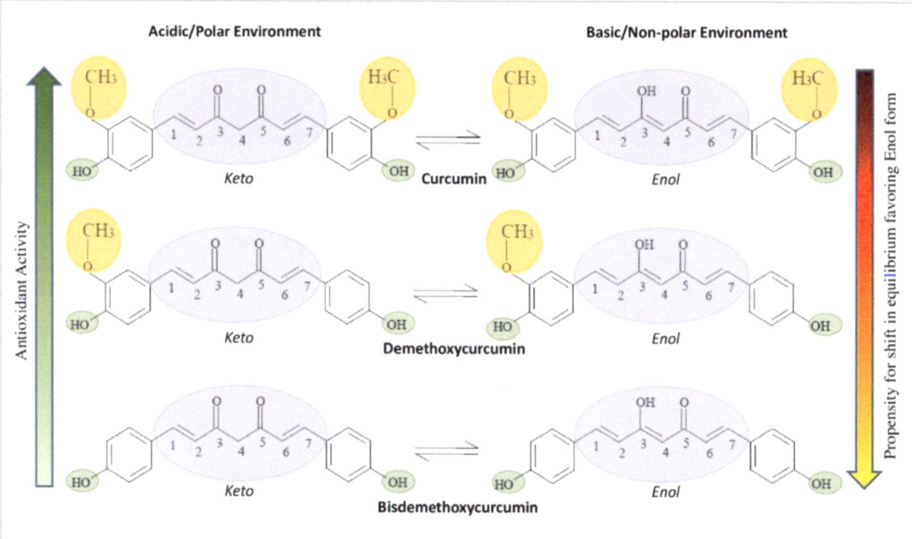

Figure 3.
Structure–function relationship of Curcuminoids.

Demethoxycurcumin has greater antioxidant activity than bisdemethoxycurcumin, which lacks a methoxy group.

5. Pharmacology of curcumin: role of degradation products

Curcumin is poorly bioavailable and fairly unstable in tissue under normal physiologic conditions. As a result, it is very likely that the metabolically transformed curcumin products, which are relatively more water-soluble, are responsible for the observed health benefits of curcumin. It has been shown that 90% of curcumin degrades within 30 minutes in phosphate buffer (pH 7.4) into various products such as, trans-6-(4hydroxy-3-methoxyphenyl)-2,4-dioxo-5-hexanal, ferulic aldehyde, ferulic acid, feruloyl methane, vanillin, and a few others [29]. Degradation occurs in basic medium via nucleophilic attack of the basic -hydroxide ion. The alkaline hydrolysis of curcumin produces feruloylmethane and ferulic acid. Further hydrolysis of the feruloylmethane results in the formation of vanillin and acetone. Thus, under basic conditions, the heptadienone moiety is broken, resulting in the disappearance of the active methylene group that contributes tothe majority of curcumin's antioxidant activity. Depending on the conditions it is subjected to, Curcumin can also undergo autoxidation or photooxidation to give rise to different degradation products (**Figure 4**).

Furthermore, it is unclear how curcumin exerts its inhibitory effects on such a large number of different enzymes whose binding pockets are unable to bind curcumin specifically. By comparing the biological activities of curcumin and its degradation products against diseases such as Alzheimer's and cancer, as well as their preferential inhibition of certain enzymes, it appears as though the bioactive degradation products may play a significant role in contributing to curcumin's observed pharmacological effects [30]. On the other hand, when curcumin enters the bloodstream, it forms complexes with proteins such as Albumin etc. and gets stabilized [31]. As a result, the rapid degradation of curcumin

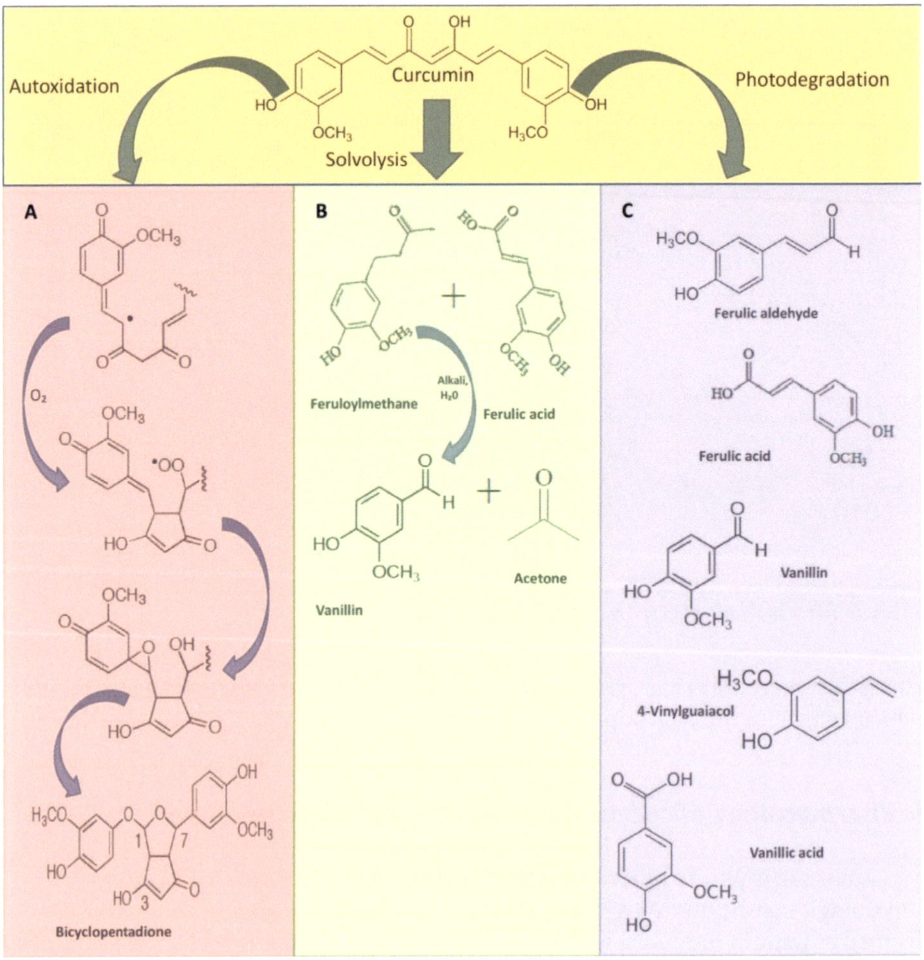

Figure 4.
Different paths for degradation of curcumin.

observed in the absence of proteins may not be occurring to the same extent in the tissue. This possibility should be investigated further in order to understand curcumin's pharmacokinetics and beneficial effects in the treatment of various diseases.

6. Biosynthesis of curcuminoids in the rhizome

Three polyketide synthases (PKS) isoforms, CURS1, CURS2, and CURS3, found in the leaves and rhizomes of *Curcuma longa* are involved in catalyzing the synthesis of various curcuminoids using various feruloyldiketide-CoAs as starter substrates [32]. The Curcuminoid Biosynthetic Pathway in *Curcuma longa* rhizome was investigated using 13C-labeled precursors and the enzyme involved in the process. It has been demonstrated that CURS1 exclusively utilizes feruloyl-CoA as a starting substrate and converts feruloyldiketide-CoA esters to curcumin. Similarly, CURS2 produces both curcumin and demethoxycurcumin using feruloyl-CoA as a starter substrate, whereas CURS3 produces all three curcuminoids, curcumin, demethoxycurcumin, and bisdemethoxycurcumin, using either feruloyl-CoA or 4-coumaroyl-CoA as the starter substrate [32].

Heterologous production of Curcuminoids has been attempted in *E. coli* and *Saccharomyces cerevisiae*. Katsuyama et al. prepared an *E. coli* strain with artificial biosynthetic pathway by combining enzyme-encoding genes such as 4-coumarate-CoA ligase (4CL) from *Lithospermumerythrorhizon* (Le4CL1), curcuminoid synthase (CUS)from *O. sativa* and Acetyl-CoA carboxylase (ACC) from *Corynebacterium glutamicum* which generated a new set of gene clusters which produced curcuminoids [33]. Using this approach and by adding two different unnatural carboxylic acids, 9 new curcuminoids which are not found in nature could also be produced [34]. This precursor-driven biosynthetic approach allowed the production of unnatural novel polyketides. This way of producing unnatural curcuminoids may provide novel drug candidates.

The production of curcumin and its derivatives by CURS may be an adaptive mechanism employed by the *Curcuma longa* plant to both protect against and respond to a variety of threats. Curcumin is a potent antioxidant that acts as a scavenger of free radicals, removing them from the plant's cells. Curcumin's bitter taste may also serve as a deterrent to herbivores.

7. Can curcuminoids be lead molecules to be a drug?

In a spirited article Kathryn *M. nelson* et al. have pointed out that "curcuminods which constitute about ~5% of turmeric has been classified as pan-assay interference (PAINS) compounds as well as invalid metabolic panaceas (IMPS) candidate [35]. Further curcuminoids are nonbioavailable, unstable and reactive compounds. Therefore they arehighly improbable lead for development of any drug. They pointed out and I quote "To our knowledge, compound 1 has never been shown to be conclusively effective in a randomized, placebo-controlled clinical trial for any indication. Curcumin is best typified, therefore, as a missile that continually blows up on the launch pad, never reaching the atmosphere or its intended target (s). These results have given curcumin the label of pharmacodynamically fierce (hits many targets) yet pharmacokinetically feeble (does not get to its targets). While these failures would normally end further research on its use as a therapeutic, they apparently have not deterred researchers interested in its development."

Responding to this paper by Nelson et al., Padmanaban G. and Nagaraj V. wrote a paper entitled "Curcumin May Defy Medicinal Chemists" to remind Dr. Nelson that just taking 4 clinical trials on curcuminoids into consideration it is not proper to suggest that all research on Curcuminoids should be suspended [36]. They wrote and I quote ". With over 10,000 papers published and 120 clinical trials under various stages of progress using curcumin, the review is a huge dampener, considering the projected potential of curcumin and other natural products as a panacea. Even if 1% of the papers published make sense, it would still be a sizable number to warrant against passing a negative verdict on the whole field. The review has picked four clinical trials and concluded that given its low systemic bioavailability, it is doubtful whether oral curcumin would ever be effective in human clinical trials."

After this paper by Padmanaban et al. was published, Nelson et al. responded without realizing that their arguments are based on wrong interpretation of data generated by others [37]. Soon another paper was published pointing out that while some of the arguments about curcuminoids are true, many of the conclusions drawn by Nelson et al. on the basis of referred papers are hard to accept as they were never made by the authors of these referred papers. The issue of curcuminoids being PAINS compounds was insignificant unless it actually interferes with the high-throughput screening employed. What actually matters at the end of the human clinical trials and case studies is whether human life could be saved for which nature has designed these molecules [38]. In a recent letter to editor of Nature Michal Heger writes not to discount all the curcumin trial data. He points out that out of 49 clinical trials conducted recently 17 have shown efficacy. Therefore the molecular targets and the mechanisms of action of curcumin should be examined further [39]. Curcuminoids are wonderful molecules and can be developed to play significant role as adjunct therapy against inflammatory diseases. The pace of research on curcumin has not slowed down in spite of the two papers by Nelson et al.

It has been demonstrated that when curcumin was bound to chitosan nano particles and delivered orally to mice infected with *Plasmodium yoelii* parasite, the treated mice survived longer than the infected untreated mice [40]. Curcumin alone could not do so. When it was adsorbed on to chitosan nano particles and fed orally it's bioavailability increased and it entered into infected RBC and prevented hemozoin synthesis which killed the parasite.

In another experiment it was demonstrated that when nano curcumin alone was given orally to *Mycobacterium tuberculosis* infected mice it did not kill the *Mycobacteria* and the infected animals did not survive. But when it was administered in the presence if INH it helped to cure the infected mice in five weeks while INH alone could cure only in 8 weeks [41]. Therefore the combination of nano curcumin with INH was more effective than INH alone.

In a third experiment it has been shown that nano curcumin when administered orally to mice can modulate memory T cells and induced immune response against BCG in a manner which does not happen in the absence of nano curcumin [42]. These papers showed that curcumin can modulate immune memory mechanisms which was effective in prevention of death.

8. Human clinical trials with curcumin demonstrating efficacy of treatment

8.1 Curcumin for the prevention of colorectal neoplasia

Inhibition of the procarcinogenic eicosanoids prostaglandin E2 (PGE2) and 5-hydroxyeicosatetraenoic acid (5-HETE) has been shown in rodent models to have the potential to suppress carcinogenesis. In a nonrandomized, open-label clinical trial involving 44 patients, Robert E. et al. evaluated the effects of oral curcumin administration (2 g or 4 g per day for 30 days) on PGE2 within aberrant crypt foci (ACF), 5-HETE, ACF number, and proliferation [43]. To be eligible, men and women had to be at least 40 years old, a current smoker with a smoking history of more than three pack-years, and have at least eight rectal ACF detected using magnification chromoendoscopy. Subjects were excluded if they used nonsteroidal antiinflammatory drugs (NSAIDs), such as acetylsalicylic acid (ASA, or aspirin), for more than 10 days per month, unless they completed a 30-day washout period, or if they had a history of chronic inflammatory bowel disease, prior pelvic irradiation, or a history of endoscopically confirmed peptic ulcer disease within 5 years of enrollment. Neither dose of curcumin reduced PGE2 or 5-HETE in ACF or normal mucosa, nor did it reduce Ki-67 in normal mucosa, but the group receiving 4 g oral curcumin experienced a significant decrease in the number of ACF. After treatment, the reduction in ACF in this group was associated with a fivefold increase in serum curcumin or curcumin conjugates levels.

8.2 Effects of curcumin supplementation in patients with polycystic ovary syndrome

Heshmati et al. investigated the effect of curcumin supplementation on fasting blood glucose, insulin resistance, and androgen levels in patients with polycystic ovary syndrome [44]. In a randomized double-blind placebo-controlled trial, 72 women with polycystic ovary were enrolled. The study included women with PCOS aged 18–49 years (considered to be of reproductive age) who had a definitive diagnosis of PCOS for at least two years (made by a specialist physician during the mild to moderate phase), had impaired glucose tolerance (IGT), were a user of only one of the metformin or clomiphene drug groups, and had a body mass index (BMI) greater than 25 but less than 30. Patients were excluded if they had any of the following: a) Other hormonal diseases/disorders, autoimmune diseases, cancer, inflammatory disease, infections, pregnancy, or lactation, b) use of multivitamin-mineral, omega3, polyphenolic, or antioxidant supplements, as well as anticoagulants such as heparin and warfarin or aspirin, blood cholesterol-lowering drugs (statins), or non-steroidal anti-inflammatory drugs (NSAIDs). Curcumin capsules containing 500 mg curcumin powder were given to the intervention group, while maltodextrin capsules containing 500 mg maltodextrin were given to the placebo group. For 12 weeks, participants took three capsules daily (1500 mg total). The trial's primary outcomes were changes in fasting plasma glucose (FPG), fasting insulin (FI), sex hormones (Estradiol, Dehydroepiandrosterone (DHEA), Follicle-Stimulating Hormone (FSH), and Luteinizing Hormone (LH), and the modified Ferriman-Gallwey (mFG) hirsutism questionnaire. Changes in waist circumference (WC), weight, and body mass index were secondary outcomes of this study (BMI). At the conclusion of the study, it was observed that FPG and Dehydroepiandrosterone levels had decreased significantly, whereas Estradiol levels had increased statistically non-significantly in the intervention group following oral curcumin administration, in comparison to the placebo control group. At the end of the study, the authors concluded that curcumin is a safe and useful supplement for the treatment of PCOS-associated symptoms.

8.3 Curcumin in radiation dermatitis

One of the most common side effects experienced by patients suffering from cancers of sarcoma, breast, lung, and head and neck cancer and receiving radiotherapy (RT) is radiation dermatitis. Because the skin is a highly proliferative and self-renewing organ, it is particularly susceptible to damage from ionizing radiation, and as a result, the majority of patients undergoing radiotherapy develop radiation-induced skin reactions. Following dose- and time-dependent standard fractionation regimens in conventional radiotherapy, an accumulation of basal keratinocyte loss and impairment of the epidermal skin barrier occurs. The severity of radiation dermatitis varies from mild to severe erythema to dry or moist desquamation and ulceration. The current clinical guidelines for radiation-induced skin reactions include the following: 1) washing with lukewarm water and a mild soap; 2) applying unscented, lanolin-free, water-based moisturizers; and 3) IMRT. There is, however, no consensus regarding an agent capable of effectively reducing or preventing radiation dermatitis. Due to the fact that curcumin is a potent antioxidant and anti-inflammatory agent that has long been used to treat skin conditions and wound healing, Ryan et al. conducted a randomized, double-blind, placebo-controlled clinical trial to evaluate curcumin's ability to reduce the severity of radiation dermatitis in 30 breast cancer patients [45]. Individuals over the age of 18 years who have been diagnosed with noninflammatory breast cancer or carcinoma in situ and have been prescribed RT without concurrent chemotherapy were included in the study. Patients were excluded if they had bilateral breast cancer; had received prior radiation to the chest or breast area; had undergone breast reconstruction and/or expanders prior to RT; were on anticoagulant (warfarin, coumadin, or heparin) or anti-epidermal growth factor receptor (EGFR) therapy; or had received partial breast irradiations. All patients received standard fractionated radiotherapy (1.8–2.4 Gy per session) for four to seven weeks, with or without boost, for a total dose of 42 Gy. The intervention group received four 500 mg curcumin capsules (Curcumin C3 complex, Sabsina) three times daily during the course of RT prescribed. The control group received identical placebo capsules containing dicalcium phosphate 500 mg, excipients, and a yellow food coloring. Curcumin treatment was found to be more effective than placebo at reducing Radiation Dermatitis Severity (RDS) at the conclusion of treatment.

8.4 Curcumin in oral leukoplakia

Oral leukoplakia is a potentially malignant lesion of the oral cavity, for which no effective treatment is available. Kuriakose et al. conducted a Phase IIB Randomized Double-Blind Placebo-Controlled Trial to determine the efficacy of Curcumin in the treatment of Oral Leukoplakia [46]. After establishing eligibility and performing a baseline clinical examination, all subjects underwent lesion incision biopsy using a 5 mm punch biopsy. Subjects with a clinical and histologic diagnosis of leukoplakia, as well as other inclusion/exclusion criteria, were randomly assigned to receive either placebo or curcumin (three 600 mg capsules) twice daily after food for six months. At the conclusion of the study, physical examinations and laboratory tests, including complete blood count, serum biochemistry, and urine analysis, were performed at baseline, six months after randomization, and twelve months after randomization, respectively. The study concluded at the conclusion of the study period that curcumin was well tolerated, with combined clinical and histologic response assessments indicating a significantly better response with curcumin treatment compared to placebo.

8.5 Efficacy of curcumin in cancer patients

Saghatelyanet al. conducted a randomized, double-blind, placebo-controlled, parallel-group clinical trial to determine the efficacy and safety of an intravenous infusion of curcumin in combination with paclitaxel in patients with metastatic or advanced breast cancer [47]. The eligible patients were randomly assigned to one of two study groups: curcumin + paclitaxel (curcumin group) or paclitaxel + placebo (placebo group). Paclitaxel (80 mg/m2) plus curcumin (CUC-1*, 300 mg solution, once weekly) were administered intravenously to the curcumin group for 12 weeks with a 3-month follow-up. For the same period, the placebo group received paclitaxel plus a solution of riboflavin (200 mg in 20 ml). The study concluded that curcumin treatment had a significantly higher Objective Response Rate than placebo at four weeks of follow-up and was even better for patients who completed the treatment. Curcumin had a superior effect over placebo in both patients who completed the treatment and 3 months later. There were no other significant differences between the curcumin and placebo groups except that patients self-reported significantly greater physical performance with curcumin than with placebo during treatment and at the end of the follow-up, implying improved Paclitaxel tolerance in the curcumin group.

Choi et al. conducted a randomized, double-blind, placebo-controlled trial to determine the effect of curcumin on the duration of the first off-treatment, the change in PSA and testosterone levels, the rate of PSA progression, and health-related quality of life scores in patients with prostate cancer receiving intermittent androgen deprivation (IAD) [48]. The study included patients with prostate cancer who were treated with IAD for I biochemical recurrence (BCR) following localized therapy (eg, radical prostatectomy, radiation therapy, and high intensity focused ultrasound) or (ii) metastatic prostate cancer at initial diagnosis. All participants in this study received at least six months of treatment with an LHRH agonist and anti-androgens and entered the ADT withdrawal (off-treatment) period after a minimum of three months of maintaining a stable PSA nadir level. Exclusion criteria included prior use of an IAD for prostate cancer, hypersensitivity to curcumin, prior use of dietary supplements containing curcumin or turmeric to treat or prevent prostate cancer within the preceding six months of enrollment, and serious medical or psychological conditions (including impaired liver, kidney, cardiac, or hematopoietic functions) other than prostate cancer. The patients were randomly assigned to receive either a placebo or curcumin (240 mg of curcuminoid powder in capsule form), which was administered as two capsules three times daily (1440 mg/day) for six months following the cessation of ADT. The study concluded that during the six-month active treatment period, the proportion of patients with PSA progression was significantly lower in the Curcumin treatment group than in the placebo treatment group. The change in PSA, testosterone levels, and HRQOL scores after six months were comparable between the curcumin and placebo groups, but adverse events were more prevalent in the placebo group than in the curcumin group.

8.6 Effect of curcumin treatment in arthritis

Amalraj et al. conducted a randomized, double-blind, placebo-controlled, three-arm, parallel-group study to compare the efficacy of two different doses of curcumin to that of a placebo in patients with active rheumatoid arthritis (RA) [49]. For 90 days, twelve patients in each group received a placebo, 250 or 500 mg of the curcumin product, respectively. The American College of Rheumatology (ACR) response, visual analogue scale (VAS), C-reactive protein (CRP), Disease Activity Score 28 (DAS28), erythrocyte sedimentation rate (ESR), and rheumatoid factor (RF) values were used to assess the patients' responses. At the conclusion of the study, RA patients who received the curcumin product at low and high doses reported statistically significant improvements in their clinical symptoms. Significant changes in ESR, CPR, and RF values were observed in patients receiving the study product when compared to baseline and placebo. The results indicate that this novel curcumin in a turmeric matrix acts as an analgesic and anti-inflammatory agent in the treatment of rheumatoid arthritis at a dose as low as 250 mg twice daily, as demonstrated by significant improvement in ESR, CRP, VAS, RF, DAS28, and ACR responses when compared to placebo. Both doses of the study product were well tolerated and were associated without any adverse events.

Fifty patients with Kellgren–Lawrence grade II or III knee osteoarthritis and a minimum age of 40 years were enrolled in a prospective, randomized, double-blind, placebo-controlled clinical study [50]. For eight weeks, either a placebo or Theracurmin containing 180 mg/day of curcumin was administered orally. Blood biochemistry analyses were performed before and after each intervention for the purpose of monitoring adverse events. The Japanese Knee Osteoarthritis Measure, the knee pain visual analogue scale (VAS), the Japanese Orthopedic Association's knee scoring system, and the need for nonsteroidal anti-inflammatory drugs were used to evaluate the patients' knee symptoms at 0, 2, 4, 6, and 8 weeks. At 8 weeks after treatment initiation, theracurmin-treated patients had significantly lower VAS scores for knee pain than placebo-treated patients, except for those with initial VAS scores of 0.15 or less. Theracurmin significantly reduced celecoxib dependence compared to placebo. There were no significant adverse effects associated with Theracurmin treatment.

Osteoarthritis (OA) is a degenerative joint disease that is characterized by chronic and acute inflammation. Numerous studies have demonstrated curcumin's anti-arthritic properties in humans with OA and rheumatoid arthritis (RA). In a six-week randomized double-blind placebo-controlled trial, 40 subjects with mild-to-moderate knee OA were randomly assigned to receive either curcuminoid (500 mg/day in three divided doses, n = 19) with 5 mg piperine added to each 500-mg dose or a matched placebo (n = 21) [51]. Additionally, there was a reduction in systemic oxidative stress in subjects receiving the treatment compared to those receiving the placebo, as measured by serum SOD activity and concentrations of reduced GSH and malonedialdehyde (MDA). In a longer-term (eight months) randomized control trial, 50 subjects diagnosed with OA were randomly assigned to receive standard treatment plus two 500-mg tablets (Meriva®) daily containing a natural curcuminoid mixture (20%), phosphatidyl-choline (40%) and microcrystalline cellulose (40%) [52]. When comparing baseline to follow-up, the treatment group demonstrated significant decreases in all inflammation markers (soluble CD40 ligand (sCD40L), interleukin 1 beta (IL-1), interleukin 6 (IL-6), soluble vascular cell adhesion molecule 1 (sVCAM-1), and erythrocyte sedimentation rate (ESR), whereas the control group did not.

8.7 Effect of curcumin on inflammatory and metabolic disorders

Chronic low-grade inflammation is associated with the release of pro-inflammatory cytokines, which results in Metabolic syndrome (MetS), which is defined by insulin resistance, hyperglycemia, hypertension, low high-density lipoprotein cholesterol (HDL-C), elevated low-density lipoprotein cholesterol (LDL-C), elevated triglyceride levels, and obesity, particularly visceral obesity. These cytokines are thought to be at the root of diabetes and cardiovascular disease complications. For eight weeks, 117 subjects with MetS received either 1 g curcumin plus 10 mg piperine to increase absorption or a placebo plus 10 mg piperine in a randomized double-blind placebo-controlled trial with a parallel-group design. Following curcumin supplementation, serum concentrations of TNF- α, IL-6, transforming growth factor beta (TGF-b), and monocyte chemoattractant protein-1 (MCP-1) were significantly decreased. TGF-b serum levels were decreased in the placebo group, but not those of IL-6, TNF- α, or MCP-1. Between-group comparisons indicated that the curcumin group significantly reduced serum concentrations of TNF- α, IL-6, TGF-b, and MCP-1. Curcuminoids were found to be more effective than a placebo at lowering serum LDL-C, non-HDL-C, total cholesterol, triglycerides, and lipoprotein a (Lp (a)), as well as elevating HDL-C concentrations. Additionally, there was a significant improvement in serum SOD activity, reduced MDA, and C-reactive protein (CRP) concentrations in the group receiving curcumin with piperine compared to the placebo group, and the authors concluded that short-term supplementation with a curcuminoid-piperine combination significantly improves oxidative and inflammatory status [53–55].

A double-blind, randomized pilot study was conducted on 31 hemodialysis HD patients and divided them into two groups: the curcumin group (receiving 100 mL of orange juice with 12 g of carrot and 2.5 g of turmeric after each dialysis session/week for three months) and the control group (receiving the same juice without curcumin). After three months of supplementation, the curcumin group demonstrated a significant decrease in NF-kB mRNA expression (AU) and plasma high sensitivity C-reactive protein (hsCRP) levels [56].

Cicero et al. conducted a randomized double-blind placebo-controlled trial in which 80 overweight subjects with suboptimal fasting plasma glucose were randomly assigned to receive 2 capsules of 800 mg phytosomal curcumin (Curserin®: 200 mg) [57]. The study included individuals aged 18 to 70 years, with a body mass index (BMI) of between 25 and 30 kg/m2, and FPG levels of between 100 and 125 mg/dL. Subjects were excluded if they had a personal history of cardiovascular disease or a risk factor for coronary heart disease, were taking glucose-lowering medications (oral antidiabetics, insulins), lipid-lowering medications (statins, fbrates, ezetimibe, omega-3 polyunsaturated fatty acids), or were taking drugs that affect lipid metabolism (i.e., full-dose thiazides, corticosteroids, or immunosuppressants), or After 56 days of treatment, it was observed that the curcumin-treated group had a significant improvement in fasting plasma insulin (FPI), HOMA index, waist circumference, blood pressure, triglycerides (TG), HDL-C, liver transaminases, gamma-GT, index of liver steatosis, and serum cortisol, when compared to the baseline. Additionally, FPI, TG, liver transaminases, fatty liver index, and serum cortisol levels improved significantly when compared to the placebo-treated group. In comparison to the baseline, the placebo group improved only in FPG and TG at the study's conclusion. In conclusion, the trial demonstrated that supplementation with a phytosomal curcumin preparation containing phosphatidylserine and piperine could improve glycemic factors, hepatic function, and serum cortisol levels in overweight subjects with impaired fasting glucose.

Satoskar et al. investigated the effect of curcumin on spermatic cord edoema following surgery. Forty-five patients (ages 15–68) received 400 mg curcumin (Group A), 250 mg lactose powder placebo (Group B), or 100 mg phenylbutazone (Group C) thrice daily for six days following inguinal hernia or hydrocele repair [58]. The spermatic cord edoema, spermatic cord tenderness, operative site pain, and operative site tenderness were all recorded and graded on a scale of 0-3 (0, absent, 1, mild, 2, moderate, 3, severe). The overall effect of treatment was determined by calculating the intensity score (TIS) for each group ranging from 0 to 12. Curcumin treatment resulted in an 84.2% reduction in TIS. TIS was reduced by 61.8% and 86%, respectively, with placebo and phenylbutazone treatments. Although phenylbutazone treatment reduced TIS to a comparable extent on day 6, it did not alleviate tenderness at the operative site. In comparison, Curcumin treatment was superior because it resulted in a decrease in all four inflammatory parameters.

Holt et al. studied ten patients aged 28 to 54 years to determine curcumin's therapeutic effect in the treatment of inflammatory bowel disease (IBD) [59]. Crohn's disease (CD) and ulcerative colitis (UC) are the two most common types of inflammatory bowel disease (IBD). Both are characterized by abdominal pain, vomiting, diarrhea, bloody stools, and weight loss, as well as secondary complications such as arthritis, pyoderma gangrenosum, and primary sclerosing cholangitis. Five patients with rectal UC were given 550 mg curcumin twice daily for one month and then three times daily for another month. The remaining five Crohn's disease patients received 360 mg curcumin three times daily for one month and then four times daily for an additional month. At baseline and at the end of the study period, hematological and biochemical blood analysis, erythrocyte sedimentation rate (ESR), C-reactive protein (CRP), sigmoidoscopy, and biopsy were performed on the first group of patients. The second group of patients had their Crohn's Disease Activity Index (CDAI), CRP, ESR, hematological blood analysis, and kidney function evaluated. All five patients in the first group improved by the end of the study period, as measured by a global score, and all five subjects had normal ESR, CRP, and serologic indices of inflammation after two months of curcumin treatment. CDAI scores decreased by an average of 55 points in the CD group, and CRP and

ESR levels decreased in four of five patients. CDAI scores decreased by an average of 55 points in the second group, while CRP and ESR levels decreased in four of five patients.

8.8 Efficacy of curcumin in the treatment of neurological and brain disorders

For an 18-month period, forty subjects (aged 51–84 years) were randomly assigned to receive a bioavailable form of curcumin [Theracurmin® containing 90 mg of curcumin twice daily (N = 21)] or a placebo (N = 19). Verbal (Buschke Selective Reminding Test [SRT]) and visual (Brief Visual Memory Test-Revised [BVMT-R]) memory were used as primary outcomes, while attention (Trail Making A) was used as a secondary outcome to evaluate the efficacy and progress of treatment. FDDNP-PET signals in the amygdala, hypothalamus, medial and lateral temporal lobes, posterior cingulate, parietal, frontal, and motor regions were determined to measure the treatment outcomes and it was observed that in non-dementia adults, daily oral Theracurmin improves memory and attention. The FDDNP-PET results indicated that symptom improvement was associated with decreases in amyloid and tau accumulation in brain regions associated with mood and memory [60].

Numerous studies have confirmed curcumin's antidepressant properties in patients with major depressive disorder. In one study, for 12 weeks, 123 individuals with major depressive disorder were randomly assigned to one of four treatment conditions: placebo, low-dose curcumin extract (250 mg), high-dose curcumin extract (500 mg), or a combination of low-dose curcumin extract and saffron (15 mg). Depressive symptoms were assessed for changes or improvements in comparison to placebo. The active drug treatments (when used in combination) were associated with significantly greater improvements in depressive symptoms and superior improvements in Spielberger State–Trait Anxiety Inventory STAI-state and STAI-trait scores compared to placebo. Active drug treatments were also more effective in people with atypical depression than in the general population. The study concluded that active drug treatments containing varying doses of curcumin and a combination of curcumin were effective at alleviating depressive and anxiolytic symptoms in people with major depressive disorder, with no significant differences observed between the varying curcumin doses [61].

Another study enrolled forty patients who had just experienced their first episode of depression in a 5-week, double-blind, randomized, placebo-controlled clinical trial. Subjects received either 500 mg/d curcumin or a placebo in combination with antidepressants (escitalopram or venlafaxine). The Clinical Global Impression—Severity Scale, Hamilton Depression Rating Scale, and Montgomery-Asberg Depression Rating Scale were used as outcome measures. The analysis of variance revealed that both groups experienced significant positive changes in all scales of measurement from baseline to the end of the study. These changes became noticeable following the first visit following seven days of treatment. There was no statistically significant difference between curcumin and a placebo. However, patients in the curcumin group experienced a trend toward a faster resolution of depressive symptoms than those in the placebo group [62].

In a population of community-dwelling older adults, a 12-month, randomized, placebo-controlled, double-blind study was conducted to determine the ability of a curcumin formulation to prevent cognitive decline. For 12 months, participants (n 96) were randomly assigned to receive placebo or 1500 mg/d BiocurcumaxTM. At baseline and at the 6-month and 12-month follow-up assessments, a battery of clinical and cognitive measures was administered. Although no differences in clinical or cognitive measures were observed between the groups, a significant time treatment group interaction was observed for the Montreal Cognitive Assessment (repeated measures analysis), which revealed a decline in function in the placebo group at 6 months that was not observed in the curcumin treatment group [63].

A 24-week, double-blind, randomized, placebo-controlled study with thirty-eight patients with chronic schizophrenia was conducted [64]. Subjects received either 3000 mg/d curcumin or a placebo in combination with antipsychotics. Positive and Negative Symptoms Scale (PANSS) and Calgary Depression Scale for Schizophrenia were used as outcome measures. The analysis of variance revealed that both groups experienced significant improvements in all scales of measurement from the baseline period to the study's conclusion. Within six months, curcumin produced a significant improvement in the total PANSS and the negative symptoms subscale. There were no differences between the treatment and placebo groups in terms of the positive and general PANSS subscales, as well as the Calgary Depression Scale for Schizophrenia scores.

A study examining the efficacy of curcumin oral supplementation in Amyotrophic Lateral Sclerosis randomly assigned patients to one of two groups: one that received a placebo for three months, followed by three months of curcumin oral supplementation (600 mg/day, Brainoil); and the second group that received curcumin oral supplementation (600 mg/day, Brainoil) for six months [65]. The evaluations were conducted at baseline (T0), three months after receiving either Brainoil or a placebo, and three months after the open-label phase. During an incremental forearm exercise test, clinical evaluations and measurement of oxidative stress biomarkers such as oxidative protein products (AOPPs), ferric reducing ability (FRAP), total thiols (T-SH), and lactate were compared to a control group and the study found that the ALS-FRS-r score in the first group decreased, whereas the second group maintained a stable ALS-FRS-r score. Additionally, while FRAP exercise values remained stable in the second group, they decreased in the first group without treatment, after 3 months into the study. The entire ALS population demonstrated increased oxidative stress when compared to controls, with those treated with curcumin in the second group exhibiting decreased exercise AOPPs with values comparable to controls.

9. Conclusion

Turmeric has been used in our traditional system of medicine for centuries in treating some of the common health related problems in children and elderly individuals. For example when children catch cold and cough and get fever thousands of mothers and grandmothers have given them a tea spoon full of turmeric suspended in milk to drink in the night before going to bed and invariably most of the children recover overnight. This has become an age old practice in Indian house hold for hundreds of years and there is no record how many children and elderly persons have benefited by this. At that time no one knew how turmeric worked and the modern medicine which the medicinal chemists think is their contribution was not even born. But since it had worked, even today a mother in an Indian village would prefer to give turmeric rather than an antibiotic to their children to control fever and cold. When children get infested with worms and their health deteriorates, mothers again give them turmeric orally for few days and children get cured and remain healthy. The modern medicinal chemistry has provided medicines like Albindazole which of course works but is toxic and children tend to get reinfected. Turmeric modulates the immune system and provides protection against reinfection. When children get wounded while playing mothers apply a paste of turmeric in some oil to the wound and it heals the wound very efficiently. Now modern science has to give us answers to how this works rather than dismissing all these observations just because curcumin is unstable and cannot be a lead candidate. Even clinical trials, several of which have worked under double blind and placebo controlled conditions illustrate that curcuminoids, inspite of being unstable, can alleviate inflammatory conditions in several chronic disease conditions in humans. Therefore there is an intensive need to study Curcuminoids further and develop formulations which will help humans to combat severe overwhelming diseases.

Author details

Sitabja Mukherjee[1] and Santosh K. Kar[2*]

1 KIIT School of Biotechnology, KIIT University, Bhubaneswar, Odisha, India

2 Nano Herb Research Laboratory, KIIT TBI, KIIT University, Bhubaneswar, Odisha, India

*Address all correspondence to: santoshkariis@rediffmail.com

References

[1] Hay E, Lucariello A, Contieri M, Esposito T, De Luca A, Guerra G, Perna A. Therapeutic effects of turmeric in several diseases: An overview. Chem Biol Interact. 2019 Sep 1; 310: 108729.

[2] Gupta SC, Patchva S, Aggarwal BB. Therapeutic roles of curcumin: lessons learned from clinical trials. AAPS J. 2013 Jan; 15(1): 195-218. doi:10.1208/s12248-012-9432-8.

[3] Vogel, Pelletier J. Examen chimique de la racine de Curcuma. J. Pharm. 1815; i: 289-300.

[4] Vogel A., Jr. Journal de Pharma. et de Chemie. 1842; 3: 20.

[5] Milobedzka J, Kostanecki S, Lampe V. Zur Kenntnis des Curcumins. Ber. Deut. Chem. Ges. 1910; 43: 2163-2170.

[6] Lampe V, Milobedzka J. Studienuber Curcumin. Ber. Deut. Chem. Ges. 1913; 46: 2235-2237.

[7] Srinivasan, K.R. The coloring matter in turmeric. Curr. Sci. 1952; 21: 311-312.

[8] Srinivasan KR. A chromatographic study of the curcuminoids in Curcuma longa, L. J Pharm Pharmacol. 1953; 5: 448-457.

[9] Nair A, Amalraj A, Jacob J, Kunnumakkara AB, Gopi S. Non-Curcuminoids from Turmeric and Their Potential in Cancer Therapy and Anticancer Drug Delivery Formulations. Biomolecules. 2019 Jan 2; 9(1): 13. doi:10.3390/biom9010013.

[10] Fu M, Chen L, Zhang L, Yu X, Yang Q. Cyclocurcumin, a curcumin derivative, exhibits immune-modulating ability and is a potential compound for the treatment of rheumatoid arthritis as predicted by the MM-PBSA method. Int J Mol Med. 2017 May; 39(5): 1164-1172.

[11] Priyadarsini KI. Chemical and structural features influencing the biological activity of curcumin. Curr Pharm Des. 2013;19(11):2093-2100. doi: 10.2174/138161213805289228.

[12] Amalraj A, Pius A, Gopi S, Gopi S. Biological activities of curcuminoids, other biomolecules from turmeric and their derivatives - A review. J Tradit Complement Med. 2016;7(2):205-233. doi: 10.1016/j.jtcme.2016.05.005.

[13] Olotu F, Agoni C, Soremekun O, Soliman MES. An Update on the Pharmacological Usage of Curcumin: Has it Failed in the Drug Discovery Pipeline? Cell BiochemBiophys. 2020;78(3):267-289.

[14] *Curcuma longa* L. Plants of the World Online. Kew Science. http://www.plantsoftheworldonline.org/taxon/urn:lsid:ipni.org:names:796451-1

[15] Acevedo-Rodríguez, P. & Strong, M.T. (2012). Catalogue of seed plants of the West Indies Smithsonian Contributions to Botany 98: 1-1192.

[16] Sasikumar B. Genetic resources of Curcuma: Diversity, characterization and utilization. Plant Genetic Resources. 2005; 3:1479-2621.

[17] Esatbeyoglu T, Huebbe P, Ernst IM, Chin D, Wagner AE, Rimbach G. Curcumin--from molecule to biological function. AngewChemInt Ed Engl. 2012;51(22):5308-32.

[18] Kumar A, Singh AK, Kaushik MS, et al. Interaction of turmeric (*Curcuma longa* L.) with beneficial microbes: a review. 3 Biotech. 2017;7(6):357.

[19] Sahne F, Mohammadi M, Najafpour G, Moghadamnia A. Extraction of bioactive compound curcumin from turmeric (*Curcuma*

longa L.) via different routes: A comparative study.2016;13: 173-180.

[20] Degot P, Huber V, Hofmann E, Hahn M, Touraud D, Kunz W. Solubilization and extraction of curcumin from *Curcuma longa* using green, sustainable, and food-approved surfactant-free microemulsions. Food Chem. 2021;336:127660.

[21] Valizadeh Kiamahalleh M, Najafpour-Darzi G, Rahimnejad M, Moghadamnia AA, Valizadeh Kiamahalleh M. High performance curcumin subcritical water extraction from turmeric (*Curcuma longa* L.). J Chromatogr B Analyt Technol Biomed Life Sci. 2016;1022:191-198.

[22] Kim YJ, Lee HJ, Shin Y. Optimization and validation of high-performance liquid chromatography method for individual curcuminoids in turmeric by heat-refluxed extraction. J Agric Food Chem. 2013 Nov 20;61(46):10911-8.

[23] Chen W, Fan-Havard P, Yee LD, et al. A liquid chromatography-tandem mass spectrometric method for quantification of curcumin-O-glucuronide and curcumin in human plasma. *J Chromatogr B Analyt Technol Biomed Life Sci*. 2012;900:89-93.

[24] Pabon H. Synthesis of curcumin and related compounds. Recueil des TravauxChimiques des Pays-Bas. 2010;83:379 - 386.

[25] Chao IC, Wang CM, Li SP, Lin LG, Ye WC, Zhang QW. Simultaneous Quantification of Three Curcuminoids and Three Volatile Components of *Curcuma longa* Using Pressurized Liquid Extraction and High-Performance Liquid Chromatography. Molecules. 2018 Jun 28;23(7):1568.

[26] Mondal S, Ghosh S, Moulik SP. Stability of curcumin in different solvent and solution media: UV-visible and steady-state fluorescence spectral study. J Photochem Photobiol B. 2016;158:212-8.

[27] Pandey A, Chaturvedi M, Mishra S, Kumar P, Somvanshi P, Chaturvedi R. Reductive metabolites of curcumin and their therapeutic effects. Heliyon. 2020;6(11):e05469.

[28] Karthikeyan A, Senthil N, Min T. Nanocurcumin: A Promising Candidate for Therapeutic Applications. Front Pharmacol. 2020;11:487.

[29] Wang YJ, Pan MH, Cheng AL, Lin LI, Ho YS, Hsieh CY, Lin JK. Stability of curcumin in buffer solutions and characterization of its degradation products. J Pharm Biomed Anal. 1997;15(12):1867-76.

[30] Shen L, Ji HF. The pharmacology of curcumin: is it the degradation products? Trends Mol Med. 2012;18(3):138-44.

[31] Leung MH, Kee TW. Effective stabilization of curcumin by association to plasma proteins: human serum albumin and fibrinogen. Langmuir. 2009;25(10):5773-7.

[32] Katsuyama Y, Kita T, Horinouchi S. Identification and characterization of multiple curcumin synthases from the herb *Curcuma longa*. FEBS Lett. 2009;583(17):2799-803.

[33] Katsuyama Y, Matsuzawa M, Funa N, Horinouchi S. Production of curcuminoids by *Escherichia coli* carrying an artificial biosynthesis pathway. Microbiology (Reading). 2008;154(Pt 9):2620-2628.

[34] Katsuyama Y, Hirose Y, Funa N, Ohnishi Y, Horinouchi S. Precursor-directed biosynthesis of curcumin analogs in *Escherichia coli*. BiosciBiotechnolBiochem. 2010;74(3):641-5.

[35] Nelson KM, Dahlin JL, Bisson J, Graham J, Pauli GF, Walters MA. The

Essential Medicinal Chemistry of Curcumin. J Med Chem. 2017;60(5):1620-1637.

[36] Padmanaban G, Nagaraj VA. Curcumin May Defy Medicinal Chemists. ACS Med Chem Lett. 2017;8(3):274.

[37] Nelson KM, Dahlin JL, Bisson J, Graham J, Pauli GF, Walters MA. Curcumin May (Not) Defy Science. ACS Med Chem Lett. 2017;8(5):467-470.

[38] Bahadori F, Demiray M. A Realistic View on "The Essential Medicinal Chemistry of Curcumin". ACS Med Chem Lett. 2017;8(9):893-896.

[39] Heger M. Drug screening: Don't discount all curcumin trial data. Nature. 2017 Mar 1;543(7643):40. doi: 10.1038/543040c.

[40] Akhtar F, Rizvi MM, Kar SK. Oral delivery of curcumin bound to chitosan nanoparticles cured *Plasmodium yoelii* infected mice. Biotechnol Adv. 2012;30(1):310-20.

[41] Tousif S, Singh DK, Mukherjee S, et al. Nanoparticle-Formulated Curcumin Prevents Posttherapeutic Disease Reactivation and Reinfection with *Mycobacterium tuberculosis* following Isoniazid Therapy. Front Immunol. 2017;8:739.

[42] Ahmad S, Bhattacharya D, Kar S, Ranganathan A, Van Kaer L, Das G. Curcumin Nanoparticles Enhance Mycobacterium bovis BCG Vaccine Efficacy by Modulating Host Immune Responses. Infect Immun. 2019;87(11):e00291-19.

[43] Carroll RE, Benya RV, Turgeon DK, Vareed S, Neuman M, Rodriguez L, Kakarala M, Carpenter PM, McLaren C, Meyskens FL Jr, Brenner DE. Phase IIa clinical trial of curcumin for the prevention of colorectal neoplasia. Cancer Prev Res (Phila). 2011 Mar;4(3):354-64. doi: 10.1158/1940-6207.CAPR-10-0098. Erratum in: Cancer Prev Res (Phila). 2012;5(12):1407.

[44] Heshmati J, Moini A, Sepidarkish M, Morvaridzadeh M, Salehi M, Palmowski A, Mojtahedi MF, Shidfar F. Effects of curcumin supplementation on blood glucose, insulin resistance and androgens in patients with polycystic ovary syndrome: A randomized double-blind placebo-controlled clinical trial. Phytomedicine. 2021;80:153395.

[45] Ryan JL, Heckler CE, Ling M, Katz A, Williams JP, Pentland AP, Morrow GR. Curcumin for radiation dermatitis: a randomized, double-blind, placebo-controlled clinical trial of thirty breast cancer patients. Radiat Res. 2013;180(1):34-43.

[46] Kuriakose MA, Ramdas K, Dey B, Iyer S, Rajan G, Elango KK, Suresh A, Ravindran D, Kumar RR, R P, Ramachandran S, Kumar NA, Thomas G, Somanathan T, Ravindran HK, Ranganathan K, Katakam SB, Parashuram S, Jayaprakash V, Pillai MR. A Randomized Double-Blind Placebo-Controlled Phase IIB Trial of Curcumin in Oral Leukoplakia. Cancer Prev Res (Phila). 2016;9(8):683-91.

[47] Saghatelyan T, Tananyan A, Janoyan N, Tadevosyan A, Petrosyan H, Hovhannisyan A, Hayrapetyan L, Arustamyan M, Arnhold J, Rotmann AR, Hovhannisyan A, Panossian A. Efficacy and safety of curcumin in combination with paclitaxel in patients with advanced, metastatic breast cancer: A comparative, randomized, double-blind, placebo-controlled clinical trial. Phytomedicine. 2020;70:153218.

[48] Choi YH, Han DH, Kim SW, Kim MJ, Sung HH, Jeon HG, Jeong BC, Seo SI, Jeon SS, Lee HM, Choi HY. A

randomized, double-blind, placebo-controlled trial to evaluate the role of curcumin in prostate cancer patients with intermittent androgen deprivation. Prostate. 2019;79(6):614-621.

[49] Amalraj A, Varma K, Jacob J, Divya C, Kunnumakkara AB, Stohs SJ, Gopi S. A Novel Highly Bioavailable Curcumin Formulation Improves Symptoms and Diagnostic Indicators in Rheumatoid Arthritis Patients: A Randomized, Double-Blind, Placebo-Controlled, Two-Dose, Three-Arm, and Parallel-Group Study. J Med Food. 2017;20(10):1022-1030.

[50] Nakagawa Y, Mukai S, Yamada S, Matsuoka M, Tarumi E, Hashimoto T, Tamura C, Imaizumi A, Nishihira J, Nakamura T. Short-term effects of highly-bioavailable curcumin for treating knee osteoarthritis: a randomized, double-blind, placebo-controlled prospective study. J Orthop Sci. 2014;19(6):933-9.

[51] Panahi Y, Rahimnia AR, Sharafi M, Alishiri G, Saburi A, Sahebkar A. Curcuminoid treatment for knee osteoarthritis: a randomized double-blind placebo-controlled trial. Phytother Res. 2014;28(11):1625-31.

[52] Belcaro G, Cesarone MR, Dugall M, Pellegrini L, Ledda A, Grossi MG, Togni S, Appendino G. Product-evaluation registry of Meriva®, a curcumin-phosphatidylcholine complex, for the complementary management of osteoarthritis. Panminerva Med. 2010;52(2 Suppl 1):55-62.

[53] Panahi Y, Khalili N, Hosseini MS, Abbasinazari M, Sahebkar A. Lipid-modifying effects of adjunctive therapy with curcuminoids-piperine combination in patients with metabolic syndrome: results of a randomized controlled trial. Complement Ther Med. 2014;22(5):851-7.

[54] Panahi Y, Hosseini MS, Khalili N, Naimi E, Majeed M, Sahebkar A. Antioxidant and anti-inflammatory effects of curcuminoid-piperine combination in subjects with metabolic syndrome: A randomized controlled trial and an updated meta-analysis. ClinNutr. 2015;34(6):1101-8.

[55] Ganjali S, Sahebkar A, Mahdipour E, Jamialahmadi K, Torabi S, Akhlaghi S, Ferns G, Parizadeh SM, Ghayour-Mobarhan M. Investigation of the effects of curcumin on serum cytokines in obese individuals: a randomized controlled trial. ScientificWorldJournal. 2014;2014:898361.

[56] Alvarenga L, Salarolli R, Cardozo LFMF, Santos RS, de Brito JS, Kemp JA, Reis D, de Paiva BR, Stenvinkel P, Lindholm B, Fouque D, Mafra D. Impact of curcumin supplementation on expression of inflammatory transcription factors in hemodialysis patients: A pilot randomized, double-blind, controlled study. ClinNutr. 2020;39(12):3594-3600.

[57] Cicero AFG, Sahebkar A, Fogacci F, Bove M, Giovannini M, Borghi C. Effects of phytosomal curcumin on anthropometric parameters, insulin resistance, cortisolemia and non-alcoholic fatty liver disease indices: a double-blind, placebo-controlled clinical trial. Eur J Nutr. 2020;59(2):477-483.

[58] Satoskar RR, Shah SJ, Shenoy SG. Evaluation of anti-inflammatory property of curcumin (diferuloyl methane) in patients with postoperative inflammation. Int J ClinPharmacolTherToxicol. 1986;24(12):651-4.

[59] Holt PR, Katz S, Kirshoff R. Curcumin therapy in inflammatory bowel disease: a pilot study. Dig Dis Sci. 2005;50(11):2191-3.

[60] Small GW, Siddarth P, Li Z, Miller KJ, Ercoli L, Emerson ND, Martinez J, Wong KP, Liu J, Merrill DA, Chen ST, Henning SM, Satyamurthy N, Huang SC, Heber D, Barrio JR. Memory and Brain Amyloid and Tau Effects of a Bioavailable Form of Curcumin in Non-Demented Adults: A Double-Blind, Placebo-Controlled 18-Month Trial. Am J Geriatr Psychiatry. 2018;26(3):266-277.

[61] Lopresti AL, Drummond PD. Efficacy of curcumin, and a saffron/curcumin combination for the treatment of major depression: A randomised, double-blind, placebo-controlled study. J Affect Disord. 2017;207:188-196.

[62] Bergman J, Miodownik C, Bersudsky Y, Sokolik S, Lerner PP, Kreinin A, Polakiewicz J, Lerner V. Curcumin as an add-on to antidepressive treatment: a randomized, double-blind, placebo-controlled, pilot clinical study. ClinNeuropharmacol. 2013;36(3):73-7.

[63] Rainey-Smith SR, Brown BM, Sohrabi HR, Shah T, Goozee KG, Gupta VB, Martins RN. Curcumin and cognition: a randomised, placebo-controlled, double-blind study of community-dwelling older adults. Br J Nutr. 2016;115(12):2106-13.

[64] Miodownik C, Lerner V, Kudkaeva N, Lerner PP, Pashinian A, Bersudsky Y, Eliyahu R, Kreinin A, Bergman J. Curcumin as Add-On to Antipsychotic Treatment in Patients With Chronic Schizophrenia: A Randomized, Double-Blind, Placebo-Controlled Study. ClinNeuropharmacol. 2019;42(4):117-122.

[65] Chico L, Ienco EC, Bisordi C, Lo Gerfo A, Petrozzi L, Petrucci A, Mancuso M, Siciliano G. Amyotrophic Lateral Sclerosis and Oxidative Stress: A Double-Blind Therapeutic Trial After Curcumin Supplementation. CNS NeurolDisord Drug Targets. 2018;17(10):767-779.

Chapter 7

Herbs and Spices—New Processing Technologies. *Syzygium aromaticum*: Medicinal Properties and Phytochemical Screening

Vikrant Kumar, Deepak Mishra, Mukesh Chandra Joshi, Priyanka Mishra and Megha Tanwar

Abstract

All over the world, Plants have found to be a valuable source of herbs and spices for a long period of time to maintain the human health. Varieties of herbs and spices have been used to impart an aroma and taste to food for last few centuries. Several applications of plants species have been reported as antioxidative, anti-inflammatory, antidiabetic, antihypertensive and antimicrobial activities. Currently efforts are focused on their scientific merits, to provide science-based evidence for their traditional uses and to develop either functional foods or nutraceutical behavior. India is well recognized all over the world for their variety of herbs, spices and medicinal biodiversity. The WHO has listed more than 21000 plants, which are used for their medicinal purposes either in the form of essential oil or in the form of flavor. Among these, more than 2500 species and herbs are found in India, however; among them more than 150 species are used commercially on large scale. In India, the use of spices and herbs in the form of essential oil or in the form of flavor are traditionally used in routine treatment. For example, Curcumin which is found in turmeric are frequently used in medical facilities to wound healing, rheumatic disorders, and gastrointestinal symptoms etc.

Keywords: *Syzygium aromaticum*, essential oil, Flavonoids, Eugenol, phytochemistry

1. Introduction

Herbs and Spices are seeds, fruits, roots, bark, berries, buds, or vegetable substances, which have been used from decades primarily for flavoring, coloring, or preserving food and formulation of medicinal items. Globally, India and Pakistan, have been notable for their tremendous production of spices and flavors. It is worldwide accepted that a wide range of physiological and pharmaceutical benefits can be derived from spices. Numerous health problems, like neurodegenerative diseases and oxidative stress, are controlled and restored with plant based eating regimens, because they contain various valuable chemical compounds and antioxidants [1]. Various metabolic diseases and age-related issues are associated with oxidative mechanisms in the human body are also cured by the proper use of herbs. Due to nonhazardous impact of flavors on people, they are viewed as safe for use in food with no adverse effect. Major spices and herbs are harvested and used in the subcontinent, viz. black pepper (*Piper nigrum*), cloves (*Syzygium aromaticum)*, cinnamon (*Cinnamomum verum*), seeds of flax (*Linum usitatissimum*), cardamom (*Elettaria cardamomum*), poppy (*Papaver somniferum*), fenugreek (*Trigonella foenum-graecum*), cumin (*Cuminum cyminum*), sesame, fennel, carom, ajwain, coriander, turmeric, tamarind, ginger, onion, garlic, and red chilies. These spices are secret fortune of various therapeutic components which help directly and indirectly for various health disorders. In this chapter we are focusing Clove (*Syzygium aromaticum*), which has been employed for centuries as food preservative and various medicinal purposes including its antimicrobial and antioxidant properties. The health benefits associated with the consumption of *Syzygium aromaticum* are briefly discussed below and shown in **Figure 1**.

Syzygium aromaticum is a tree which belongs to the family Myrtaceae and originate from Indonesia and is one of most valuable and second most important spice in the world trade. Various synonyms are used for the Clove, viz. *Caryophyllus aromaticus, Caryophyllus silvestris, Eugenia caryophyllus, Jambosa caryophyllus* and *Myrtus caryophyllus* [2]. The tree of *Syzygium aromaticum* attains medium size and reaches up to 20 m in height. Depending on the variety of this tree its canopy shape varies from cylindrical to pyramidal [3]. The life span period of this tree for up to 100 years and above. The tree prefers to grow in very much depleted soil with adequate soil moisture. The tree requires high atmospheric temperature in the range of 25 to 35°C with heavy sunlight, besides this well-distributed rainfall and high humidity i.e. >70% is also necessary condition for their growth [4]. In India cloves tree are harvested in deep black loamy soil of humid tropics and successfully grows in the red soils of midlands of Kerala and in the hilly territory of Western Ghats in Karnataka and Tamil Nadu [5].

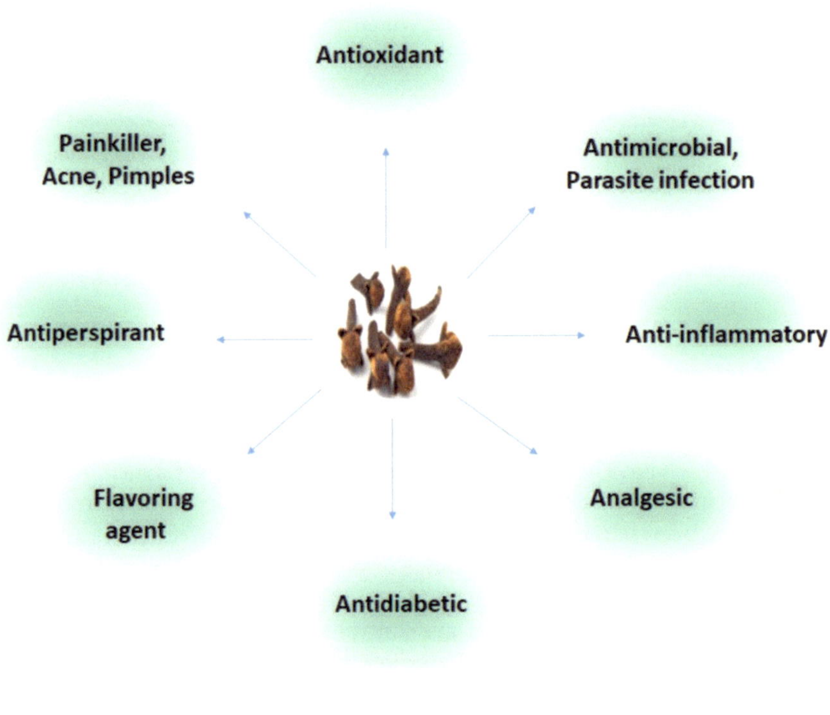

Figure 1.
Uses of S. aromaticum.

The aromatic flower buds which has characteristic odors of this plant are known as cloves and are commonly used as a spice and several therapeutic areas to treat variety of disease and infections like nausea, vomiting, cough, diarrhea, dyspepsia, flatulence, stomach distension, and gastrointestinal spasm; relieve pain; cause uterine contractions; and stimulate the nerves [6]. Because of these it makes an attraction for commercially cultivation of cloves in different part of the world like India, Pakistan, Sri Lanka, as well as in African countries. India becomes second largest consumer of clove after the Indonesia [7]. The plant is also used as a folk medicine in diuretic, odontalgic, stomachic, tonicardiac, and condiment with carminative and stimulant effects [8]. The essential oil derived from this aromatic plant not only serves as a fragrance and flavor agent, but also used as a dietary antioxidant to prevent several diseases caused by a free radical [9, 10]. Clove are rich in flavonoids, organic acids, volatile acids phenolic components like eugenol, terpenoids, tannins, and gallic acid, which have great potential for pharmaceutical, food, and agricultural applications [11]. In Brazil and other tropical countries, faces a serious health problem cause by Dengue, is countered by clove, due to its larvicidal activity [12].

1.1 Morphology of *Syzygium aromaticum*

The clove is aromatic spice tree mainly contains leaves and buds which are the common commercial part of the tree. The term clove is taken from French word 'Clove' and 'Clou' which signifies 'Nail'. Clove is conical myrtle, medium sized tree with straight trunk which grows up to 18 to 20 m in height. The branches of clove tree are grayish, thick and semi erect. Leaves are enormous elongated to elliptic, simple obovate opposite, glabrous and possess lots of essential oil glands on the lower surface. Tree started flowering bud formation in around 7 years and keeps flowering for a very long time or more after plantation. Flowers are small, crimson in color and are bisexual borne at the terminal ends of the small branches. Each peduncle carries 3 to 4 stalked flowers and inflorescence length remains between 4 to 5 cm. Initially, the color of the flower buds is pale yellow with glossy appearance and turn green to bright red on maturing. These are reaped when they become dark red ellipsoid berry [12, 13].

1.2 Chemical constituents of clove

Pharmacologically, Clove is found to be rich in pharmacophore phenolic compounds like flavonoids (quercetin), hydroxybenzoic acids, hydroxyphenylpropens, hydroxycinamic acids, eugenol and derivatives of gallic acid. [11–14]. It has also been found that 18–20% of essential oil are present in the stem, buds and leaf of clove flower with different chemical compostions having variety of applications [15, 16]. These oils are colorless or pale yellow with a particular flavor and taste [15, 16].

Alma, *et al.* in 2007 [17] extracted and reported the presence of essential oil from bud of Clove which is yellow in color and have high density than water. They extracted and characterized the components as eugenol (87%), chavibetol (19.7%), β-caryophyllene (13%), eugenol acetate (8.01%), trisiloxane-1,1,1,5,5,5-hexa-methyl-3,3-bis-[(trimethylsilyl) oxy] (1.7%), etc. [18, 19], Marya, *et al.* 2012 [20] and Kasai, *et al.* 2016 [21] further studied and reported the presence of eugenol (74.32%), β-caryophyllene (15.94%) and eugenol acetate (5.8%) as major component in a Clove bud. Another component methyl-*n*-amyl ketone which has characteristic fruity and fresh odor was also found in buds of clove (2001) [22]. Xu, *et al.* (2016) [23] studied the chemical composition of Clove bud essential oil by performing Gas Chromatography-Mass Spectrophometery (GC–MS) and reported the presence of caryophyllene oxide, α-selinene, cadinene, 2-pinene etc. with the previously reported oil. Fankem *et al* [24] confirmed the presence of oxygenated monoterpenes (89.06%), monoterpenes (0.04%), sesquiterpenes (10.6%) and linear components (0.03%) in Clove bud essential oil along with eugenol.

Essential oil also extracted from leaf of Clove and known as Clove leaf essential oil. The oil which is extracted from leaf have pleasant odor and faint yellow in color. Jirovetz, *et al.* and coworkers in 2006 [25] reported the presence of 23 other compounds along with α-humulene, eugenol and their acetate derivatives as major components. These finding suggested that eugenol, chavibetal, β-caryophyllene, eugenol acetate are the major components in the tree of Clove. These essential oils are also found in the stem of Clove [26–28].

Bao, *et al.*, 2012 [29], reported several other phenolics components from methenol extract of *S. aromaticum*, viz. biflorin, kaempferol, rhamnocitrin, myricetin, gallic acid, and ellagic acid (**Figure 2**). Bao, *et al.*, 2012 [29], also reported the presence of eighteen hydrolyzable tannins from an aqueous acetone extract of dried flower buds of *S. aromaticum* such as aromatinin A, platycaryanin A, bicornin, syzyginin A, alunusnin A, rugosin C, tellimagrandin II, casuarictin, heterophylliin D, rugosin D, rugosin F, euprostin A, 1,2-di-Ogalloyl-3-*O*-digalloyl-4,6-*O*-(*S*)-hexahydroxydiphenoy-β-D-glucose, alienanin B, squarrosanin A, casuarinin, syzyginin B, 1,2,3-tri-*O*-galloyl-β-D-glucose, and 1,2,3,6-tetra-*O*-galloyl-β-D-glucose.

1.3 Pharmacological activities of clove oil

The essential oil or chemical compounds which were extracted from different parts clove exhibit variety of pharmacological activities and several literatures have been reported in which they exhibit anticancerous, antimicrobial, antidiabetic, anti-inflammatory, antidepressant, antiulcer, antioxidant, antinoceptive, and antiprotozoal, etc. (**Figure 3**).

1.4 Antimicrobial activity

The oil isolated from Clove, has wide range of medicinal application. It is essentially used in the manufacturing of variety of Indian Ayurvedic and Chinese medicine. These oils are also used in the manufacturing of antibiotics because its antimicrobial properties. Numerous reports exhibit that its component eugenol inhibiting bacterial migration, bacterial adhesion, fimbriae formation of *Gram*-negative bacteria such as *Escherichia coli*, *Salmonella*, *Pseudomonas aeruginosa*, etc., and *Gram*-positive bacteria such as *Staphylococcus*, *Streptococcus*, *Listeria*, etc. [30].

Matan *et al.* (2012) [31] reported that Clove oil exhibit strong antimicrobial activity against *Penicillium* sp., *Aspergillus flavus* and *Staphylococcus aureus* found on dried fish (*Decapterus maruadsi*). Zengin & Baysal (2014) [32] were found that they exhibit activity against three *Gram*-positive bacteria such as *Listeria innocua, Carnobacterium divergens* and *Staphyloccous aureus* and also inhibit potential activity against four *Gram*-negative bacteria like *Salmonella typhimurium, Escherichia coli, Serratia liquefaciens* and *Shewanella putrefacians*. The data strongly proved that Clove essential oil inhibit the growth of all bacteria whether it is *Gram*- positive or *Gram*-negative, while the main constituent of the essential oil was found to be inactive towards *Shewanella* and *Listeria* [33]. Abdulwahab Kammon, *et al.* in 2020 reported antimicrobial activity of Clove oil against *Gram*-negative bacteria isolated from chickens *E. coli (1 avian pathogenic E. coli (APEC) and 2 non-pathogenic E. coli), Salmonella enteritidis, and Salmonella spp.,* which were isolated from chicken at the Department of Poultry and Fish diseases [34]. In the food industry clove essential oil have received a prime attention because of *L. monocytogenes* contamination, especially for food

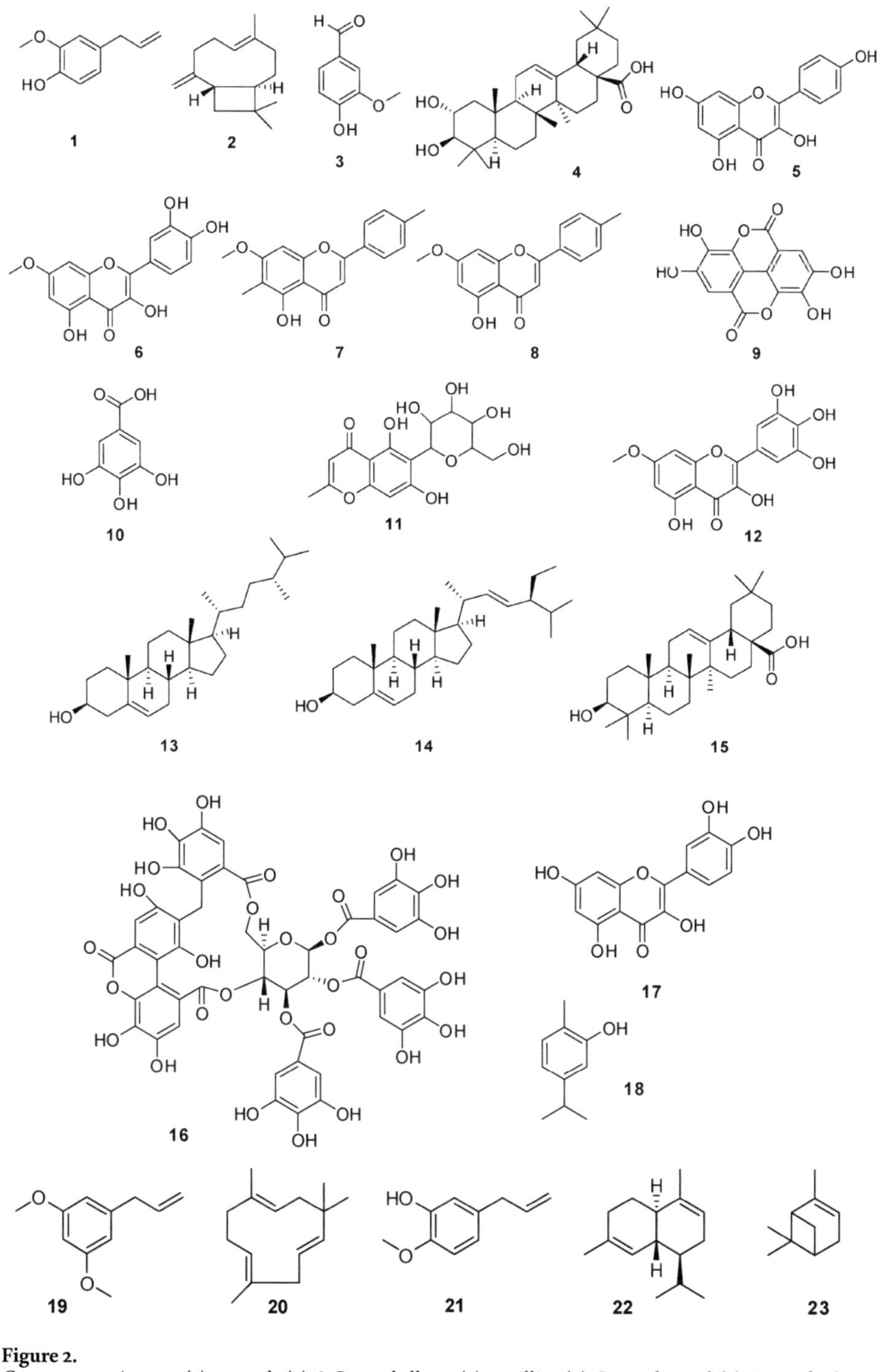

Figure 2.
Common constituents: (1) eugenol, (2) β-Caryophyllene, (3) vanillin, (4) Crategolic acid (5) Kaempferol, (6) Rhamnetin, (7) Eugenitin, (8) Eugenin, (9) Ellagic acid, (10) Gallic acid, (11) Biflorin, (12) Myricetin, (13) Campesterol, (14) Stigmasterol, (15) Oleanolic acid, (16) Bicornin, (17) quercetin (18) Carvacrol, (19) eugenol acetate, (20) α-Caryophyllene or α-humulene, (21) Chavibetol, (22) Cadinene (23) Pinene, (24).

preserved at low temperature because these bacteria multiply at low temperature and contaminate the food [35]. Singh, *et al.* (2003) [36] reported that clove oil was highly effective against *L. monocytogenes* in peptone water and reduced the bacterial population. The essential oil of Cloves (5%) reduced *L. monocytogenes*

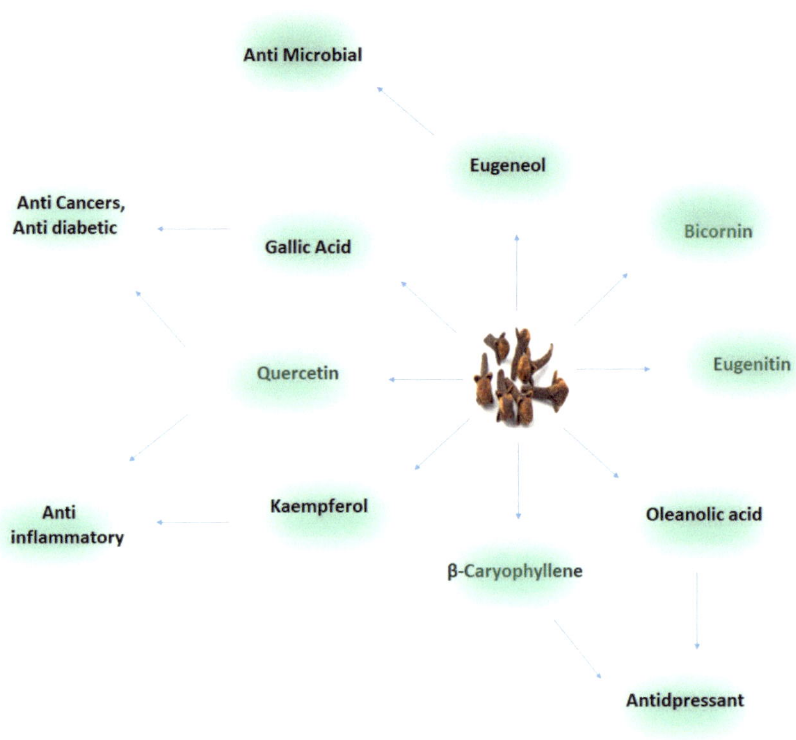

Figure 3.
Biological uses of compounds extracted from S. aromaticum.

cells to an undetectable level in ground chicken meat within one day of exposure, therefore, it can be used to control *L. monocytogenes* in ground chicken meat [37].

1.5 Antioxidant activity

In the past, oxidation mechanisms and free radical mechanism have been of great interest in living systems [38]. Oxygen uptake is essential to cell metabolism which results in the production of reactive oxygen species (ROS). The reaction of ROS with lipid molecules produces peroxyl radicals which further interact with nucleic acids and proteins results in alterations and, therefore, functional modifications [39]. ROS, include free radicals like superoxide anion radicals O_2^-, singlet oxygen, non-free-radical hydrogen peroxide and hydroxyl radicals are different forms of reactive oxygen species [40–43]. ROS are produced continuously during normal physiologic process and can easily lead to the peroxidation of lipids, which results in the accumulation of lipid peroxides. ROS is responsible for destroying crucial biomolecules like nucleic acids, proteins, lipids, as well as carbohydrates. They are also responsible for DNA damage that initiate the mutation [43, 44]. These suggest that, if the ROS are not adequately scavenged, they cause more than 100 of diseases like Alzheimer's disease, diabetes mellitus, hypertension [45, 46], prostate and colon cancers, coronary heart disease, atherosclerosis, cancer [47], cellular injury and aging process [48, 49], Therefore, to avoid the harmful effect of the ROS, can be blocked by antioxidant substances which scavenge the free radicals and detoxify the organism [50]. Antioxidants are those compounds that can protect the human body from free radicals and ROS effects and retard the progress of many chronic diseases by inhibiting the oxidation of lipid or other molecules by inhibiting the initiation or propagation of oxidizing chain reactions which suggest that Gallic acid, eugenol and eugenyl acetate have been used as an major antioxidants [51–55]. The antioxidant activity of eugenol and eugenyl acetate was found to be comparable to that of the natural antioxidant, vitamin E (α-tocopherol). Eugenol and *iso*-eugenol also found to be antioxidant and inhibit the peroxidation of lecithin induced by the Fe^{2+}-H_2O_2 system [56].

Gülçin, *et al.* [57] compare the scavenging of the DPPH radical of clove oil with some artificial antioxidant agents like α-tocopherol, BHT, Trolox, and butylated hydroxyanisole, and illustrated that the clove oil antioxidant activity declined as follows: Clove oil > BHT > α-tocopherol > butylated hydroxyanisole > Trolox. Numerous *in vitro* protocol including DPPH, oxygen radical absorbance capacity, ferric reducing antioxidant power, 2-deoxiguanosine, 2,20-azino-bis-(3-ethylbenzo-thiazoline-6-sulphonic acid) (ABTS), and xanthine oxidase have been employed to examine the antioxidant activity of aqueous *S. aromaticum* extract. After this studies, they illustrated that the potential antioxidant property of aqueous *S. aromaticum* extract may be due to the strong hydrogen donating ability, scavenging of hydrogen peroxide, free radicals and superoxide and metal chelating ability [58]. Therefore, the high antioxidant activity shown by clove oil is due the presence of phenolic compounds eugenol, thymol and eugenol acetate [59–61].

1.6 Antifungal activity

Several reports have been published which exhibit the antifungal activity of Clove oil which is further due to the presence of phenolic compound eugenol and carvacrol [62]. Pinto, *et al.* in 2009 [63] reported that Clove oil reduces the amount of specific fungal cell membrane ergosterol which cure the spread of fungal infection. Eugenol also inhibit the growth of filamentous fungi, yeast as human pathogenic fungi and fungal species born from food [64–66]. Kumar *et al.* in 2012 [67] reported that the phenolic compound carvacrol possess maximum antifungal activity against the *Candida fungal* species like *Candida albicans Candida tropicalis* and *Candida guilliermondii*. They also exhibited some antifungal activity contaminate bakery products by fungus such as *Eurotium spp., Aspergillus spp. and Penicillium spp*. These findings strengthen the possibility of using plant essential oils as an alternative to chemicals, to preserve bakery products [68]. Viuda-Martos, *et al.* [69] also reported the antifungal activity of Clove oil against food spoilage fungi *Aspergillus flavus* and *Aspergillus niger* by using agar dilution method and it was found that it exhibit stronger inhibition activity against *Aspergillus niger* than *Aspergillus flavus*. Bansod & Rai, in 2008 [70] further studied the comparative antifungal activity of different essential oils including Clove oil against *Aspergillus fumigates* and *Aspergillus niger* by using three different methods, disc diffusion method, broth dilution method and agar dilution method. Their studied further support the strong antifungal activity of Clove oil among all other oil. Estrada-Cano, *et al.*, 2017 [71] report the strong antifungal inhibitory action of encapsulated Clove oil against *Fusarium oxysporum* by oxford cup method. Based on the experimental observation they conclude that naked Clove oil had greatest inhibitory action against *Fusarium oxysporum* in beginning. But, after 8 hours the efficiency of microcapsulated Clove oil was maximum.

1.7 Anticancer activity

Cancer is the major public health problem in the worldwide and the number of patient increases continuously [72]. It is the second largest leading cause of death. When cancer is diagnosed at an advanced stage, chemotherapy is the most effective option to improve the patient's life to prolong time survival [73]. Recent literature survey revealed that some natural products have significant role as an antitumor agent. It is found that almost 30–40% drugs used globally for the treatment of cancer are derived from plant sources [74]. The dried buds of Cloves contain a wide range of bioactive compounds, which include eugenol, β-caryophyllene, humulene, chavicol, methyl salicylate, α-ylangene, and eugenone; the flavonoids eugenin, rhamnetin, kaempferol, and eugenitin; triterpenoids like oleanolic acid, stigmasterol, and campesterol; and several sesquiterpenes were screened as an anticancer agent. Haizhou Liu, *et al.* [75] reported that extract of Cloves displayed potent cytotoxic activity against several human cancer cell lines. They were performed *in vivo* antitumor activity of Clove extract by a number of experiments on variety of cancerous cell like human cancer cells, including ovarian cancer cells (SKOV-3), cervical epithelial cells (HeLa), liver cancer cells (BEL-7402), colon cancer cells (HT-29), breast cancer cells (MCF-7), pancreatic cells (PANC-1), normal colon epithelial cells (CCD 841 CoN), and normal lung fibroblasts (IMR-90) in order to identify the bioactive compounds. They were reported that the inhibition power of dried Clove powder in human colon cancer HT-29 cells by using the MTT assay was approximately 2.2 mg/mL. The antiproliferative effects was enhance by upto an approximate 10-fold by the use of the ethanol extract of Clove powder against a panel of human cancer cell lines, including breast (MCF-7), ovarian (SKOV-3), cervical (HeLa), liver (BEL-7402), pancreatic (PANC-1), and colon (HT-29) cells. After identification of inhibition activity, they were extract the bioactive compound from ethyl acetate extract of Cloves and found that oleanolic acid was the one of the bioactive component which has *in vitro* antiproliferative and *in vivo* antitumor activity. Kumar, *et al.* (2014) [76] reported the anticancer bioactive component of various concentrations of water, ethanol extract and essential oil of Clove *in vitro* through MTT and brine shrimp lethality test (BSLT) assay against MCF-7 human breast cancer cells. In both MTT and BSLT essential Clove oil showed excellent cytotoxic effect. In another study Lesgards, *et al.* (2014) [77] reported that Clove essential oil contains phenylpropanoids and terpenoids shows antitumor activity on both cell line and tumors in animals. Dwivedi, *et al.* (2011) [78] performed the comparative study of anticancer potential of Clove oil, its ethanol and water extract towards prostate cancer DU-145, cervical cancer HeLa, esophageal cancer TE-13, MDA-MB-231 (ER-ve) and breast cancer MCF-7 (ER + ve) along with normal human peripheral blood lymphocytes for antiproliferation by using MTT assay. Maximum cytotoxic activity and maximum cell deaths were observed in TF-13 cells within 24 hours by using essential Clove oil up to 300 μl/mL, whereas minimal cell death in DU-145 cells but with same dose no cytotoxicity was found in human peripheral blood mononuclear cells.

1.8 Anti-inflammatory activity

Cloves are well known for their anti-inflammatory effects. Traditional use of clove oil as a lotion or drinking of cloves in tea with daily routine may help to reduce inflammation caused by Arthritis. Past studies [79] have shown eating them on the daily could lead to major health benefits. Susan, *et al.* have concluded that DNA strand breaks and inflammatory biomarkers are a good functional measure of a food's bioavailability. Han, *et al.* [80] has recently provides important evidence of Clove essential Oil (CEO)-induced anti-inflammatory and tissue remodeling activity in human dermal fibroblasts. CEO at 0.011% concentration exhibit robust antiproliferative effects on human dermal fibroblasts. It significantly inhibited the increased production of several proinflammatory biomarkers such as vascular cell adhesion molecule-1 (VCAM-1), interferon-inducible T-cell α-chemoattractant

(I-TAC), interferon γ-induced protein 10 (IP-10), and monokine induced by γ interferon (MIG). CEO also significantly inhibited tissue remodeling protein molecules, namely, collagen-I, collagen-III, macrophage colony-stimulating factor (M-CSF), and tissue inhibitor of metalloproteinase-2 (TIMP-2). Furthermore, it significantly modulated global gene expression and altered signaling pathways critical for inflammation, tissue remodeling, and cancer signaling processes. CEO significantly inhibited VCAM-1 and collagen-III at both protein and gene expression levels. This study also supports the anticancer properties of CEO and its major active component eugenol. Barboza *et al.* [81] have reported that the eugenol a constituent of Clove exerts a beneficial action on oxidative stress through the inhibition of enzymes and oxidative processes, which is related to the anti-inflammatory drug profile of this compound. Sugihartini*et al.* [82] have also reported the activity of eugenol an essential oil component of Clove in absorption base ointment can be increased with the addition of enhancer. Its activity was better than natrium diclofenac in positive control. However, the formula containing propylene glycol needs to be evaluated for its anti-inflammatory activity for a longer duration to ensure its effectivity. Banerjee *et al.* [83] have reported that Clove oil emulsion can substitute chemical based topical products for anti-inflammatory and wound healing applications. Nikoui et al. [84] have also reported that clove oil administration has anti-inflammatory and antipyretic properties in dogs after surgery. Leem et al. [85] have reported that, among the volatile distillate extracts of 8 herbal medicines, the distillate extract of cloves exhibited the strongest antioxidant activity (IC_{50} = 8.85 μg/mL) and COX-2 inhibitory activity (inhibition rate was 58.15% at 10 μg/mL concentration), whereas 15-LOX inhibitory activity (inhibition rate was 86.15% at 25 μg/mL concentration) was the second highest after Angelica. They also measured an antioxidant and anti-inflammatory activities of eugenol and its derivatives (methyl eugenol and acetyl eugenol), eugenol (IC_{50} = 5.99 μg/mL), which exhibited the highest antioxidant activity, whereas methyl eugenol and acetyl eugenol exhibited a little activity. In the case of COX-2, eugenol (85.35%) at a concentration of 20 μg/mL showed the strongest inhibitory activity, whereas in 15-LOX, methyl eugenol (83.29%) at a concentration of 20 μg/mL showed the strongest inhibitory activity, whereas in 15-LOX, methyl eugenol (83.29%) at a concentration of 20 μg/mL showed the highest inhibitory activity.

1.9 Antidiabetic activity

Kroda *et al.* [86] have reported that Clove (*Syzygium aromaticum* flower buds) EtOH extract significantly suppressed an increase in blood glucose level in type 2 diabetic KK-A(y) mice. The results indicate that clove has potential as a functional food ingredient for the prevention of type 2 diabetes and that 2–4 mainly contribute to its hypoglycemic effects via PPAR-γ activation. *In-vitro* evaluation exhibited the extract had human peroxisome proliferator-activated receptor (PPAR)-γ ligand-binding activity in a GAL4-PPAR-γ chimera assay. They isolated 8 compounds, of which dehydrodieugenol and dehydrodieugenol B had potent PPAR-γ ligand-binding activities and also showed to stimulate 3 T3-L1 preadipocyte differentiation through PPAR-γ activation, whereas major constituent oleanolic acid in the EtOH extract, had moderate activity. Topal [87] reported that Isoeugenol (2-methoxy-4-(prop-1-en-1-yl)phenol), a constituent of clove oil exhibited excellent inhibitory effects against some metabolic enzymes viz. acetylcholinesterase (AChE) enzymes, α-glycosidase, and α-amylase. Isoeugenol has the IC_{50} values of 411.5, 19.25 and 77.00 nM for α-amylase, α-glycosidase and AChE, respectively. The K_i values of isoeugenol were found as 21 ± 9 and 16 ± 3 nM against α-glycosidase and AChE, respectively, whereas, tacrine as standard AChE inhibitor exhibited IC_{50} value of 20.38 nM. α-Glycosidase inhibitors, commonly referred to as starch blockers, are anti-diabetic drugs that help reduce edible blood glucose levels. Chaudhry *et al.* [88] reported that Clove extract has glucose lowering effect in STZ induced diabetic rats and this effect is dose related and the dose of 750 mg/kg body weight has produced maximum effect. Abdulrazak et al. [89] have evaluated the effects of clove and fermented ginger supplements on blood glucose, serum insulin, insulin receptor and Leptin levels of high fat diet-induced type-2 diabetes mellitus in rabbits. They found a significantly ($P < 0.05$) decrease in blood glucose levels was recorded in the supplements treated groups compared to diabetic control group. Clove supplement has been most effective and sustaining in antihyperglycemic activity, also appears with a significant decreasing effect on leptin levels compared to diabetic control group. A significant increase in insulin levels was also detected in the fermented ginger treated group along with higher levels of Leptin compared as compared to control group. Thus overall, the study reveals that clove and fermented ginger supplementation possesses anti-diabetic properties and may help in the control of hyperleptinaemia in type 2 diabetes.

1.10 Herbicidal activity

Clove oil also exhibit herbicidal activity against the many herbicides. Tworkoski (2002) [90] investigated the herbicidal of different essential oils including Clove and Cinnamon oil on detached leaves of dandelion. Clove and Cinnamon essential oil were applied using dandelion leaf disk assay and whole plant assay with Johnson grass, common lambsquarters and common ragweed in green house. The observed that shoot death occurred from one hour to one day after the application of oil. Bainard, *et al.* (2006) [91] investigated the herbicidal activity of Clove oil and its primary constituent eugenol on *Amaranthus retroflexus* (redroot pigweed), *Chenopodium album* (common lambsquarters) and effect on leaf cell membrane integrity and seedling growth. They observed that Clove oil and its major constituent eugenol caused reduction in cell membrane integrity and inhibition of seedling growth. Evans, *et al.* (2009) [92] performed their studies on herbicidal effect of Clove oil and vinegar on *Abutilon theopharst* (velvet leaf) and *Amaranthus retroflexus* (redroot pigweed). In their studies they were found that redroot pigweed was easier to control with both products than velvetleaf. Park, *et al.* (2011) [93] further investigate the herbicidal action of Clove oil on the cucumber seedlings in light and dark conditions. Clove oil treatment increased superoxide dismutase (SOD) activity and decreased catalase activity whereas SOD and catalase activity decreased in the paraquat treatment. They reported that the Clove oil exhibit herbicidal action through a mechanism different from that of parquet.

Besides this they also exhibit insecticidal activity, anesthetic activity and several literatures are available on that. Rom these studies we observed that the essential oil present in Clove are beneficial and are in use for treatment of variety of disease.

2. Conclusion

Overall, *Syzygium aromaticum*, is an essential herb which contains many essential oils, terpenoids, flavonoids, polyphenols, eugenol and many other active pharmacaphores. These leading pharmacophore made *S. aromaticum* a special plant to treat many disease like cancer, Alzhimer and many body infections and dis-regulations. Traditional use of this is widely known whereas, it is scientifically proved as well. It can be used as antimicrobial, antibacterial, antifungal, antioxidant, anticancerous, antiherbicidal, antidiabetic, anti-inflammatory, antidepressant, antiulcer, antinoceptive, and antiprotozoal etc.

Author details

Vikrant Kumar[1*], Deepak Mishra[2], Mukesh Chandra Joshi[3], Priyanka Mishra[4] and Megha Tanwar[1]

1 Department of Chemistry, Acharya Narendra Dev College (University of Delhi), New Delhi, India

2 Department of Chemistry, SRM University, Delhi-NCR, Haryana, India

3 Department of Chemistry, Motilal Nehru College (University of Delhi), New Delhi, India

4 Department of Botany, Zakir Hussain Delhi College (University of Delhi), New Delhi, India

*Address all correspondence to: vikrantkumar@andc.du.ac.in

References

[1] Carlsen, M.H., Halvorsen, B.L., Holte, K., Bohn, S.K., Dragland, S., Sampson, L., Willey, C., Senoo, H., Umezono, Y., Sanada, C., Barikmo, I., Berhe, N., Willett, W.C., Phillips, K.M., Jacobs, J.R., Blomhoff, R., The total antioxidant content of more than 3100 foods, beverages, spices, herbs and supplements used worldwide. Nutr. J. 2010; 9:1-3.

[2] Soh W.K., Parnell J. A revision of Syzygium gaerth (Myrtaceace) in Indochina (Cambodia, Laos and Vietnam). Adansonia. 2015; 37:179-275.

[3] Nurdjannah, N., Bermawie, N., 2012. 11—Cloves. In: Peter, K.V. (Ed.), Handbook of Herbs and Spices. Second ed. Woodhead Publishing, Cambridge, UK, pp. 197-215.

[4] Danthu P., Penot E., Ranoarisoa K.M., Rakotondravelo J.C., Michel I., Tiollier M *et al*. The clove tree of Madagascar: a success story with an unpredictable future. Bois et Forets des Tropiques. 2014; 320:83-96.

[5] Byng. Revision of Eugenia and Syzygium (Myrtaceae) from Comoro archipelago. Phytotaxa. 2016; 252:162-184.

[6] Shrivastava K., Sahu S., Mishra S., De, K. In vitro antimicrobial activity and phytochemical screening of *Syzygium aromaticum*. Asian J. Res. Pharm. Sci. 2014; 4(1):12-15.

[7] Board N. Handbook on Spices. Asia Pacific Business Press Inc, Delhi, 2010; 199-213.

[8] Pandey A., Singh P. Antibacterial activity of syzygium aromaticum (clove) with metal ion effect against food borne pathogens. Asian J. Plant Sci. Res., 2011; 1(2):69-80.

[9] Cai, L., Wu, C.D.,. Compounds from *Syzygium aromaticum* possessing growth inhibitory activity against oral pathogens. J. Nat. Prod. 1996; 59(10):987-990.

[10] Halliwell, B., 1999. Free radicals in biology and medicine. Oxford University Press, Oxford.

[11] Shan, B., Cai, Y.Z., Sun, M., Corke, H. Antioxidant capacity of 26 spice extracts and characterization of their phenolic constituents. J. Agric. Food Chem. 2005; 53:7749-7759.

[12] Cortés-Rojas, D.F., De-Souza, C.R., Oliveira, W.P. Clove (*Syzygium aromaticum*): a precious spice. Asian Pac. J. Trop. Biomed.2014; 4:90-96.

[13] Kamatou GP, Vermaak I, Viljoen AM. Eugenol from Maluka Islands to the international market place: A review of a remarkable and versatile molecules. Molecules. 2010; 17:6953-6981.

[14] Neveu, V.; Perez-Jiménez, J.; Vos, F.; Crespy, V.; du Cha_aut, L.; Mennen, L.; Knox, C.; Eisner, R.; Cruz, J.; Wishart, D.; et al. Phenol-Explorer: An online comprehensive database on polyphenol contents in foods. Database 2010.

[15] Verzar-Petri G, Then M, Meszaros S. formation of essential oil in clary sage under different condition. In: Proceeding of the 15th International Symposium on Essential Oils, Svendsen AB, Scheffer JJC (eds). Martinus Nijhoff/Dt W,Junk Publishers, Boston, 19-21.

[16] Arslan N, Gurbuz B, Sarihan EO. Variation in essential oil content and xcomposition in Turkish anise (*Pimpinella anisum* L.) populations. Turkish Journal of Agricultural Forestry. 2004; 28:173-177.

[17] Alma M.H., Ertas M., Nitz S., Kollmannsberger H. Chemical

composition and content of essential oil from the bud of cultivated Turkish clove (*Syzygium aromaticum* L.). Bio. Resources. 2007; 2:265-269.

[18] Khan M.S., Zahin M, Hasan S, Husain F.M. Inhibition of quorum sensing regulated bacterial functions by plant essential oils with special reference to clove oil. Letters Applied Microbiology. 2009; 49:354-360.

[19] Matta FB. Essential oils from six herbal pkants for biocontrol of the maize weevil. Hort. Science. 2010; 45:592-598.

[20] Marya CM, Satija G, Avinash J, Nagpal R, Ahmad A. *In vitro* inhibitory of clove essential oil and its two active principles on tooth decalcification by apple juice. International Journal of Dentistry. 2012. http://dx.doi.org/10.1155/2012/759618.

[21] Kasai H, Shirao M, Ikegami-Kawai M. Analysis of volatile compounds of clove (*Syzygium aromaticum*) buds as influenced by growth phase and investigation of antioxidant activity of clove extract. Flavour and Fragrance Journal. 2016; 31:178-184.

[22] Pruthi JS. Minor Spices and Condiments Crop Management and Post-Harvest Technology. Indian Council of Agricultural Research, New Delhi, India, 2001; 308-331.

[23] Xu JG, Liu T, Hu QP, Cao XM. Chemical composition, antibacterial properties and mechanism of action of essential oil from clove buds against *Staphylococcus aureus*. Molecules. 2016; 21:1-13.

[24] Fankem P.M., Kwanga S.N., Sameza M.L., Tchoumbougnang F, Tchabong R, Ngoune T *et al*. Antioxidant and antifungal activities of cocoa butter (*Theobroma cacao*), essential oil of *Syzygium aromaticum* and a combination of both extracts against three dermotophytes. American Scientific Research Journal for Engineering Technology and Sciences. 2017; 37:255-272.

[25] Jirovetz L, Buchbauer G, Stoilova I, Stoyanova A, Krastanov A, Schmidt E. Chemical composition and antioxidant properties of clove leaf essential oil. Journal of Agricultural and Food Chemistry. 2006; 54:6303-6307.

[26] Srivastava AK, Srivastava SK, Syamsundar KV. Bud and leaf essential oil composition of *Syzygium aromaticum* from India and Madagascar. Flavour and Fragrance Journal. 2005; 20:51-53.

[27] Kapahi BK, Thappa RK. Some essential oil bearing plants under cultivation in Andaman Island. Pafabi. 1989; 11:23-24.

[28] Patil DA, Dhale DA. Spices and Condiments Origin, Histroy and Application. Daya Publishing House, New Delhi, India, 2013, 76-80

[29] Bao, L.-M., Eerdunbayaer, Nozaki, A., Takahashi, E., Okamoto, K., Ito, H.,. Hydrolysable tannins isolated from *Syzygium aromaticum*: structure of a new C-glucosidic ellagitannin and spectral features of tannins with a tergalloyl group. Heterocycles. 2012; 85(2):365-381.

[30] Qiao Hu, Meifang Zhou, Shuyong wei. Progress on the antimicrobial activity research of clove oil and eugenol in the food antisepsis field. 2018; 83(6):1476-1483.

[31] Matan M. Antimicrobial activity of edible film incorporated with essential oils to preserve dried fish (*Decapterus maruadsi*). International Food Research Journal. 2012; 19:1733-1738.

[32] Zengin H, Baysal H. Antioxidant and antimicrobial activities of thyme and clove essential oils and application

in minced beef. Journal of Food Processing and Preservation. 2014; 39:1261-1271.

[33] Gupta A, Duhan J, Tewari S, Sangwan P, Yadav A *et al*. Comparative evaluation of antimicrobial efficacy of *Syzygium aromaticum*, *Ocimum sanctum* and *Cinnamomum zeylanicum* plant extracts against *Enterococcus faecalis*: A preliminary study. International Endodontic Journal. 2013; 46:775-783.

[34] Kammon A., Almaeyoufi A., Asheg A., In Vitro antimicrobial activity of clove oil against gram negative bacteria isolated from chickens. Appro Poult Dairy & Vet Sci 6(2). APDV.000635.2019. DOI.org/10.31031/APDV.2019.06.000635.

[35] Juntila Jr, Niemela Si, Hirn J. Minimum growth temperature of *Listeria monocytogenes* and non-hemolytic *Listeria*, *J. Appli. Bacteriol.*, 1988; 65:321-7.

[36] Singh A., Singh R.K., Bhunia A.K., Singh N. Efficacy of plant essential oils as antimicrobial agents against *Listeria monocytogenes* in hotdogs, Lebensm.-Wiss. U.-technol, 2003; 36:787-794.

[37] Hoque M.M., Bari M.L., Juneja V.K., Kawamoto S. Antimicrobial activity of cloves and cinnamon extracts against food borne pathogens and spoilage bacteria, and inactivation of *Listeria monocytogenes* in ground chicken meat with their essential oils, J. Food Sci. Technol., 2007; 72:9-21.

[38] Halliwell, B.; Gutteridge, J.; Aruoma, O. The deoxyribose method: A simple "test tube" assay for determination of rate constants for reaction of hydroxyl radicals. Anal. Biochem. 1987; 165:215-219.

[39] Chaillou, H.I., Nazareno, M. New method to determine antiox-idant activity of polyphenols. J. Agric. Food Chem. 2006; 54:8397-8402.

[40] Buyukokuroglu M.E., Gulcin I., Oktay M., Kufrevioglu O.I. In vitro antioxidant properties of dantrolene sodium. Pharmacol. Res. 2001; 44:491-495.

[41] Gulcin I., Buyukokuroglu M.E., Oktay M., Kufrevioglu O.I. Antioxidant and analgesic activities of turpentine of Pinus nigra Arn. Subsp. pallsiana (Lamb.) Holmboe. J. Ethnopharmacol. 2003a; 86:51-58.

[42] Gulcin I., Elias R., Gepdiremen A., Boyer L. Antioxidant activity of lignans from fringe tree (Chionanthus virginicus L.). Eur. Food Res. Technol. 2006a; 223:759-767.

[43] Gulcin I. Antioxidant and antiradical activities of L-carnitin. Life Sci. 2006a; 78:803-811.

[44] Gulcin I., Berashvili, D., Gepdiremen, A. Antiradical and antioxidant activity of total anthocyanins from Perilla pankinensis decne. J. Ethnopharmacol. 2005; 101:287-293.

[45] Halliwell, B., Gutteridge, J.M.C. Role of free radicals and catalytic metal ions in human disease: An overview. Method. Enzymol. 1990; 186:1-85.

[46] Gulcin I., Buyukokuroglu, M.E., Oktay M., Kufrevioglu, O.I. Antioxidant and analgesic activities of turpentine of Pinus nigra Arn. Subsp. pallsiana (Lamb.) Holmboe. J. Ethnopharmacol. 2003a; 86:51-58.

[47] Madhavi D.L., Deshpande S.S., Salunkhe D.K. Food Antioxidants: Technological, Toxicological. 1996, Health Perspective. Marcel Dekker, New York

[48] Halliwell, B., Gutteridge, J.M.C., 1989. Free Radicals in Biology and Medicine. Clarendon Press, Oxford, pp. 23-30.

[49] Gulcin I., Buyukokuroglu M.E., Oktay M. Kufrevioglu O.I. On the in vitro antioxidant properties of melatonin. J. Pineal Res. 2002a; 33:167-171.

[50] Kumaran, A., Karunakaran, R.J. Antioxidant and free radical scavenging activity of an aqueous extract of Coleus aromaticus. Food Chem. 2006, 97:109-114.

[51] Velioglu Y.S., Mazza G., Gao L., Oomah B.D. Antioxidant activity and total phenolics in selected fruits, vegetables, and grain products. J. Agric. Food Chem. 1998; 46:4113-4117.

[52] Lai, L.S., Chou, S.T., Chao, W.W. Studies on the antioxidative activities of Hsian-tsao (Mesona procumbens Hemsl) leaf gum. J. Agric. Food Chem. 2001: 49:963-968.

[53] Gulcin, I. Comparison of in vitro antioxidant and antiradical activities of l-tyrosine and l-Dopa. Amino Acids, 2007; 32:431-438.

[54] Kramer R.E. Antioxidants in clove, J. Am. Oil Chem. Soc., 1985; 62:111-113.

[55] Lee K.G., Shibamoto T. Inhibition of malonaldehyde formation from blood plasma oxidation by aroma extracts and aroma components isolated from clove and eucalyptus, Food Chem. Toxicol., 2001a; **39**:1199-1204.

[56] Toda S., Ohnishi M., Kimura M., Toda T. Inhibitory effects of eugenol and related compounds on lipid peroxidation induced by reactive oxygen, Planta Medica, 1994; 60:282.

[57] Gülçin I., Elmastas M., Aboul-Enein H.Y. Antioxidant activity of clove oil–A powerful antioxidant source. Arab. J. Chem. 2012; 5:489-499.

[58] Gülçin, Ì.; Şat, İ.G.; Beydemir, Ş.; Elmastas, M.; Küfrevioglu, Ö.I. Comparison of antioxidant activity of clove (Eugenia caryophylata Thunb) buds and lavender (*Lavandula stoechas* L.). Food Chem. 2004; 87:393-400.

[59] Yadav AS, Bhatnagar D. Free radical scavenging activity, metal chelation and antioxidant power of some of Indian spices. Biofactors. 2007; 31:219-227.

[60] Dai JP, Zhao XF, Zeng J, Wan QY, Yang JC, Li WZ *et al*. Drug screening for autophagy inhibitors based on dissociation of Beclin1-Bcl2 complex using BiFC technique and mechanism of eugenol on anti-influenza a virus activity. Plos One. 2013; 8:1-9.

[61] Najm H, Kim MM. Eugenol with antioxidant activity inhibits MM-9 related to metastasis in human fibrosarcomacells. Food Chemical Toxicology. 2013; 55:106-112.

[62] Chami N, Bennis S, Chami F, Aboussekhra A, Remmal A. Study of anticandidal activity of carvacrol and eugenol *in vitro* and *in vivo*. Oral Microbiology Immunology. 2005; 20:106-111

[63] Pinto E, Vela-Silva L, Cavelerio C, Salgueiro L. Antifungal activity of clove essential oil from *Syzygium aromaticim* on *Candida, Aspergillus* and dermatophyte specis. Journal of Medical Microbiology. 2009; 58:1454-1462.

[64] Gayoso C.W., Lima E.O., Oliveria V.T., Pereira F.O., Souza E.L., Lima I.O. *et al.* Sensitivity of fungi isolated from onychomycosis to *Eugenia caryopyllata* essential oil and eugenol. Journal of Fitoterapia. 2005; 76:247-249.

[65] Hammer K.A., Carson C.F., Riley T.V. Antimicrobial activity of essential oils and other plant extracts. Journal of Applied Microbiology. 1999; 86:985-990.

[66] Eugenia P, Luis VS, Carlo C, Ligia S. Antifungal activity of the clove essential oil from *Syzygium aromaticum* on

Candida, Aspergillus and dermatophyte species. Journal of Medical Microbiology. 2009; 58:1454-1462.

[67] Kumar A, Thakur S, Thakur VC, Kumar A, Patil S, Vohra MP. Antifungal activity of some natural essentiall oils against *Candida* species isolated from blood stream infection. Journal of Krishna Institute of Medical Sciences University. 2012; 1:61-66.

[68] Guynot M.E., Martin S., Setu L., Sanchis V. Ramos A.J. Screening for antifungal activity of some essential oils against common spoilage fungi of bakery products, Food Sci. Technol. Int., 2005; 11(1):25-32

[69] Viuda-Martos M, Ruiz-Navajas Y, Fernandes-Lopez J, Perez-Alvarez JA. Antifungal activity of thyme, clove and oregano essential oils. Journal of Food Safety. 2007; 27:91-101.

[70] Bansod S, Rai M. Antifungal activity of essential oils from Indian medicina; plants against human pathogenic *Aspergillus fumigates* and *A. niger*. World Journal of Medical Science. 2008; 3:81-88.

[71] Estrada-Cano C, Anaya-Castro MA, Munoz-Castellanos L, Amaya-Olivas N, Garcia-Triana A, Hernandez-Ochoa L. Antifungal activity of microcapsulated clove (*Eugenia caryophyllata*) and Mexican oregano (*Lippia berlandieri*) essential oils against *Fusarium oxysporum*. Journal of Microbiology and Biochemical Technology. 2017; 9:567-571.

[72] Jemal A, Bray F, Center MM, Ferlay J, Ward E, Forman D. Global cancer statistics. CA Cancer J. Clin. 2011; 61:69-90.

[73] Wyld L, Reed M. The role of surgery in the management of older women with breast cancer. Eur. J. Cancer. 2007; 43:2253-2263.

[74] Newman DJ, Cragg GM, Snader KM. Natural products as sources of new drugs over the period 1981-2002. J. Nat. Prod. 2003; 66:1022-1037.

[75] Liu H., Schmitz J.C., Wei J., Cao S., Beumer J.H., Strychor S., Cheng L., Liu M., Wang C., Wu N., Zhao X., Zhang Y., Liao J., Chu E., Lin X. Clove extract inhibits tumor growth and promotes cell cycle arrest and apoptosis. Oncol Res. 2014; 21(5):247-259.

[76] Kumar P.S., Febriyanti R.M., Sofyan F.F., Luftimas D.E., Abdulah R. Anticancer potential of *Syzygium aromaticum* L. in MCF-7 human breast cancer cell lines. Pharmacognosy Research. 2014; 6:350-354.

[77] Lesgards J.F., Baldovini N., Vidal N., Pietri S. Anticancer activities of essential oils constituents and synergy with conventional therapies: A review. Phytotherapy Research. 2014; 28:1423-1446.

[78] Dwivedi V, Shrivastava R, Husain S, Ganguly, Bharadwaj M. Comparative anticancer potential of clove (*Syzygium aromaticum*) – an Indian species – against cancer cell lines of various anatomical origin. Asian Pacific Journal of Cancer Prevention. 2011; 12:1989-1993.

[79] Percival S.S., Heuvel J.P.V., Nieves C.J., Montero C., Migliaccio A.J., Meadors J. Bioavailability of herbs and spices in humans as determined by ex vivo inflammatory suppression and DNA strand breaks. J. Am. Coll. Nutr. 2012;v31(4):288-94.

[80] Han X., Parker T. L. Anti-inflammatory activity of clove (Eugenia caryophyllata) essential oil in human dermal fibroblasts. Pharm. Biol. 2017; 55(1):1619-1622.

[81] Barboza J. N., Carlos da Silva Maia Bezerra Filho, Silva R.O., Medeiros J.V.R., de Sousa D.P., An

Overview on the Anti-inflammatory Potential and Antioxidant Profile of Eugenol. Oxidative Medicine and Cellular Longevity 2018, Article ID 3957262).

[82] Sugihartini N. Prabandari R., Yuwono T., Rahmawati D.R. The anti-inflammatory activity of essential oil of clove (Syzygium aromaticum) in absorption base ointment with addition of oleic acid and propylene glycol as enhancer.International J. Appl. Pharma.. 2019; 11(5):106-109.

[83] Banerjee K., Madhyastha H.K., Sandur R., Manikandanath V., Thiagarajan N.T., Thiagarajan N.P. Anti-inflammatory and wound healing potential of a clove oil emulsion. Colloids and Surfaces B: Biointerfaces 2020; 193:111102.

[84] Nikoui V., Ostadhadi S., Bakhtiarian A., Abbasi-Goujani E., Habibian-Dehkordi S., Rezaei-Roshan M., Foroohandeh M., Giorgi M., The anti-inflammatory and antipyretic effects of clove oil in healthy dogs after surgery. Pharma Nutrition. 2017; 5(2):52-57.

[85] Leem H.H., Kim E.O., Seo M.J., Choi S.W., Antioxidant and anti-inflammatory activities of eugenol and its derivatives from clove (Eugenia caryophyllata Thunb.) J. Korean Soc. Food Sci. Nutri. 2011; 40(10): 1361-1370.

[86] Kuroda M., Mimaki Y., Ohtomo T., Yamada J., Nishiyama T., Mae T., Kishida H., Kawada T. Hypoglycemic effects of clove (*Syzygium aromaticum* flower buds) on genetically diabetic KK-Ay mice and identification of the active ingredients. J Nat Med. 2012; 66(2):394-399.

[87] Topal F. Anticholinergic and antidiabetic effects of isoeugenol from clove (*Eugenia caryophylata*) oil. 2019; 22(1):583-592.)

[88] Chaudhry Z.R., Chaudhry S.R., Naseer A., Chaudhry F.R., Effect of *Syzygium aromaticum* (clove) extract on blood glucose level in streptozotocin induced diabetic rats. Pak Armed Forces Med. J. 2013; 63(3):323-328)

[89] Abdulrazak A., Tanko Y., Mohammed A., Mohammed K. A., Sada N.M., Dikko A.A.U. Effects of clove and fermented ginger on blood glucose, leptin, insulin and insulin receptor levels in high fat dietinduced type 2 diabetic rabbits. Niger. J. Physiol. Sci. 2018; 33:089-093.

[90] Tworkoski T. Herbicidal effects of essential oils. Weed Science. 2002; 50:425-431.

[91] Bainard Luke D, Isman M.B., Upadhayaya M.K. Phtyotoxicity of clove oil and its primary constituent eugenol and the role of leaf epicuticular wax in the susceptibitlity to these essential oils. Weed Science. 2006; 54:833-837.

[92] Evan G.J., Bellinder R.R., Giffinet M.C. Herbicidal effects of vinegar and a clove oil product on redroot pigweed (*Amaranthus retroflexus*) and velvetleaf (*Abutilon theophrasti*). Weed Technology. 2009; 23:292-299.

[93] Park, Woong K, Choi S.H., Ahn J.Y., Sohn Y.G., Kim C.G. *et al*. Herbicidial action of the clove oil on cucumber seedlings. Weed Biology and Management. 2011; 11:235-240.

Chapter 8

Garlic as a Potential Nominee in Functional Food Industry

Mavra Javed, Waqas Ahmed, Rehan Mian and Abdul Momin Rizwan Ahmad

Abstract

Functional and nutraceuticals products provide a bigger prospect to one's health by permitting health costs and supporting economic growth in lower and middle developed countries. Because of this reason, mostly diversion of people is going towards functional food and these Phyto-based foods are turning out to be popular universal in the red to the number of statements from researchers for their therapeutic applications. Garlic is one of the ancient vegetables that is used worldwide in different aspects which includes seasoning, culinary purposes, flavoring, and medical purposes. The consumption of garlic word wide increases due to its convenience, tackiness, health benefits, and low side effects. Garlic has been utilized for thousands of years because of its rich active components, phytochemicals, and other Sulfur containing components. It has so much rich history to contribute to the food industry. It has been used as a food stabilizer to prevent the development of pathogens to the prevention of many diseases. The claimed vigor reimbursements of garlic are abundant, including, anticarcinogenic, antibiotic, anti-hypertensive, and cholesterol-lowering properties, the risk of cardiovascular disease lowering the effects of hypolipidemic, antithrombotic, anti-diabetic, antioxidant, antimicrobial, immunomodulatory, antimutagenic, and prebiotic activities. The present attempt of the chapter is to explore garlic history along with its active component's involvement in the prevention of diseases and threats.

Keywords: garlic, history, garlic as functional food, active components, prevention of diseases

1. Introduction

Healthy and nutraceutical food varieties are developing mainstream the whole around the world inferable from their wellbeing advancing points of view [1] There are a few conventional plants, utilized as a remedial transporter for various physiological health problems. Analysis by way of food-based treatments, clarify the meaning of these Medicinal plants involving garlic, onion, dark cumin, green tea, ginger, nut and so on, nonetheless, a few hidden benefits from plant sources are yet to be investigated for scientists [2]. Pakistan being assorted in native rich land, has such kinds of therapeutic plants that are adding to wellbeing. Utilitarian food sources are huge in this milieu attributable to simple availability, low cost and associated wellbeing advancing viewpoints [3]. In the present situation, many plant-based foods, grains, nuts, and pulses and so forth are imperative since they have helpful potential because of certain naturally dynamic synthetic substances known as phytochemicals. These are the organically significant compound atoms in plant food that are basically maintained different metabolic pathways, similar to free extremist rummaging, antimicrobial properties and giving assurance against sicknesses [4]. The variety in human eating pattern cannot be detected up to the mark as economic and natural components lead to broad variations in the dietary example of the worldwide populace. The unexpected expansion in clinical consideration expenses and human's craving for upkeep of one's wellbeing bring about more noteworthy consideration for nutritionists and general wellbeing researchers to clarify the eating routine wellbeing linkages [5]. Eating Habits and wellbeing relationships are associating as customer string is shifted and presently, they are more cognizant towards nourishing and practical properties of food. Be that as it may, various procedures are required, to investigate supplements thick sources, their likely usage, and applications, and particularly their method of activities [6]. In any case, vegetables are one of the significant food of human eating routine since antiquated occasions and stand firm on interesting foothold in all dietary direction frameworks. The American Dietician Association suggested day by day 4–5 portions of vegetables to meet the prerequisites of required nutrition. Vegetables are wealthy source of bioactive components like carotenoids, chlorophylls, anthocyanins and flavonoid [7]. All these bioactive compounds can focus on basic level successfully by managing protein energy, arrival of cytokines, and sign transduction. Among the practical food varieties, utilization of garlic is mounting step by step due to its wellbeing advancing expected other than fundamental nourishment [8]. The medicinal usage of different spices have been demonstrated tentatively as lifesaving substances, related with personal fitness, assertions attributable to their abundant phytochemicals profile. Beneficial outcomes of garlic are principally authorized to its sulfur containing compounds essentially allicin and S-allyl cysteine (SAC). Including organosulfur composites, thiosulfates, ajoenes and allicin (diallyl thiosulphate) are the most important bioactive parts in garlic for relieving different physical abnormalities [9]. Connections of essential significance have been established between nutritional parts and individual wellbeing security. There are confirmations that utilization of various vegetables is significant for human wellbeing as they are generally excellent for colon health due to enrichment of fiber, antioxidants, carotenoids, sulfur containing mixtures, nutrients, and minerals. Epidemiological examinations directed worldwide have uncovered that liberal utilization of vegetables particularly rich in nutraceuticals is related with an assurance of anticipation and decrease of wellbeing related persistent issues [10].

2. Garlic

In summary, Garlic (*A. sativum* L.) is one of the leading used potted plant, applied both for healing reasons and gastronomic enhancement as giving spice and palate to the ultimate product. It is assumed to be started from Central Asia around 6 000 a long time earlier and has been expanded on the way to West, South and East [11]. Be that as it may, whole garlic as well as its components/segments is applied since long time ago in Chinese medications certainly 3000 a long time while Egyptians reinforced garlic to pyramid troop to boost their insusceptibility in this manner render secure from different diseases and progress their great execution [12]. Garlic wellbeing advancing viewpoints have been exhibited and it is advised around the area as a nutritional supplement. It is additionally developed for its therapeutic esteem owing to an increment in its utilization equally in culinary and therapeutic. Recently, a wide-ranging offer of its cookery associated

Phytochemicals	Per 100 g	Reference
Energy	149 kcal	These nutrition values of garlic per 100 g is adapted from https://fdc.nal.usda.gov/ndb/foods
Carbohydrates	33.06 g	
Sugars	1 g	
Dietary fiber	1.2 g	
Protein	6.34 g	
Fat	0.5 g	
Vitamins		
Thiamine	0.2 mg	
Riboflavin	0.11 mg	
Niacin	0.7 mg	
Pantothenic acid	0.59 mg	
Vitamin B_6	1.2 mg	
Folate	3 μg	
Vitamin C	31.2 mg	
Minerals		
Calcium	181 mg	
Iron	1.7 mg	
magnesium	25 mg	
Manganese	1.67 mg	
Magnesium	153 mg	
Phosphorus	401 mg	
Potassium	17 mg	
Sodium	1.16 mg	
Zinc	14.2 mg	

Table 1.
Nutrition value of garlic per 100 g.

and recuperative procedures arrive their availability in market (**Table 1**). In numerous nations, wellbeing opportunities of garlic and its unique items have been established [13].

3. Lifestyle ailments

Poor eating behaviors and changing daily routine regularly led to various physiological dangers which includes heart diseases with its impediments, immune dis-functions and development of tumor [14] It is projected that 30–40% of one-of-a-kind illnesses are curable with a full of life way of life and nutritional segments. Pathophysiological impediment scheme must encompass dietary and exercising strategies; specific embattled dietary factors could be a segment of this tactic Diet and wholesome ingredients have a sizeable influence on the immunity workable of the body and fight deficiency of nutrients, like vitamins, polyphenols that minimize the risk of a number of problems such as hyperglycemia and atherosclerosis [15] Plants wealthy in phytochemicals profile have the capacity to fight off free radicals in the body and deteriorates oxidative stress due to presence of free radicals. Among these plants' essential components like phytochemicals, phytosterols, antioxidants and flavonoids have shown hypoglycemics and hypocholesterolemia potential. Functional ingredients and their active compounds have proven beneficial conceivable towards a range of organic threats such as antioxidant, anti-cancer, and immunomodulation [16]. Free radicals present in body has a reactive tendency in nature, injury to body organs. Oxidative stress in body is generated by increased level of free reactive oxygen species. Oxidative stress is an imbalance between the production of reactive oxygen species and antioxidant defense, resulting in tissue damage. Oxidative stress also leads to DNA damage, cardiovascular and neuropathy disorders, and cancers. It is advised to use natural merchandise presenting higher effectivity and safety, as replacer for drug therapy. Various herbal merchandise that may additionally be comprised of one or combination of special antioxidants have been investigated to shield against hepatic injury, having immune modulatory or antiviral residences [17].

4. Garlic in immune nutrition

Diet is an important part of human health. Foods's rich in phytochemicals are usually related to the normal functioning of the immune system. The term "immune nutrition" refers to the intake of certain nutrients that play an important role in balancing the body's immune system. Internal and external factors, but diet plays a vital role in the regulation and normal operation of the immune system [18]. The immune system is an extremely complex device that prevents infections and diseases by controlling malignant cells and foreign cells. For centuries, humans have been looking for substances that enhance immunity. In almost many cultures, garlic and garlic supplements are used as immunity-enhancing substances in addition to claimed beneficial effects. Immunonutrition is usually based on diet, which can strengthen the immune system, maintain homeostasis, and help fight foreign and malignant cells. Several compounds and classes have been identified, which play an important role in the normal function of the immune system [19]. The use of garlic mentioned in the literature can be traced back centuries. Many civilizations rely on its ability to cure various diseases, and even the Egyptians provided food for their teams to strengthen them. Garlic has many modes of action; on the one hand, it acts as an immunostimulant, on the other hand, it may have the function of immunosuppressive agents [20].

The immunostimulant results of garlic and its components/arrangements consist of growth withinside the general white blood cell (WBC) rely on and superior bone-marrow cellularity [21]. The OSC in garlic scavenge oxidizing retailers inhibiting the oxidation of fatty acids, thereby stopping the formation of pro-inflammatory messengers, through interplay with sulfur-containing enzymes. Consumption of garlic ended in inspired synthesis of NO and, in turn, IFN-alpha in humans, which might be useful in viral or proliferative diseases [22].

The ability of bioactive compound of garlic which Is allicin has an ability to prevent immune mediated, concanavalin A (ConA) damage to liver by protecting effect on T-cells and inhabitation of NF-kappa B activation along with protecting effect against adhesion molecule [23]. In different vitro studies it has been proved that adhesion of TNF-alpha-mediated components to extracellular cell and endothelial cells [24]. On human vascular endothelial cells, inhabitancy of molecule-1 TNF-alpha facilitated intracellular and vascular cell connection molecule-1 is negotiated by allicin [25] It also mediates the inhabitation of SDF-1 alpha (CXCL12) T cell migration by activating fibronectin which further helped by down-regulation of T-cell polarization, its adhesion to fibronectin and rearrangement of cortical actin [26].

Allicin may be used as a therapeutic agent to cure chronic inflammatory disorder. Cell mediated T- Helper-1 immune response is activated by cytokines involved in inflammatory bowel disease. This cell mediated T- helper-1 cells and cytokines involved in this disease can be inhabit by regulating interleukin-10 production [27]. Inflammation associated with IBD can be controlled by garlic extract. The other two main components of garlic such as Diallyl sulphide (DAS) and diallyl disulphide (DDAS) has an inhibitory effect against Methicillin-resistant *Staphylococcus aureus* (MRRSA) infection [28]. Garlic extract has ability to protect body against different types of fungi, viruses, and pathological bacteria. In vitro effect of whole extract and identification of novel immunomodulating drugs and other therapeutic alternatives for the treatment of leishmaniasis is linked to specific 10 to 14KDa fraction [29]. generally, elements of garlic such as allicin, DAS, DDAS results in development of cellular immune parameters.

It is determined that garlic extract element S-allyl-Cysteine (SAC) has capability to prevent nitric oxide assembly with the help of repression of murine macrophage, cell line fueled by IF, settlement of protein demonstration and repression of iNOS mRNA [30]. Garlic also stimulate the proliferation of lymphocytes and phagocytosis of macrophages It also induces infiltration of macrophages and lymphocytes in transplanted tumors and initiate splenic hypertrophy [31]. It increases the efficacy of killer cells and lymphokine activated killer cell, increases the production and synthesis of cytokines. All these improved functionalities in the body leads to strong immune response [32]. Garlic and aged garlic extract initiate the Th-1 cellular immune response due to repetition of cytokines [33]. Destruction of immunity due to chemotherapy and electromagnetic contamination is protected by garlic. Aged black garlic can be act an immune modifier due to its ability to maintain the balance of immune function and it is highly effective when it is included in a diet [34].

Inflammation is triggered by stimulation of neutrophils to act of reactive oxygen species and respiratory burst to get rid of the infected deadly pathogen. This is essential component of our body defensive system [35]. Garlic appear to be very helpful in preventing the free radicals' generations from rat neutrophils. This could be effective in inflammation associated pathological condition [30].

Garlic having immunomodulatory ability have been relevant to the clinical applications. Garlic and its extract have capability to enhance innate or specific cell immunity along with improvement in host resistance to toxic pathogenic invades [36]. Innate killer units movement of advanced cancer patients has been enhanced by directing aged black garlic extract [37]. Inclusion of garlic and aged black garlic in diets especially designed for patients suffering from cancer have great impact as an immune nutrition. Garlic possible health advantages have been adopted by eras old used as an resistant supporter against pathogens.

5. Effect of garlic on cardiovascular diseases

In recent history cardiovascular diseases have been a major non-communicable disease. Garlic active main component allicin has helpful effect on cardiovascular system [38]. With the support of pharma kinetics exploration, it has been noticed that sort of allicin is aquaphobic that makes it effortless for allicin to easily carry all through cell layer without any harm to the phospholipid bilayer, leading to metabolized by cell. These metabolites have health benefits and are important to cardiovascular system [39]. It has protecting effect to heart by inducing vasodilation and inhibiting different pathological conditions to CVD, which includes angiotensin, platelet aggregation, hyperlipidemia, hyperglycemia, and cardiac hypertrophy. High cholesterol, high level of homocysteine hypertension and inflammation are the major cause for cardiovascular diseases [40]. Progression of disease with age linked to high risk of dementia and Alzheimer's. oxidative damage is most highlighted cause for cardiovascular problems. Garlic and aged black garlic due to its high profile of antioxidants may be beneficial for protection from heart related problems [41]. A study was performed which proves that allicin has a major antioxidant property that protect heart cells from oxidative stress that leads to cell injury or cell death [42].

Antioxidant estate of allicin was assessed by using 1-diphenyl-2-picrylhydrazyl (DPPH) assay and cell destruction H9C2 Cardio myoblasts induced by hydrogen peroxide (H_2O_2) [43]. It is demonstrated that allicin has shielding impact compared to oxidative damage by reducing intracellular oxidative species creation. It has also defensive influence in opposition to free radical induced myocardial cell death in ischemic condition [44].

6. Effect of garlic on blood glucose levels

Exploring garlic effect on hyperglycemic is still under studied by researchers. Not so many studies have been done by scientist to prove this claim. Presence of bioactive compounds in garlic such as allicin, alliin, diallyl disulfide, diallyl trisulfide, diallyl sulfide, S-allyl cysteine, ajoene and allyl mercaptan is mainly attributed to prevent high glucose level in blood [45]. Insulin resistance can be controlled by garlic extract [46]. It has been proved that aged black garlic extract has beneficial effect on decreasing homocysteine level, lower blood pressure and increase microcirculation that is fundamental for controlling hyperglycemia [47]. Some of studies has showed in favor of hypoglycemic effect of garlic. A study was conducted that proves metformin treatment with garlic has quicker lower of blood glucose level in patients as compared to patients treated with only metformin [48]. Another study was conducted in which patients with type 2 diabetes showed significant improvement in HDL cholesterol along with decrease concentration of LDL cholesterol when they were treated with garlic [47].

7. Anti-carcinogenic effect of garlic

Garlic has countless ability to prevent cancer growth. Anticarcinogenic outcome of garlic has been characterized by diverse mechanisms including upsurge level of glutathione, collective enzymes actions such as S-transferase, catalase, and glutathione, hunting ability to minimize radicals, restoration mechanism of DNA, safety of chromosomal impairment and settlement of cytochrome p4502E1 [49]. Different studies have been proceed including anti-proliferative ability of garlic active compounds to stop the tumor growth in vitro and in vivo [50]. Protein extracted from garlic bulb has significant effect against tumor size. Different studies revealed that individual mammary endothelial and colon cancer cell propagation has been constrained by active compound of garlic allicin [51]. Breast tumor risk is increased by linoleic acid. Garlic has negative effect against linoleic acid by increasing the effect of eicosatetraenoic acid, which is a breast cancer suppressor [52]. Probability of hormone receptive cancer is repressed by Sulfur compounds of garlic such as allyl-sulfides because of its aquaphobic environment and estrogen receptors with cysteine residue in hormone binding [53]. Different studies have been done which proves garlic and organic allyl Sulfur elements has capability to prevent cancer process. Risk of chemical induced tumors in animal model can be reduced by using water soluble component S-allyl-Cysteine which is present in garlic. Proliferation of neoplasms can be reduced by treating with oil soluble compounds such as diallyl disulphide [54].

8. Cholesterol lowering potential

All over the globe mortality and morbidity rate is increasing due to prominent cause of cardiovascular diseases. Atherosclerosis development is associated with mainly low-density lipoproteins (LDLs). Toxic Radicals initiate and increases the lipids peroxidation that further leads to increase in concentration of free radicals that disturb normal physiology of body including atherosclerosis. To colonize effect of cardiovascular disorders cholesterol controlling therapy is major vital to this [39]. Nearly All of the time patients having high-level percentage of cholesterol with other disorder is treated with drug which has side impact along with prerequisite of time. People are diverting their intentions to the natural sources to cure diseases. Garlic has been being used in natural medicine to cure lipid profile [55]. Different supplements have been invented that presents remarkable positive effect on regulating cholesterol, LDL cholesterol, and high-density lipoprotein (HDL) cholesterol and contributed to inhibit progression of disease [56].

Garlic and garlic supplements along with specific preparations have benefits to lowering cholesterol levels, blood pressure with decreasing platelets aggregation and inhibition LDL oxidation [57]. Garlic oil and extracts have also been used to lower the cholesterol level due to presence of bioactive component. A study was done to check the efficacy of garlic against cholesterol which showed decline in total cholesterol level as compared to garlic preparations such as oil [58]. Effect of garlic on lipid profile showed significant decrease of triglycerides level. Aqueous extract of garlic has sufficiency of decreasing cholesterol synthesis up to 75% without any cellular toxicity mediated by 4-alpha-methyl oxidase. It is effective against reducing coronary calcium progression [59].

In isoproterenol induced myocardial ischemia activity of lecithin acyl transferase was substantially improved along with control of 3-hydroxy-3methylgutaryl-coA reductase enzyme by garlic element S-allyl cysteine sulfoxide [60]. According to scientists observations, cholesterol synthesis can be controlled up to 40–60% by SAC, S-propyl cysteine and S-ethyl cysteine [61]. Garlic has capability to increase sulfhydryl oxidation that apparently hinder production of 3-hydroxy 3-methyl glutaryl-CoA reductase enzyme activity [62]. Yet there is not any significant mechanism to evaluate the process of reducing atherosclerosis disease progression. Further establishment should be managed to develop the relation among other garlic preparations, their antioxidant status and blood lipid profile.

9. Atherosclerosis and hyperlipidemia

The pathogenesis of atherosclerosis also includes defectiveness of microvascular perfusion, which further leads to impaired wound healing. Nitric Oxide (NO) is a crucial modulator for endothelial regeneration, vasorelaxation and leucocytic chemotaxis inhibition. The poor microvascular perfusion is due to impaired release of NO because of reduced local endothelial NO synthase (eNOS) induced by atherosclerosis linked endothelial damage. Aged garlic extract (AGE) has been shown positive therapeutic effects in wound healing through NO dependent pathways, enhancing vascular elasticity and endothelial function. In a cohort of 93 patients with confirmed atherosclerosis, 2400 mg daily ACE for a year showed a significant improvement in peripheral tissue perfusion and increase microcirculation, thus, facilitated wound healing [63]. Cardiovascular disease (CVD) leads to serious secondary manifestations such as Coronary atherosclerosis, a subsequent of hyperlipidemia, which can be further modifies if started with calcium disposition, known as calcification atherosclerotic lesions. Coronary artery calcification (CAC) is a well validated prognostic marker for the risk of ischemic heart diseases. Randomized Clinical Trial (RCT) showed a significant decrease in CAC progression with the introduction of AGE. It was also noted during experiments that AGE has had a major advantageous impact on inflammation by decreasing Interlukin-6 in patients with atherosclerosis [64, 65]. It is also evident that the high organosulfur properties of black garlic has an antioxidant effect to reduce atherosclerosis [61]. Bacterial Infections: The antibacterial activity attributed to allicin component makes garlic effective against numerous antibiotic-resistant, gram positive and gram-negative bacteria such as Shigella, *Escherichia coli*, *Staphylococcus aureus*, *Pseudomonas aeruginosa*, Streptococcus mutants, *S. faecalis*, *S. pyogenes*, *Salmonella enterica*, *Klebsiella aerogenes*, Vibrio, Mycobacteria, *Proteus vulgaris*, and *Enterococcus faecalis*. The garlic extracts such as aqueous, methanolic, and ethanolic have been reported for inhibitory effects against *E. coli* and Sal. Typhi strains and other pathogenic bacteria cause diarrheal infections in humans. Garlic also showed effectiveness in preventing the toxins produced by bacteria, and towards methicillin-resistant *S. aureus* (MRSA) infections. Allicin chemical interaction with thioredoxin reductase, RNA polymerase, and alcohol dehydrogenase makes it as an effective component in antibacterial activity. Allicin can act as a biocide in killing all eukaryotic cells by influencing cysteine proteinase metabolism [66]. Encouraging findings have been attained by the use of allicin as an antimicrobial macrophage enhancer in handling drug susceptible or drug resistance *Mycobacterium tuberculosis* infection [67]. The characteristic of forming a biofilm helps resist bacteria against certain antibiotics drugs, which has become a global concern in treatment of bacterial infection. Hydrophobic compounds such as allicin found to be as an acting agent in inhibition of bacterial biofilm formation. Other hydrophobic garlic components such as vinyl dithiins, ajoenes and diallyl polysulfides showed similar biofilm formation suppressing effects help prevent drug resistance and enhance the efficacy of existing antibiotics [68]. For example, the anti-biofilm activity of fresh garlic extract (FGE) showed 35–59% less biofilm formation in Shiga toxin producing *Escherichia coli* (STEC) samples when studied in vitro [69]. Garlic was also being used as an effective antibacterial agent for the prevention of gas gangrene during World War II [70].

10. Fungal and parasitic infections

Garlic is an excellent antifungal agent against Candida, Torulosis, Trichophyton, Cryptococcus, Aspergillus, Trichopteran, and Rhodotorula species. It is evident that the components present in garlic extracts namely aqueous, ethanolic, methanolic, and petroleum ether act as antifungal agents against different human pathogenic fungal species such as Trichophyton verrucosum, T. mentagrophytes, *T. rubrum*, Botrytis cinerea, Candida species, Epidermophyton floccose, Aspergillus niger, *A. flavus*, Rhizopus stolonifera, Microspore gypsum, M. audouinii, Alternaria alternate, Neofabraea alba, and Penicillium expansum. The mechanism involves the irreversible ultrastructural changes that eventually leads to fungal cells death. Saponin components present in garlic showed effective antifungal properties against Botrytis cinerea and Trichoderma harzianum [71]. It has been observed that the garlic could inhibit the fungal growth as equally as the antifungal drugs such as ketoconazole. There is an evidence of an effective antiparasitic activity of garlic against parasites such as *Schistosoma mansoni*, Hymenolepis diminuta, *H. microstoma*, and Taenia taeniaeformis, *Fasciola hepatica*, Plasmodium falciparum and Trypanosoma brucei, and Echinostoma caproni. The mechanism of action involves helping create antioxidants which eventually leads to reduced number of parasite eggs and low birth rate of new worms. Garlic is also helpful in treating human intestinal parasitic infection caused by *Entamoeba histolytica* and *Giardia lamblia* (chronic giardiasis) [72]. Garlic also possesses anthelmintic characteristics helpful in discarding injurious parasites in the intestine [73]. Sulphureous components of garlic make it an effective eliminating agent for intestinal tapeworms. Viral Infections: Garlic is found to be an effective herb against numerous viral infections and diseases. The antiviral components in garlic against influenza B, Human Immunodeficiency Virus (HIV), vesicular stomatitis virus, herpes simplex virus (types 1 and 2) has been demonstrated. The Ajoene component present in garlic prevents Human Immunodeficiency Virus (HIV) induced destruction of CD+ cells and boost cellular immunity, induces apoptosis of infected cells in Human cytomegalovirus (HCMV), inhibits adhesive interactions and fusion of leukocytes in HIV infected platelet aggregation and fusion assays, inhibits HIV cell attachment, and occludes HIV-induced CD4 T-cells destruction. Allicin, allyl methyl thiosulfate, and methyl allyl thiosulfate inhibit numerous virus particles entry via disruption of viral envelope and cell membrane. The lectins present in garlic help inhibit HIV-1 replication and also inhibit the early and the late infectious cycle in severe acute respiratory syndrome (SARS-CoV) [74] The antiviral potential of garlic against a number of viruses like influenza B, HIV (type 1), vesicular stomatitis virus, herpes simplex virus (types 1 and 2), coxsackievirus species, and gamma retrovirus was earlier demonstrated. The recent data has revealed that chymotrypsin-like protease (3CLpro) is a common main protease in both type 1 and type 2 SARS-CoV. The inhibition of 3CLpro in SARS-CoV was most possibly considered by seven alliin derived organosulfur compounds (OSCs). Detailed analysis revealed that alliin has the highest antiviral potency in preventing COVID-19. There is a possibility of SARS-CoV-2 elimination with the lowest side effects and toxicity by using garlic based bioactive components alone or in combination.

11. Conclusion

Garlic is one of the most vital herbaceous herbal that have been discovered next to a variety of lifetime associated ailments. Its richness in phytochemicals helps body go through abnormalities. Garlic includes magnesium, calcium, selenium, vitamin B_1 and vitamin B_6 tryptophan and protein. These components provide harmonious effect against various physiological disorders to increase preventive measure effects. More research should be designed to clarify claim of diseases. It has been identified that sulfur containing compounds in garlic has major role to prevent diseases and to insure pharmacological effect. Globally, it is consumed in different forms such as powder, extract, oil, and capsules. It should be added more frequently in diet due to its unique phytochemical's moieties. Garlic has wide application such as anti-inflammatory, antidiabetic, anticarcinogenic, antihyperlipidemic, antifungal, antiviral, and antiatherosclerosis.

Conflict of interest

The authors proclaim not any contradiction.

Author details

Mavra Javed[1*], Waqas Ahmed[1], Rehan Mian[2] and Abdul Momin Rizwan Ahmad[3]

1 Department of Food Science and Human Nutrition, University of Veterinary and Animal Sciences, Lahore, Pakistan

2 The Healthy World Organization, Lahore, Pakistan

3 Department of Human Nutrition and Dietetics, National University of Medical Sciences (NUMS), Rawalpindi, Pakistan

*Address all correspondence to: javedmavra@gmail.com

References

[1] Hueda MC. Functional Food: Improve Health through Adequate Food: BoD–Books on Demand; 2017.

[2] Rezai G, Teng PK, Shamsudin MN, Mohamed Z, Stanton JLJJoAiD, Economies E. Effect of perceptual differences on consumer purchase intention of natural functional food. 2017.

[3] Ali A, Rahut DBJIJofs. Healthy foods as proxy for functional foods: consumers' awareness, perception, and demand for natural functional foods in Pakistan. 2019;2019.

[4] Vicentini A, Liberatore L, Mastrocola DJIJoFS. Functional foods: trends and development of the global market. 2016;28(2).

[5] Küster-Boluda I, Vidal-Capilla IJSJoM-E. Consumer attitudes in the election of functional foods. 2017;21:65-79.

[6] Pappalardo G, Lusk JLJFq, preference. The role of beliefs in purchasing process of functional foods. 2016;53:151-158.

[7] Gul K, Singh A, Jabeen RJCrifs, nutrition. Nutraceuticals and functional foods: The foods for the future world. 2016;56(16):2617-2627.

[8] Wang H, Huang DJJoFF. Dietary organosulfur compounds from garlic and cruciferous vegetables as potent hypochlorite scavengers. 2015;18:986-993.

[9] Locatelli DA, Nazareno MA, Fusari C, Camargo ABJFc. Cooked garlic and antioxidant activity: Correlation with organosulfur compound composition. 2017;220:219-224.

[10] del Río-Celestino M, Font R. The health benefits of fruits and vegetables. Multidisciplinary Digital Publishing Institute; 2020.

[11] Locatelli DA, Altamirano JC, González RE, Camargo ABJJoFF. Home-cooked garlic remains a healthy food. 2015;16:1-8.

[12] Takagi H. Garlic *Allium sativum* L. Onions and allied crops: CRC Press; 2020. p. 109-146.

[13] S Bisen P, Emerald MJCN, Science F. Nutritional and therapeutic potential of garlic and onion (Allium sp.). 2016;12(3):190-9.

[14] Shafiq M, Qadir A, Ahmad SJAEER. Biofortification: A sustainable agronomic strategy to increase selenium content and antioxidant activity in Garlic. 2019;17(2):1685-1704.

[15] Noce A, Romani A, Bernini R. Dietary Intake and Chronic Disease Prevention. Multidisciplinary Digital Publishing Institute; 2021.

[16] Papas AM. Antioxidant status, diet, nutrition, and health: CRC press; 2019.

[17] Armstrong D, Stratton RD. Oxidative stress and antioxidant protection: The science of free radical biology and disease: John Wiley & Sons; 2016.

[18] Venter C, Eyerich S, Sarin T, Klatt KCJN. Nutrition and the immune system: a complicated tango. 2020;12(3):818.

[19] Lindsay KJN. Nutrition for immune health. 2021.

[20] Khodadadi SJIP. Role of herbal medicine in boosting immune system. 2015;1(1):e01.

[21] Mamatha T, Kazmi SJJoPS, Research. Garlic: an updated review on

multipotential medicinal applications. 2017;9(10):1874-1881.

[22] Upadhyay RKJIJoGP. Garlic: A potential source of pharmaceuticals and pesticides: A review. 2016;10(1).

[23] Xia ZJJoTCVM. Effects of garlic polysaccharide on the levels of GPT and GOT in serum and liver of mice with liver-injury. 2011:04.

[24] Ohtani M, Nishimura TJBr. Sulfur-containing amino acids in aged garlic extract inhibit inflammation in human gingival epithelial cells by suppressing intercellular adhesion molecule-1 expression and IL-6 secretion. 2020;12(3):99-108.

[25] Chakraborty D, Majumder AJBRT. Garlic (Lahsun)–an immunity booster against SARS-CoV-2. 2020;2(8):755-7.

[26] Khuda-Bukhsh AR, Saha SK, Das S, Saha SS. Molecular approaches toward targeted cancer therapy with some food plant products: On the role of antioxidants and immune microenvironment. Cancer: Elsevier; 2021. p. 191-202.

[27] Arsenijevic D, Stojanovic B, Milovanovic J, Arsenijevic A, Simic M, Pergal M, et al. Hepatoprotective Effect of Mixture of Dipropyl Polysulfides in Concanavalin A-Induced Hepatitis. 2021;13(3):1022.

[28] Putri UM, Rochmanti M, Wahyunitisari MR, Setiabudi RJJIJoFM, Toxicology. The Antibacterial Effect of Ethanol Extract of Garlic (*Allium sativum* L.) on Methicillin Resistant *Staphylococcus aureus* (MRSA) In Vitro. 2021;15(2).

[29] Zhang M, Zhong J, Xiong Y, Song X, Li C, He ZJV. Development of Broad-Spectrum Antiviral Agents—Inspiration from Immunomodulatory Natural Products. 2021;13(7):1257.

[30] Albrakati AJES, Research P. Aged garlic extract rescues ethephon-induced kidney damage by modulating oxidative stress, apoptosis, inflammation, and histopathological changes in rats. 2021;28(6):6818-6829.

[31] Kaur G, Gupta RJPA. GARLIC: NATURE'S PROTECTION AGAINST WOUNDS. 2021;21(1):2446-2455.

[32] Imran M, Rauf A, Khalil AA, Bawazeer S, Patel S, Shah ZA. Anti-Inflammatory Properties of Bioactive Compounds from Medicinal Plants. Health Benefits of Secondary Phytocompounds from Plant and Marine Sources: Apple Academic Press; 2021. p. 81-108.

[33] Shirgholami Z, Borji H, Mohebalian H, Heidarpour MJEP. Effects of *Allium sativum* on IFN-γ and IL4 concentrations in mice with cystic echinococcosis. 2021;220:108042.

[34] Ogbuewu I, Okoro V, Mbajiorgu CJAFS, Technology. Meta-analysis of the responses of laying hens to garlic (*Allium sativum*) supplementation. 2021:114866.

[35] Deretic VJI. Autophagy in inflammation, infection, and immunometabolism. 2021;54(3):437-53.

[36] Pawar Y, Patil AJBRT. Garlic: An Immunity Booster Spice during Pandemic Situation. 2020;2(9):978-980.

[37] Sembiring NB, Iskandar YJMOT. A Review of Component and Pharmacology Activities of Black Garlic. 2019;24(3):178-183.

[38] Q Alali F, El-Elimat T, Khalid L, Hudaib R, Saleh Al-Shehabi T, H Eid AJCpd. Garlic for cardiovascular disease: prevention or treatment? 2017;23(7):1028-41.

[39] Sobenin IA, Myasoedova VA, Iltchuk MI, Zhang D-W, Orekhov

ANJCjonm. Therapeutic effects of garlic in cardiovascular atherosclerotic disease. 2019;17(10):721-728.

[40] Siddiqui MF, Ahmed A, Bano BJIjobm. Insight into the biochemical, kinetic and spectroscopic characterization of garlic (*Allium sativum*) phytocystatin: Implication for cardiovascular disease. 2017;95:734-42.

[41] Hosseini A, Hosseinzadeh HJJoei. A review on the effects of *Allium sativum* (Garlic) in metabolic syndrome. 2015;38(11):1147-1157.

[42] Atkin M, Laight D, Cummings MHJJoD, Complications i. The effects of garlic extract upon endothelial function, vascular inflammation, oxidative stress and insulin resistance in adults with type 2 diabetes at high cardiovascular risk. A pilot double blind randomized placebo controlled trial. 2016;30(4): 723-727.

[43] Ma L, Chen S, Li S, Deng L, Li Y, Li HJE-BC, et al. Effect of allicin against ischemia/hypoxia-induced H9c2 myoblast apoptosis via eNOS/NO pathway-mediated antioxidant activity. 2018;2018.

[44] Barteková M, Adameová A, Görbe A, Ferenczyová K, Pecháňová O, Lazou A, et al. Natural and synthetic antioxidants targeting cardiac oxidative stress and redox signaling in cardiometabolic diseases. 2021;169:446-477.

[45] Shabani E, Sayemiri K, Mohammadpour MJPcd. The effect of garlic on lipid profile and glucose parameters in diabetic patients: A systematic review and meta-analysis. 2019;13(1):28-42.

[46] Maeda T, Miki S, Morihara N, Kagawa YJE, medicine t. Aged garlic extract ameliorates fatty liver and insulin resistance and improves the gut microbiota profile in a mouse model of insulin resistance. 2019;18(1):857-866.

[47] Zhu Y, Anand R, Geng X, Ding YJNr. A mini review: garlic extract and vascular diseases. 2018;40(6): 421-425.

[48] Fadheel QJJRJoP, Technology. A Comparative Study of the effect of Metformin and Metformin plus Garlic on Blood Glucose Level in patients with Type 2 Diabetes Mellitus in Iraq. 2019;12(4):1806-10.

[49] Zhang Y, Liu X, Ruan J, Zhuang X, Zhang X, Li ZJB, et al. Phytochemicals of garlic: Promising candidates for cancer therapy. 2020;123:109730.

[50] Kanamori Y, Dalla Via L, Macone A, Canettieri G, Greco A, Toninello A, et al. Aged garlic extract and its constituent, S-allyl-L-cysteine, induce the apoptosis of neuroblastoma cancer cells due to mitochondrial membrane depolarization. 2020;19(2):1511-1521.

[51] Amani M, Shokati E, Entezami K, Khorrami S, Jazayeri MH, Safari EJPB. The Immunomodulatory Effects of Low Molecular Weight Garlic Protein in Crosstalk between Peripheral Blood Mononuclear Cells and Colon Cancer Cells. 2021.

[52] Desai G, Schelske-Santos M, Nazario CM, Rosario-Rosado RV, Mansilla-Rivera I, Ramírez-Marrero F, et al. Onion and garlic intake and breast cancer, a case-control study in Puerto Rico. 2020;72(5):791-800.

[53] Sheikh Raisuddin SA, Fatima M, Dabeer SJAoP. Toxicity of anticancer drugs and its prevention with special reference to role of garlic constituents. 2018;7(1):13-26.

[54] Agbana YL, Ni Y, Zhou M, Zhang Q, Kassegne K, Karou SD, et al. Garlic-derived bioactive compound S-allylcysteine inhibits cancer progression through diverse molecular mechanisms. 2020;73:1-14.

[55] Ansary J, Forbes-Hernández TY, Gil E, Cianciosi D, Zhang J, Elexpuru-Zabaleta M, et al. Potential health benefit of garlic based on human intervention studies: A brief overview. 2020;9(7):619.

[56] Poli A, Visioli FJHBP, Prevention C. Pharmacology of nutraceuticals with lipid lowering properties. 2019;26(2):113-118.

[57] Zeb F, Safdar M, Fatima S, Khan S, Alam S, Muhammad M, et al. Supplementation of garlic and coriander seed powder: Impact on body mass index, lipid profile and blood pressure of hyperlipidemic patients. 2018;31(5).

[58] Utami M, Pantaya D, Agus A, editors. Addition of garlic extract in ration to reduce cholesterol level of broiler. Journal of Physics: Conference Series; 2018: IOP Publishing.

[59] Nazeri Z, Azizidoost S, Cheraghzadeh M, Mohammadi A, Kheirollah AJAJoP. Increased protein expression of ABCA1, HMG-CoA reductase, and CYP46A1 induced by garlic and allicin in the brain mouse and astrocytes-isolated from C57BL/6J. 2021.

[60] Islam D, Shanta MB, Akhter S, Lyzu C, Hakim M, Islam MR, et al. Cardioprotective effect of garlic extract in isoproterenol-induced myocardial infarction in a rat model: assessment of pro-apoptotic caspase-3 gene expression. 2020;6(1):1-9.

[61] Saryono, Proverawati A, editors. The potency of black garlic as anti-atherosclerotic: Mechanisms of action and the prospectively. AIP Conference Proceedings; 2019: AIP Publishing LLC.

[62] El-Sebaey AM, Abdelhamid FM, Abdalla OAJES, Research P. Protective effects of garlic extract against hematological alterations, immunosuppression, hepatic oxidative stress, and renal damage induced by cyclophosphamide in rats. 2019;26(15): 15559-15572.

[63] Lindstedt S, Wlosinska M, Nilsson AC, Hlebowicz J, Fakhro M, Sheikh RJIWJ. Successful improved peripheral tissue perfusion was seen in patients with atherosclerosis after 12 months of treatment with aged garlic extract. 2021.

[64] Wlosinska M, Nilsson A-C, Hlebowicz J, Hauggaard A, Kjellin M, Fakhro M, et al. The effect of aged garlic extract on the atherosclerotic process–a randomized double-blind placebo-controlled trial. 2020;20(1):1-10.

[65] Wlosinska M, Nilsson A-C, Hlebowicz J, Fakhro M, Malmsjö M, Lindstedt SJE-BC, et al. Aged garlic extract reduces IL-6: A double-blind placebo-controlled trial in females with a low risk of cardiovascular disease. 2021;2021.

[66] El-Saber Batiha G, Magdy Beshbishy A, G Wasef L, Elewa YH, A Al-Sagan A, El-Hack A, et al. Chemical constituents and pharmacological activities of garlic (*Allium sativum* L.): A review. 2020;12(3):872.

[67] Dwivedi VP, Bhattacharya D, Singh M, Bhaskar A, Kumar S, Fatima S, et al. Allicin enhances antimicrobial activity of macrophages during *Mycobacterium tuberculosis* infection. 2019;243:111634.

[68] Nakamoto M, Kunimura K, Suzuki JI, Kodera YJE, medicine t. Antimicrobial properties of hydrophobic compounds in garlic: Allicin, vinyldithiin, ajoene and diallyl polysulfides. 2020;19(2):1550-1553.

[69] Bhatwalkar SB, Gound SS, Mondal R, Srivastava RK, Anupam RJIjom. Anti-biofilm and antibacterial activity of *Allium sativum* against drug resistant shiga-toxin producing *Escherichia coli* (STEC) isolates from

patient samples and food Sources. 2019;59(2):171-179.

[70] Gudalwar BR, Nimbalwar MG, Panchale WA, Wadekar AB, Manwar JV, Bakal RLJGAR, et al. *Allium sativum*, a potential phytopharmacological source of natural medicine for better health. 2021;6(3):220-232.

[71] El-Saber Batiha G, Magdy Beshbishy A, L GW, Elewa YHA, A AA-S, Abd El-Hack ME, et al. Chemical Constituents and Pharmacological Activities of Garlic (*Allium sativum* L.): A Review. Nutrients. 2020;12(3).

[72] Khanmohammadi M, Rasi-Bonab F. Garlic and its effects on parasitic diseases2018.

[73] Mayekar VM, Ali A, Alim H, Patel NJPST. A review: Antimicrobial activity of the medicinal spice plants to cure human disease. 2021;8(3): 629-46-–46.

[74] Rouf R, Uddin SJ, Sarker DK, Islam MT, Ali ES, Shilpi JA, et al. Antiviral potential of garlic (Allium sativum) and its organosulfur compounds: A systematic update of pre-clinical and clinical data. Trends in food science & technology. 2020;104:219-234.

Chapter 9

Phyto-Potential of *Allium cepa* and *Allium sativum*

Rubi Gupta and Prashant Kaushik

Abstract

Garlic and onion are either cooked like a vegetable because of their green leaves or are also used as a condiment. Many scientific studies affirm the positives of both for their anti-inflammatory, antioxidant, and antimicrobial potential. Moreover, garlic and onion are regularly employed to treat cardiovascular illnesses, strokes, atherosclerosis, hypertension, hyperlipidemias, and thrombosis, and are also proved effective against Alzheimer's, diabetes, and cancers. Here we have compiled a piece of information regarding the compounds present in garlic and onion along with their pharmacological properties. Although much more studies are required to refine the utilization and enhance garlic and medicine's effectiveness. We hope this work will provide helpful information regarding their pharmacological aspects.

Keywords: antioxidants, compounds, garlic, onion, pharmacological

1. Introduction

The members of family Alliaceae both Garlic (*Allium sativum*) and onion (*Allium cepa*) are beneficial for human health because of high content of nutraceutical compounds. Moreover, they are extensively cultivated and are readily available. Moreover, there is a continuous rise in garlic and onion production within the past 10 years. This escalation in these plants' development might be connected to the dietary and therapeutic attributes of these plants. *Allium sativum* as well as *Allium cepa*, have been known for the therapeutic value. Most classical Egyptian records also highlight onion and garlic for their medicinal and therapeutic effect. The Father of Ayurvedic medication, Charaka, has also applied the advantages of onion in maintaining blood pressure and balance of good cholesterol. Similarly, garlic use can be an all-natural option for managing parasite infection, esophagus infections, digestive problems, and fungal diseases.

Garlic and onion have a high amount of carbohydrates. While garlic comprises of 33.06% carbohydrate, onion possesses around 9.34% of carbohydrates. The volume of soluble fiber in garlic and onion are 2.1% along with 1.7%, respectively. A small amount of monounsaturated and polyunsaturated fatty acids may additionally be found in garlic and onion. In this direction, the volume of Quercetin is more as when as opposed with various other flavanols. Garlic is plentiful in organosulfur mixture alliin (Sallylcysteine sulfoxide). Enzyme alliinase can flip alliin into allicin. Onion bulb has ()-S-alk(en)yl-L-cysteine sulfoxide and -glutamyl peptide cysteine within an astonishing amount. These factors are responsible for 70% of the whole sulfur in onion. Garlic can incorporate all-natural selenium elements in addition to steroidal saponins.

2. Compounds present in onion and garlic

2.1 Onion

Majority (80–95%) of the fresh weight of onion is water. Non-structural carbohydrates like glucose, fructose, sucrose, and fructo-oligosaccharides (FOS) consist of up to 65% of onion's dry weight. Kestose (GF2), fructofuranosylnystose (GF4), and nystose (GF3) are the main FOS in onion bulb. The significant phenolics in onions are the flavonoids [1]. Quercetin and kaempferol are the most abundant flavonoids present in onions. Quercetin 4′-glucoside and quercetin 3,4′-diglucoside are reported as the main onion flavanols of the flesh whereas quercetin aglycon is found in higher concentration in the skin of onions. Major phenolic compounds present in onion are Gallic acid, Ferulic acid, Quercetin, Kaempferol and Chlorogenic acid. Onion is also an important source of phytonutrients, the important phytochemicals present in onions are inulin, kestose, nystose, and fructo-furanosylnystose [2]. Onion is also composed of several aldehydes and ketones. Aldehydes present in onion are propionaldehyde, Methyl-2-pentenal, Furfuraldehyde, 5-Methyl-2-furfuraldehyde ketonic compound present are 1,2-Cyclopentanedione, Butyrolactone. The most unique component of onions are the sulfur-containing compounds, such as 1-Propanethiol, Propylene sulfide, Dimethyl sulfide, Methyl propyl disulfide, cis-Methyl-1-propenyl disulfide, Methyl-1,3-thiazole, trans-Methyl-1-propenyl disulfide, 4-Dimethyl thiophene, Methyl-2-propenyl disulfide, Dipropyl disulfide, 1,2,4-Trithiolane, trans-Propenyl propyl disulfide, cis-Propenyl propyl disulfide, Methyl propyl trisulfide, Dipropyl trisulfide.

2.2 Garlic

Garlic has been reported to be composed of higher concentration of sulfur compounds. Among the sulfur compounds, Allicin or S-allyl-cysteine sulfoxide (ACSO) is the most important constituent of garlic [3, 4]. Methyl allyl disulfide, *trans*-Propenyl methyl disulfide, dimethyl trisulfide, diallyl disulfude, methyl allyl trisulfide, 2-Vinyl-1.3-dithiane, 1.4-dimethyl tetrasulfide, 1.4-dimethyl tetrasulfide, diallyl trisulfide, eugenol, α-Caryophyllene, α-Guaiene, aromadendrene, α-Bisabolene, γ-Cadinene, diallyl tetrasulfide, elemicin are the sulfur containing compounds present in garlic. Other compounds, such as ajoenes, and other sulfur-containing compounds, such as 1,2-vinyldithiin, allixin and S-allyl-cysteine present in garlic are reported to have bioactive properties.

3. Pharmacological activities of garlic and onion

3.1 Antiviral

Flavonoids found in onion and garlic have a strong inhibitory effect on virus multiplication. Phytochemicals found in these plants have been observed to block the improvement of genetic material and protein within the disease. Onion has Quercetin and kaempferol as main flavanols. These factors are found to impact the improvement of huge viruses. Onion extracts were efficient in reducing infection of New Castle Disease illness. Nevertheless, Coxsackie Bl condition was not affected by the addition of garlic extracts. In another analysis, garlic was observed to significantly decrease the common cold virus's occurrence. Chemicals such as ajoene, diallyl disulphide in garlic can act against HIV infected cells. In an experimental evaluation, compounds like diallyl disulphide (DADS), diallyl sulphide (DAS) and alliin substantially reduced inflammation during dengue disorders disease.

Onion and garlic could provide an alternative treatment for viral illness and protection against severe disease development. Viruses demand several enzymes for replication. Viruses are dependent on cellular machinery for a selection of replication processes. Antiviral drugs generally focus on the process of virus cycle as connection, uncoating, replication of genetic material, interpretation, and release. Quercetin may be the central combination in onion connected with an anti-infective and anti-replicative effect over the illness.

Many researchers have performed research to elucidate the mechanism of quercetin effectivity against viruses. Quercetin is ascertained to inhibit viral entry or perhaps inhibitinterferingents required for viral replication. Since onion is a rich source of Quercetin, therefore onion may be utilized to lessen viral infection. In an exciting study, Quercetin was observed to interact with Haemagglutinin protein-rich foods, which led to the inhibition of viral replication into the cellular. This was due to a decrease in viral RNA Polymerase, an enzyme needed to replicate the viral genome. Similarly, Quercetin was observed to stop the translation process of the hepatitis C disorders. A lot more intriguing analysis suggests that Quercetin can induce mitochondrial biogenesis in cells, that might further minimize susceptibility to influenza. Quercetin inhibits the Human Immunodeficiency Virus integrase and overturn transcriptase enzymes in HIV infected cells. Quercetin also provides the chance to disturb the activation of RNA polymerase by lessening the processing of polyprotein by Rhinovirus proteases.

Few authors have identified strategies by which allicin and garlic prevent viral illness, although these strategies are much more focused on modifications in a multitude of cellular machinery. Allicin can modulate the body 's immune system in response to viral infection. Allicin comes with an amazing amount of selenium and sulfur and thus imparts antioxidant activity by responding with intracellular thiol components... Since onion is a natural resource of Quercetin, for that main reason, it ought to be further investigated to produce a great medicine against the disease.

3.2 Antifungal activity

Study on the efficacy of garlic extract on candida colonies has been reported to be substantially effective. Moreover, ajoene, present in garlic plays an excellent role as a topical antifungal agent. The study even revealed that garlic stimulated phagocytic activity. Garlic induces the body 's very own defenses which helps in the control of fungal infections. Besides, external application of garlic oil allows in the treatment of ringworm, warts, and skin parasites (Mikali et al., 2013). Oil extract from onion has been demonstrated to exhibit an inhibitory effect on *Aspergillus niger* and Penicillium. In contrast, the fungicidal effect was viewed on the growth of *Aspergillus carbonarius*, *Aspergillus wentii*, *Aspergillus versicolor*, *Penicillium brevicompactum*, *Penicillium* glabrum, *Penicillium chrysogenum*, and *Fusarium* spp. The application of onion essential oil has also reported to cause changes in macro-morphology and micro-morphology of fungi (Tanackov et al., 2016).

3.3 Antiparasitic activity

A study by [5], on the antiparasitic activity of Allicin indicated that it is effective against *Plasmodium falciparum* and *Trypanosoma brucei*. Ajoene isolated from *A. sativum* has also been reported to show antiparasitic actions [6, 7]. Alchinal, preparation of three different substances, *Echinacea purpurea*, *A. sativum* extracts and cocoa, has been demonstrated to significantly decreases the number of larvae of Trichinella spiralis. Moreover, garlic oil is also reported to be effective against some microorganisms like *Plasmodium* spp., *Trypanosoma* spp., *Leishmania* spp., *Giardia* spp., and *Cochlospermum planchonii* [8]. Also, Hymenolepiasis and giardiasis were demonstrated to be affected by garlic extract [9].

3.4 Anti-diabetic activity

Several experiments on mice and rats have demonstrated the efficacy of garlic in decreasing blood sugar in streptozotocin-induced and alloxan-induced diabetes mellitus. According to published reports, *S*-methyl L-cysteine from garlic and onion effectively treats and controls diabetes. Diallyl disulphide of garlic oil has a hypolipidemic effect and reduces the morbidity in diabetes. The *S*-allyl-mercaptocaptopril has proven to be a promising antidiabetic and cardiovascular protective agent integrates the antihypertensive feature between allicin and captopril. Garlic improves metabolic syndrome such as abdominal obesity, hypertension, dyslipidemia, and hyperglycemia disorders, and prevents obesity by the downregulation of gene expression patterns (Kim et al., 2011). Various reports on onion components, such as *S*-methylcysteine and flavonoids, have demonstrated their antidiabetic effect. These compounds decrease blood glucose levels, serum lipids, oxidative stress, and lipid peroxidation, while increasing insulin secretion and antioxidant enzyme activity. A study by Gautam et al., 2015 showed that the ethanolic extract of onion controls diabetes by the phosphatidylinositol-4,5-bisphosphate 3-kinase/Akt dependent pathway.

3.5 Anti-inflammatory and antioxidative effects

Garlic and onion have shown to have anti-inflammatory and antioxidant activity [29]. Allicin from garlic have been reported to show a significant protective effect against endothelial cell injury induced by PM2.5. Allicin from garlic may help reduce oxidative stress, inflammation, vascular dysfunction, and the aortic pathology . Diallyl trisulfide found in Garlic is now being studied as an important therapeutic candidate for inflammation related neurodegenerative diseases treatment. It is also a potential therapeutic agent for periodontal inflammation (Fu et al., 2015). It downregulates the AKT1/TGF-β-activated kinase-mediated NFκB and MAPK signaling pathways that leads to an anti-inflammatory effect. Research on the effect of onion stalk extract on inflammatory diseases has reported it to be a potential agent used to reduce atherosclerosis and regulate inflammatory response. It has been known that fresh garlic and onion extracts enhances immune function. Many immunological disorders like ulcerative colitis, Crohn's disease, and intestinal inflammation are reported to be treated by allyl methyl disulfide from fresh garlic extract. Moreover, the recalcitrant multiple common warts have better cure using lipid garlic extract as immunotherapy. Garlic is also reported to stimulate macrophages, lymphocytes, natural killer (NK) cells, eosinophils, and dendritic cells, thus enhancing the immune system functioning. Garlic extract modulates cytokine secretion, immunoglobulin production, phagocytosis, and macrophage activation to boost the immune system.

3.6 Anticancer activity

Compounds found in garlic are demonstrated to have anti-cancerous activity. As reported, allicin improves the immune function and inhibits tumor vessel formation, it helps in inhibiting the development and metastasis of colorectal cancer. It induces the expression of surviving genes to promote apoptosis of cancer cells, leading to inhibition of tumor formation [10]. Allicin inhibits H2O2-induced senescence in human umbilical vein endothelial cells through activation of *SIRT1* [11]. Chhabria et al. in 2015 demonstrated the use of allicin as a therapy to improve pancreatic cancer, which suppresses cancer cell growth by reverse gene silencing [12]. Allicin is also useful in treating human gastric carcinoma cells by inducing the apoptosis of MGC 803, thus inhibiting the proliferation [13]. Allicin induced apoptosis SKOV3 cells by activating JNK and translocation of mitochondrial Bax shows an essential therapy for human ovarian cancer [14].

S-allyl-mercapto cysteine including allicin, was found, including many man anti-tumor activities including neuroblastoma, adenocarcinoma, and breast cancer [15]. S-benzyl-cysteine, a structural analog of S allylcysteine, triggers the reliant mitochondrial apoptosis through p53 as well as Bax/Bcl two routes in male gastric cancer cells, thus indicating the possibility of its being an anti-tumor compound [16, 17]. Z-ajoene from garlic has the capacity to cure glioblastoma by focusing on its cancer stem cells, like the allyl mercaptan from garlic is open including anticancer methods. Garlic's components can cause genes linked to immunity and apoptosis and, thus, its use is negatively in touch with cancer and cardiovascular disease. Onion A from onions was proven to manage the protumour activation of strong cytotoxicity and tumor-associated macrophages against cancer cells, enabling it to be viewed as an invaluable prospect for combating people with ovarian cancers [18–20]. The flavonoid fisetin (3,7,3,4 tetrahydroxyflavone) from onion is a promising cancer treatment representative [21]. The quercetin plus diosgenin as an outcome of targeting neuropilin one receptor and inhibiting the development of cancer cells that are different may be used as an excellent anticancer therapy [22, 23].

Cardioprotective pastime Garlic like a dietary supplement to improve cardiovascular health has become a preferred choice among individuals with cardiovascular problems, in ischemic cardiovascular disease. Garlic extracts happen to be discovered displaying cardioprotective characteristics against cardiotoxicity, ischemia–reperfusion injury, arrhythmia, cardiac, hypertrophy, myocardial infarction and mitochondrial dysfunction [24–29]. Allicin from garlic can display anti myocardial fibrosis outcome and the mechanism connected with TGF β/Smads signal transduction [24].

4. Conclusions

Garlic and onions are pantry staples for many home cooks. Despite their quantities consumed experts believe they are quite nutritious. All varieties of onions are high in vitamin C, vitamin B6, potassium, folate, and magnesium, whereas garlic is high in vitamin C, vitamin B6, thiamin, potassium, calcium, phosphorous, copper, and manganese. Numerous traditional healing systems, such as Ayurveda, consider garlic and onions, to be medicinal foods due to their abundance of health benefits. Certain experimental studies have confirmed that the chemopreventive properties of Allium vegetables increase in relation to their organosulphur content. To sum up, the promising clinical data indicate that regular consumption of garlic and onion may help to help prevent prostate cancer. The anticarcinogenic activity of organosulphor compounds found in onions, at least in part, may be due to their structure. The uniqueness of garlic and onion is believed to be clinically relevant, as it is expected that they are safe to consume over the long term.

Author details

Rubi Gupta[1] and Prashant Kaushik[2]*

1 Department of Agricultural Biotechnology, Assam Agricultural University, Jorhat, India

2 Instituto de Conservación y Mejora de la Agrodiversidad Valenciana, Universitat Politècnica de València, Valencia, Spain

*Address all correspondence to: prakau@doctor.upv.es

References

[1] R. M. Perez-Gregorio, M. S. García-Falcon, J. Simal-Gándara, A. S. Rodrigues, and D.P.F. Almeida, "Identification and quantification of flavonoids in traditional cultivars of red and white onions at harvest," Journal of Food Composition and Analysis, vol. 23, no. 6, pp. 592-598, 2010.

[2] V. Benitez, E. Molla, M. A. Mart et al., "Study of bioactive compound content in different onion sections," Plant Foods for Human Nutrition, vol. 66, no. 1, pp. 48-57, 2011

[3] McRae MP. A review of studies of garlic (Allium sativum) on serum lipids and blood pressure before and after 1994: does the amount of allicin released from garlic powder tablets play a role? J Chiropr Med 2005; 4:82-90

[4] Ankri S, Mirelman D. Antimicrobial properties of allicin from garlic. Microbes Infect 1999; 2:125-129.

[5] Waag T, Gelhaus C, Rath J, Stich A, Leippe M, Schirmeister T. Allicin and derivates are cysteine protease inhibitors with antiparasitic activity. Bioorg Med Chem Lett 2010; 20:5541-5543

[6] Gallwitz H, Bonse S, Martinez-Cruz A, Schlichting I, Schumacher K, Krauth-Siegel RL. Ajoene is an inhibitor and subversive substrate of human glutathione reductase and Trypanosoma cruzi trypanothione reductase: crystallographic, kinetic, and spectroscopic studies. J Med Chem 1999; 42:364-372

[7] Bany J, Zdanowska D, Zdanowski R, SkopińskaRózewska E. The effect of herbal remedy on the development of Trichinella spiralis infection in mice.Pol J Vet Sci 2003; 6:6-8.

[8] Anthony JP, Fyfe L, Smith H. Plant active components - a resource for antiparasitic agents? Trends Parasitol 2005; 21:462-468.

[9] Soffar SA, Mokhtar GM. Evaluation of the antiparasitic effect of aqueous garlic (Allium sativum) extract in hymenolepiasis nana and giardiasis. J Egypt Soc Parasitol 1991; 21:497-502.

[10] X. K. Wang, X. Wang, and J. Huang, "Effects of allicin on experimental colorectal cancer in rats and its mechanism," *Product Research & Development*, vol. 28, pp. 943-948, 2016.

[11] H. J. Hu, Y. Q. Pan, X. J. Fan, X. M. Hu, W. W. Zou, and X.L. Lin, "Allicin inhibits H2O2-induced senescence in human umbilical vein endothelial cells through activation of SIRT1," Chinese Journal of Biochemistry and Molecular Biology, vol. 32,no. 5, pp. 536-543, 2016.

[12] S.V.Chhabria, M. A. Akbarsha,A. P. Li, P. S. Kharkar, andK. B.Desai, "In situ allicin generation using targeted alliinase delivery for inhibition of MIA PaCa-2 cells via epigenetic changes, oxidative stress and cyclin-dependent kinase inhibitor (CDKI) expression," Apoptosis, vol. 20, no. 10, pp. 1388-1409, 2015.

[13] X. Zhang, Y. Zhu,W. Duan, C. Feng, and X.He, "Allicin induces apoptosis of the MGC-803 human gastric carcinoma cell line through the p38 mitogen-activated protein kinase/caspase-3 10 Evidence-Based Complementary and Alternative Medicine signaling pathway," Molecular Medicine Reports, vol. 11, no. 4, pp. 2755-2760, 2015.

[14] L. Xu, J. Yu, D. Zhai et al., "Role of JNKactivation andmitochondrial Bax translocation in allicin-induced apoptosis in human ovarian cancer SKOV3 cells," *Evidence-Based Complementary and Alternative Medicine*, vol. 2014, Article ID 378684, 6 pages, 2014.

[15] J. Zhuang, Y. Li, and Y. Chi, "Role of p38 MAPK activation and mitochondrial cytochrome-c release in allicin-induced apoptosis in SK-N-SH cells," Anti-Cancer Drugs, vol. 27, no. 4, pp. 312-317, 2016.

[16] B. Czepukojc, A.-K. Baltes, C. Cerella et al., "Synthetic polysulfane derivatives induce cell cycle arrest and apoptotic cell death in human hematopoietic cancer cells," Food and Chemical Toxicology, vol. 64, pp. 249-257, 2014.

[17] K.-C. Lai, C.-L. Kuo, H.-C. Ho et al., "Diallyl sulfide, diallyl disulfide and diallyl trisulfide affect drug resistant gene expression in colo 205 human colon cancer cells *in vitro* and *in vivo*," Phytomedicine, vol. 19, no. 7, pp. 625-630, 2012.

[18] H. Nian, B. Delage, J. T. Pinto, and R. H. Dashwood, "Allyl mercaptan, a garlic-derived organosulfur compound, inhibits histone deacetylase and enhances Sp3 binding on the P21WAF1 promoter," Carcinogenesis, vol. 29, no. 9, pp. 1816-1824, 2008.

[19] Y. Jung, H. Park, H.-Y. Zhao, R. Jeon, J.-H. Ryu, and W.-Y. Kim, "Systemic approaches identify a garlic-derived chemical, Z-ajoene, as a glioblastomamultiforme cancer stem cell-specific targeting agent," Molecules and cells, vol. 37, no. 7, pp. 547-553, 2014.

[20] J. Tsuboki, Y. Fujiwara, H. Horlad et al., "Onionin A inhibits ovarian cancer progression by suppressing cancer cell proliferation and the protumour function of macrophages," *Scientific Reports*, vol. 6, Article ID29588, 2016.

[21] T. Rengarajan and N. S. Yaacob, "The flavonoid fisetin as an anticancer agent targeting the growth signaling pathways,"*European Journal of Pharmacology*, vol. 789, pp. 8-16, 2016.

[22] K. Sak, "Site-specific anticancer effects of dietary flavonoid quercetin," Nutrition and Cancer, vol. 66, no. 2, pp. 177-193, 2014.

[23] T. Yasmin, M. T. Ali, S. Haque, and M. Hossain, "Interaction of quercetin of onion with axon guidance protein receptor, NRP-1 plays important role in cancer treatment: an in Silico approach," *Interdisciplinary Sciences: Computational Life Sciences*, 2015.

[24] S.-C. Li, L.-N. Ma, J. Chen, and Y.-K. Li, "Effect of allicin on myocardial fibrosis after myocardial infarction in rats and its relationship with TGFβ/ Smads signal transduction," China Journal of Chinese Materia Medica, vol. 41, no. 13, pp. 2517-2521, 2016.

[25] M. Lavu, S. Bhushan, and D. J. Lefer, "Hydrogen sulfidemediated cardioprotection: mechanisms and therapeutic potential," Clinical Science, vol. 120, no. 6, pp. 219-229, 2011.

[26] V. Br¨ull, C. Burak, B. Stoffel-Wagner et al., "Effects of a quercetin-rich onion skin extract on 24 h ambulatory blood pressure and endothelial function in overweight-to-obese patients with (pre-)hypertension: a randomised double-blinded placebo-controlled cross-over trial," British Journal of Nutrition, vol. 114, no. 8, pp. 1263-1277, 2015.

[27] L. Supakul, H. Pintana, N. Apaijai, S. Chattipakorn, K. Shinlapawittayatorn, and N. Chattipakorn, "Protective effects of garlic extract on cardiac function, heart rate variability, and cardiac mitochondria in obese insulin-resistant rats," European Journal of Nutrition, vol. 53, no. 3, pp. 919-928, 2014.

[28] T. N. Khatua, R. Adela, and S. K. Banerjee, "Garlic and cardioprotection: insights into the molecular mechanisms," Canadian Journal of

Physiology and Pharmacology, vol. 91, no. 6, pp. 448– 458, 2013.

[29] M. A. Vazquez-Prieto, C. Rodriguez Lanzi, C. Lembo, C. R. Galmarini, and R. M. Miatello, "Garlic and onion attenuates vascular inflammation and oxidative stress in fructose-fed rats," *Journal of Nutrition and Metabolism*, vol. 2011, Article ID 475216, 7 pages, 2011.

Chapter 10

Meticulous Endorsement of Black Seed and Jambolana: A Scientific Review

Nikhat Farhana

Abstract

The repository of traditional, historical and cultural heritage of natural prophylactic medicine to treat different disease, disorder and its aliment is limitless and time-immemorial. As per the hadith narrated by Ibn Abbas (RA), Prophet Muhammed (ﷺ) specifically mentioned about Sulayman (AS) recorded the name and use of many herbal medicinal remedies after construction of his castle (Ibn Asakri's Mukhtasar Tareekh Dimashq 3.393), in addition to it, Prophet Muhammed (ﷺ) use to recommend 65 different herbal prophylactic medicines which are scientifically proved to be highly effective against almost all types of ailments, among this repository of 65, while prescribing the NS Prophet Muhammed (ﷺ) narrated "use this black seeds regularly it is having the properties to cure all disease (ailment) except death (An authentic hadith narrated by Abu Hurayrah (RA) and recorded by Bukhari, Muslim Ahmad Ibn Majah). This in-depth review specially articulated to elaborate phytochemical, pharmacological and mechanistic approach to bring out the properties of not only NS but in addition, it focusing on the important properties of EJ. Preliminarily to say NS claim to have anti-inflammatory, analgesic, hepato-protective, neuro-protective, gastro-protective and other useful activity are due to two important constituents Thymoquinone (TQ) and NS oil (NSO). TQ has interaction with human serum albumin. Seeds containing volatile oils mainly Melanthin showed toxicity at larger doses. Whereas, EJ simultaneously proved its effectiveness underutilized fruit, crops are nutritious bearing wide range of pharmaceuticals properties. EJ fruit is highly perishable and is mainly used for the diabetes patients, it is well known as a traditional medicinal plant having essential bioactive compounds which are present in all parts of the plant. The major bioactive compounds present in the EJ roots are phytosterols, flavonoids, carotenoids, myricetin, oxalic acid, gallic acid, citronellol, cyanidin diglucoside, hotrienol, and polyphenols as well as micronutrients having many health benefits. It is also a good source of anthocyanin and effective against numerous health problems and act as chemo-preventive, radioprotective and demonstrating antineoplastic properties. The ripe fruits are pleasant, astringent taste and are eaten either raw or processed into different products mainly vinegar, jam, jellies and squash. The jambolana seed contains alkaloid, jambosine, and glycoside jambolin or antimellin. To be concluded, NS and EJ both bearing similar therapeutic and pharmacological endorsement with different remarkable biological active molecule, which will become future reference to find out the natural way to cure untreatable disease and its disorder such as HIV-Aids, Cancer and recent outbreak, etc. according to narration made by Prophet Muhammed (ﷺ).

Keywords: Ranunculaceae, Myrtaceae, Thymoquinone, flavonoids, pharmaceutical, HIV-Aids, Cancer

1. Introduction

Historical evidences indicates that, herbs and spices have beneficial consequences as medicine to treat different disease and its ailments, primarily they are having food valve, apart from this the composition comprised in different herbs and spices to get rid from major and minor disorder associated with the complex organic physiological system, demonstrating benefits as food by scientific mean is challenging, specially, when standards applied to assess the pharmaceutical agents. Pharmaceutical agents are special molecules which were isolated and purified in concentrated forms, whereas food is having in combination, literally in large quantity [1]. The real challenge not here to prove whether herbs and spices as food have healthy benefits but rather figuring out, one of the greatest saying by *Abu Huraira (R.A)*, may Allah be pleased with him, narrated that the *Prophet, Muhammed Sallallaahu alaihi wa sallam* (May Allah exalt his mention), said: "use this black seed regularly, because it is a cure for every disease except death" [Al-Bukhari and Muslim] [2], secondly we encounter the another black herbs called Jambolana (Black Plum) [3].

2. *Nigella sativa* (black seeds)

NS belonging to the family *Ranunculaceae* is prominent miraculous and remarkable herb with holistic, historical and religious authenticated endorsement. NS sands apart with holds promising phytochemical and wide range of therapeutic potential among the botanical repository of medicinal plants in the world, NS is popularly known by the name of black seed. NS is native to Southern Europe, North Africa and Southwest Asia and is grown in many countries around the world, including the Middle East Mediterranean region, Southern Europe, India, Pakistan, Syria, Turkey and Saudi Arabia [4].

2.1 Botanical description

NS plant germinate, flower, set seed and die all in one. Ultimately reproduce themselves to set of seeds. Grow up to height of 20–30 cm (7.10–11.9 inches) with linear lanceolate leaves. The flowers are very much dedicated bearing 10 to 5 petals with remarkable white, yellow, pale blue. Pink, pale violet in colors. NS plants fruits are large & inflated capsules bearing with 3 to 7 united follicles having enormous number of seeds, whereas seeds containing black color with flattened, angular oblong with 0.2 cm long and 0.1 cm wide funnel shaped [5].

2.1.1 NS flower taxonomy

- Domine: Plantae
- Sub-domine: Tracheobionta
- Division: Spermatophyta
- Phylum: Magnoliophyta

- Class Magnoliopsida
- Order: Ranunculales
- Family: Ranunculacese
- Genus: Nigella
- Species: Sativa

2.1.2 Common names

Wild onion seeds, Funnel flower, Black cumin, Nutmeg flower, Black caraway, black seeds, Devil in the bush, Roman coriander, Roman coriander, Damascene etc.

2.1.3 Synonyms

- **English:** Black seeds, Love-in-a-mist, nutmeg flower, Roman coriander, funnel flower black cumin
- **Arabic:** Habatut Barakha, Shooneez, Habba Sauda, Al-barka
- **Sanskrit:** Krishana-jiraka, Upakunchik
- **Germa:** schwarzkummel

2.1.4 NS seeds and oil

- Chinese: Pei hei zhong cao
- French: Cheveux de Vénus, Nigelle
- Hindi: Kalonji.
- Marathi: Kalonji Jire
- Persian: Siah Dana
- Punjabi: Kalvanji
- Urdu: Kalonji

Moreover, the NS meticulously endorsed by above mentioned taxonomical and botanical descriptions. Indeed, much uncertainty about particular name of NS seed. NS seed is called black cumin, black caraway and black onion seed in particular regions of the continent, such as Central Asia and Northern India, with different botanical and taxonomical description, NS seed or any such seed, apparently, are often the part of the stock, that is commercially available and used as adulterants [6].

2.1.5 Cultivation and collection

NS herb mostly grown during the winter season. It is annually grown on light and heavy soil. The scattering period of seeds in between October–November and get harvest in between April and May. The yield is about 350 kg/acre to 450 kg/acre.

The germination processes of the plant would be delay, if scattering of seeds on upper soil or deep inside but it should be optimal. It need not be irrigated frequently. When the fruit / capsule turns yellowish, the crop is harvested.

It can be threshed by trampling with a tractor or proper thresher after harvesting and proper drying. The seeds are stored properly in bags or containers after threshing [6].

2.2 Phytochemical description of NS

As mentioned in above point-2, NS bearing ultimately important and valuable amount of phytoconstituent which were extracted, separated, identified and reported and updated up to the limit of extent but still needs to be explored, where in contemplation to retrieve the relevant documentary evidence leads to figure out the following valuable constituents, such TQ (48%) in 25 gm, thymohydroquinone, dithymoquinone, p-cymene (15%), carvacrol (12%), 4-terpineol (7%), tanethol (5%), sesquiterpene longifolene (1 to 8%), thymol & α-pinene etc. Seeds contain dual different types of alkaloids called iso-quinoline alkaloids (indazole ring bearing alkaloids are nigellicinine, nigellicimine-N-Oxide & pyrazole alkaloids). NS seeds are also contain α-hederin which is water soluble pentacyclic triterpene and saponin (potential anticancer agent). The potential pharmacological activity of NS seeds is mainly due to Quinine constituents, whereas thymoquinone is most abundant one. NS seeds also contains micro & macromolecules that are, carbohydrates-28%, protines 27%, fats-25%, crude fibers-9%, total ash-5%, Vitamins &, minerals like Cu, P, Zn and Fe^{++} etc.: **unsaturated fatty acids** like linolic acid-60%, oilic acid-20%, eicodadienoic acid-4% & dihomolinoleic acid-10%; saturated fatty acids are present nearly about less than 30% (palmitic & stearic acid), apart from this NS also embedded with Other constituents such as α-sitosterol 44 to 54% of total sterols, Tunisian stigmasterol 6.8 to 20.92% of total sterols, the above mentioned constituents were reported apart from this some structural analysis also documented in the literatures these structures mentioned in **Figure 1** [7].

2.2.1 Reported constituent and its structures of NS

Some important steroidal monomers also reported from NS seed are nigellone, avenasterol-5-ene, avenasterol-7-ene, campesterol, cholesterol, sitrostadienol, obtusfoliol, lophenol, stigasterol, stigmasterol-7-ene, β-amirn, butyrospermol, cycloartenol, 24-methylene-cycloartenol, taraxerol, tirucallol, 3-O-[β-D-xylopyranosyl(1 → 3)-α-L-rhamnopyranosyl(1 → 2)-α-L-arabinopyranosyl]-28-O-[α-L-rhamnopyranosy](1 → 4)-β-D-glucopyranosyl(1 → 6)-β-D-glucopyranosyl]-hedera- genin, up to 1.6%-Volatile oil, fatty oil-41.6%, olic acid,

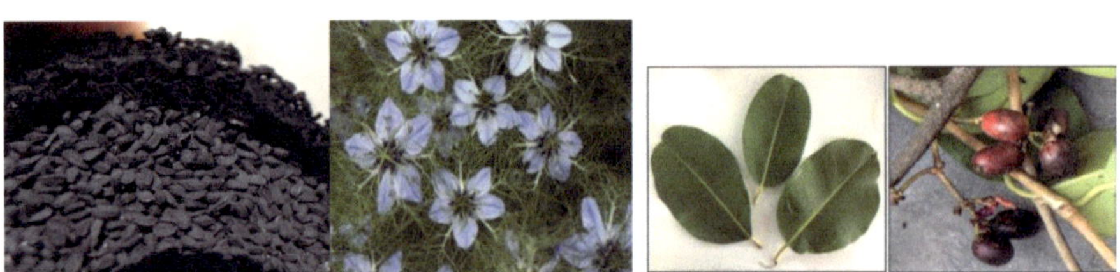

a b c

Figure 1.
a- NS seeds b- NS flowers c- EJ leaves and fruits.

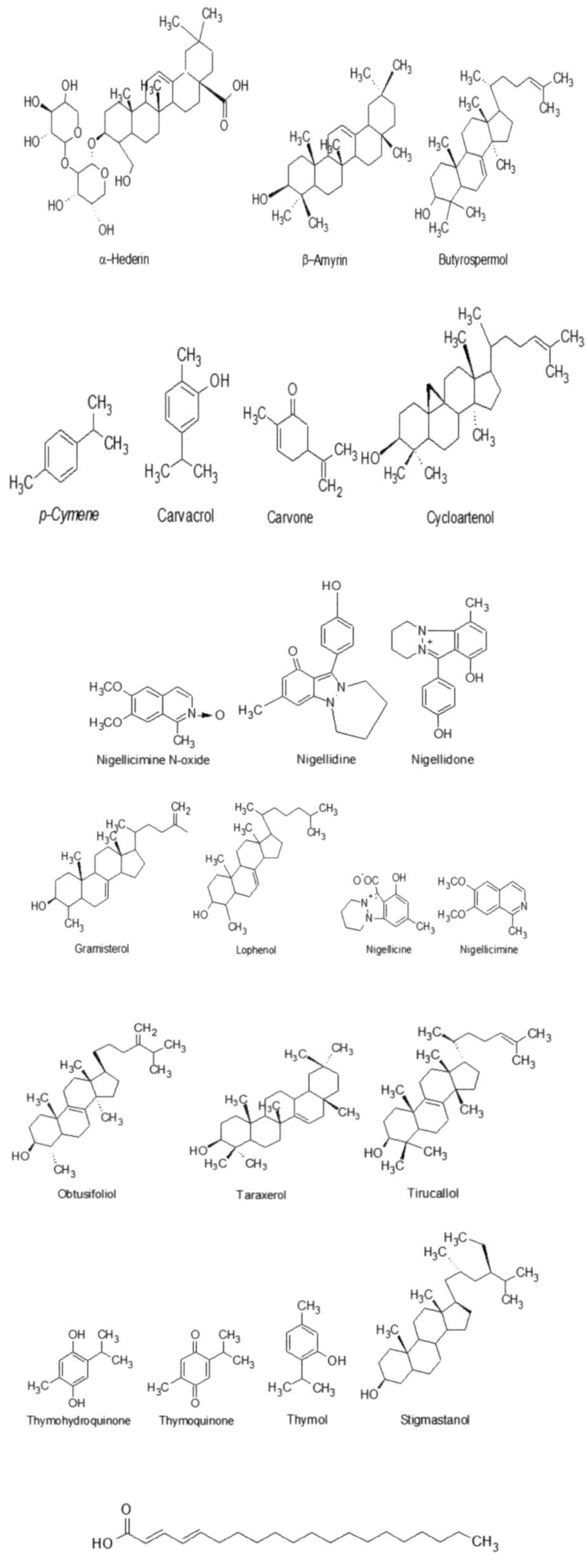

Figure 2.
Reported bioactive components of NS.

C15 esters of unsaturated fatty acid with higher terpenoids,, esters of dehydrosteric-acid & linolic acid, aliphatic alcohols like melanthin, melanthigenin etc, moreover to endorsed it also contain bitter constituents with tannin, resin, protein, reducing sugars like saponine, 3-O-[β-D-xylopyranosyl, (1 → 2)-α-L-rhambopyranosyl, (1 → 2)-β-D-glucopyranosyl]-11-methoxy-16, 23-dihydroxy-28-methyl-olean-12-enoate, stigma-5, 22-diene-3-β-D-glucopyranoside, cycloart-23-methyl-7,20,22-triene-3β, 25-diol, negellidine-4-O-sulfite, N-amines A3, A4, A5, C & A1, A2, B1 & B2 were found in seeds of NS. Hence it was assumed that, because of presence of above-mentioned bioactive constituents, NS stands apart with special category of medicinal specie, with infinite number of medicinal properties to manage bronchitis, diarrhea, rheumatism, asthma, skin disorders, it also acts as liver tonic, anti-diarrheal, appetite stimulant, digestive disorders. It also beneficial to increase milk production in nursing mothers, it also utilized to fight with parasitic infections, immunity system will be strengthened by regular utilization of NS seeds. In addition to above NS seeds are also used in food as additives, especially flavoring agent in bread and pickles coz low level of toxicity value. The NS seeds and oil also preferred in treatment of worm infestation, skin eruption, antiseptic, eternal anesthetics & roosted seeds of NS given internally to stop vomiting (**Figure 2**) [8].

3. *Eugenia jambolana* (black plum)

Next to NS another herbs which is bearing identical pharmacological properties with extra ordinary source of natural remedies and therapeutic application to treat different disease and its aliment, mid-nineteenth century was the era, which came up, with its first scientific evidence, as antidiabetic properties, apart from this the medicinal values endorsed in the ayurvedic, Unani, siddha and other folklore system of medicine [9].

3.1 Botanical and taxonomical description

Eugenia jambolana (EJ) or *Syzygium cumini* (L) Skeel was evergreen plant which grows up to 25 meters which is estimated up to 80 feet tall, it having grayish white steam with coarse & discolored lower bark, leaves are simple, elliptic, opposite to oblong, glossy smooth and somewhat leathery, midrib of the leaves is prominent yellowish, with 5 to 15 cm long and 2 to 8 cm broad, the base of the leaves are cuneate or round; apex is short, rounded or obtuse; edges are toothed; stalk is slender light yellow; veins are fine, close together parallel and gland are dotted. The petals adhere and fall together as a small disk. The stamens are many and almost the same length as calyx. The fruits are ovoid, 1-seeded berry, with a length of 2 centimeters (0.8 inch), dark purple red, shiny, with white to lavender flesh, fruit are oval to elliptic, length from 1.5 to 3.5 cm, dark purple to black in color, taste of the fruit is the combination of sweet, mildly sour with astringent flavor, it tends to color the tongue purple. Because of the dark violet color of the fruit it resembles to the olive tree fruits both shape and weight [10].

3.1.1 Taxonomical description

Kingdom: Plantae.
Subkingdom: Viridaeplantae.
Infrakingdom: Streptophyta.

Division: Tracheophyta.
Subdivision: Spermatophytina.
Infradivision: Angiospermae.
Class: Magnliopsida.
Superorder: Rosanae.
Order: Myrtales.
Family: Myrtaceae.
Genus: Syzygium.
Species: Cumini.
Scientific Name: Syzigium cumini (L) Skeel.

3.1.2 Common names

Hindi: Jamuna, Sanskrit: Mahajambu, Ksudrajambu, Assam: Jam, Bengali: Jaam, Kalajam, English: Jambul tree, Gujarat: Gambu Jamun,Tamil: Naval, Urdu: Jamun, Telegu: Neredu [11].

3.1.3 Synonyms

Brazil - Azeitona,Pakistan – Jaman, West Indies-Jambol, Nepal-Java plum, Thailand – Lukwa, Japan - Madan Madagascar – Rotra.

3.1.4 Cultivation and collection of EJ

EJ was tropical & subtropical plant grows up to 2,000 meters in the region where annual day time temperature ranges from 20 to 32°C & it tolerate 12 to 48°C, mature growth of the plant will be affected at -2°C lower, whist youngest growth is affected at -1°C. The plant grows well at annual rainfall in the range 1500 to 6,000 mm but tolerates 800–9900 mm. EJ can withstand a dry season of up to 7 months, where it prefers a sunny position, the pH prefer to range 5.5 to 7. The plants are moderately shade-tolerant, especially when young [12]. The

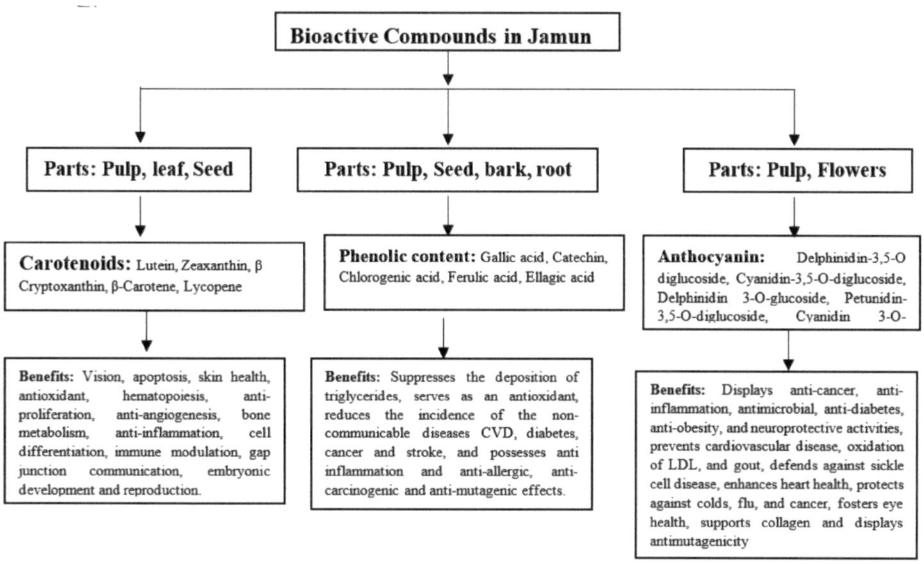

Figure 3.
Major bioactive constituents of jamun and its benefits.

versatile plant will grow on wide range of soils, even in shallow rocky soils where provided rainfall is maximum to tolerate prolonged flooding, once established, it tolerates drought in dry sites, the plant confine itself to the vicinity of water-courses & it tolerates quite strong winds, it sow-self freely and become serious pests in pasture.

In Florida EJ plant is listed as undesirable fast-growing plant, seedlings may reach up to 4 meter in 2 Years. This tree coppices remarkably well, with vigorous shoots, in large number, with minor and major stumps alike, the coppice which were stands in streams, will grew up to 4.6 meter in 4 years, and the raw material of the plant can be collected in rainy seasons to get good amount of bioactive constituents [13].

3.2 Phytochemical description of EJ

EJ is found to be rich in tannins, alkaloids, carbohydrates, flavonoids, sterols, glycosides, and among other phytoconstituents in different parts of the tree. There are many families of phytochemicals and they help the human body in a variety of ways. Phytochemicals can protect (**Figure 3**) human from diseases. Phytochemicals are nonnutritive plant chemicals that have protective or disease preventive properties. The fruits produce and determine the physical–chemical and sensory characteristics of light jambolan jelly. This fruit has intense purple color, which gave the jellies - both standard and light - a quite attractive visual aspect. The phytochemical analysis of ethanol extract of Jamun stem bark, leaf, seed and fruit pulp showed the presence of alkaloids, anthraquinone glycosides, flavonoids, tannins, saponins, phenols, cardiac glycosides, terpenoids, phytosterols, steroids and amino acids in all extracts. Terpenoids and phytosterols were absent in the leaf extract. The seeds are rich in protein and calcium. The seeds contain both micro & macromolecules as in NS. EJ also contines fats and oil such as tannins-19%, ellagic acid-2%, glycoside, jamboline, starch, myricyl alcohol in un-saponified fraction in small quantity that is 0.05% of pale yellow oil with specific gravity 20:0.926, [α] D- 5.420. The essential oils isolated from the freshly collected leaf (accounting for 82% of the oil), stem, seed, fruits contain α-Pinene, camphene, β-Pinene, myrcene, limonene, cis-ocimeme, trans-ocimeme, sterculic and vernolic acid, literature reported that huge quantity of malic acid present in fruits, i.e. thrice the weight of the fruit (0.59% wt of fruit), whereas oxalic acid present in minor amount but Gallic acid and tannin accountable for astringent taste of the fruit. The purple color of fruit is due to Cyanidin diglycosides, fruits are reach source of suger-9%, non-reducing sugars-10%. The fruits also contain monomeric sugar units such as glucose, fructose, mannose, galactose & mineral constituents were also reported to be present (mg/100 g of edible pulp) are Ca, Mg, Fe, Na, K, and Cu,. The vitamins present (in 100 g. edible pulp) are vit. A, 80 IU; thiamine, 0.03 mg, riboflavin, 0.01 mg; nicotinic acid,0.2 mg; vit. C, 18 mg; choline, 7 mg; folic acid, 3 μg. The stem bark contain friedelin, kaempferol, ellagic acid, gallotannin, betulinic acid, βsitosterol, eugenin. The leaves contain phenolic content like ferullic acid, catechin, also, n-dotricontanol, myrcetin, mycaminose, quercetin, annic acid, tocopherol and acetylated flavonol glycoside. The flowers contain oleanolic acid and other triterpenoids also acetyl oleanolin acid (0.3%) melting point (260–262°C), Eugenia- triterpenoid A (0.5%) and Eugenia triterpenoid B (0.3%). The roots contain myricetin 3-O-glucoside and myricetin 3-O-robinoside. Reported constituents (**Figure 4**) structures from different part of plant [14].

3.2.1 Reported constituent and its structure of EJ

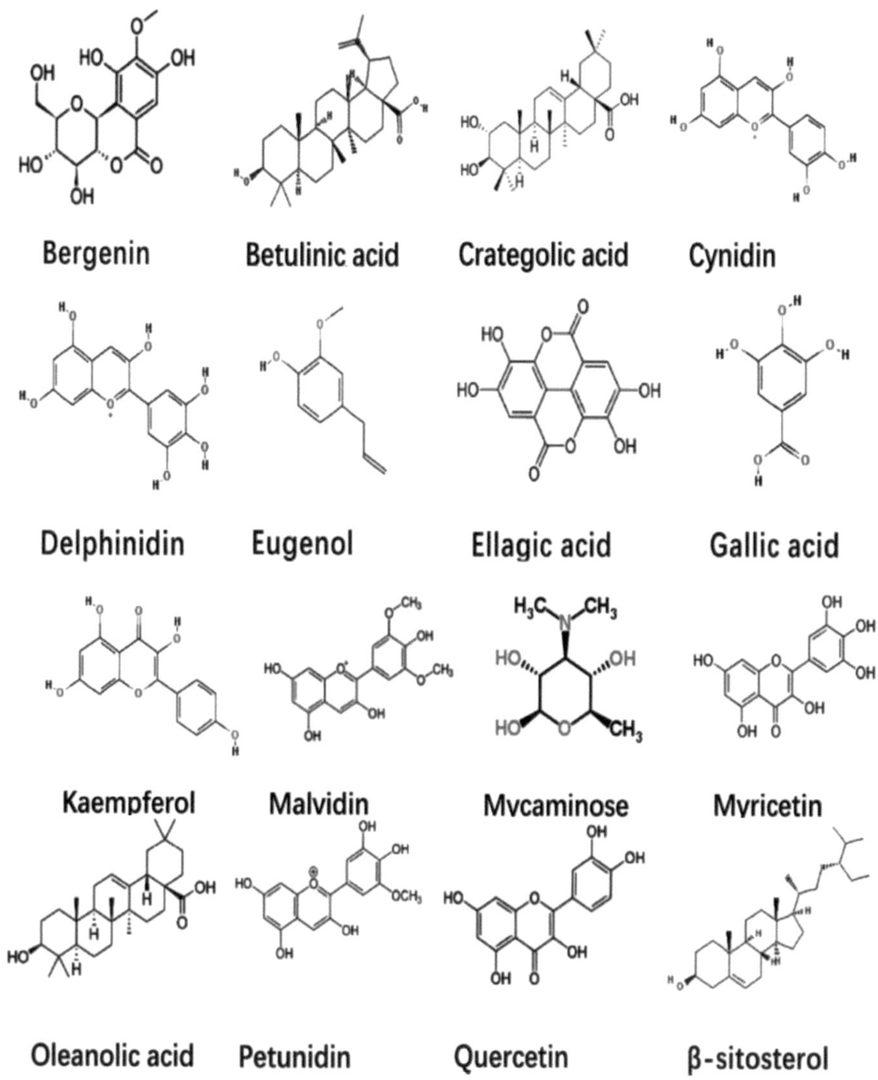

Figure 4.
Constituents from eugenia jambolana.

4. Endorsed pharmacological descriptions of ns and EJ

4.1 Pharmacological properties of NS seeds and oil

NS seeds and oil has been broadly utilized to cure different disease & its aliments associated with, leaving physiological system, which was proved by adopting modern scientific methodology. The collected research repository from different sources with regardless of time, focusing the activity done on NS, worldwide form the centuries NS seeds and oil traditionally utilized as therapeutic medicine, in Indian system of medicine (Unani & ayurvedic) the pharmacological applications are endorsed [15], further more to say our Prophet Muhammed (ﷺ) advocated the importance in one of his saying that "NS seeds is remedy for all disease accept death" on this hadith NS considered as greatest healing medicine available in the form of Herbs and species, further recommendation of use was endorsed in Tibb-e-Nabwi (Prophetic Medicine). NS bearing wide range of therapeutic & pharmacological activity such as diuretic, antidiabetic, anti-hypertensive, analgesic, immunomodulatory, antimicrobial, anthelmintic, anti-inflammatory, spasmolytic, fever, influenza, eczema, cough, headache, paralysis, hemorrhage, amenoria, anorexia, bronchodilator, GIT protective, Hepatoprotective, renal treatment and antioxidant, skin disease [16], the activity of the NS seed is due to the presence of thymoquinone (TQ) which is major bioactive component NS oil. As already mentioned NS seeds are having food value hence it does not shows any adverse effect, TQ having potent anti-microbial properties including Gram +Ve and Gram -Ve bacteria [17], it also effective in viruses, parasites schistosomes and fungal infections.

The efficacy of NS seeds and TQ are variable and depend on target species. And other study reported the use of seeds and oil to control the symptoms of COVID-19 in combination with crude extract of EJ [18].

4.2 Pharmacological properties EJ

The second herbs which is having similar pharmacological properties was *Eugenia jambolana (EJ)*, which is excellently prominent herb which utilized by ancient people of different continent to combat with the deficiency's associated with physiological system apart from this the importance of this plant is endorsed in the ancient scriptures like Siddha, Ayurveda and Unani medication for its therapeutic potentials [19].

The entire plant is used in various traditional system of medicine in India and other parts of the continent around the globe. However, the leaves and bark are regarded as most significant part. In Ayurveda, the bark is acrid, sweet, digestive and astringent to the bowels, anti-helminths. Besides it is used to cure sore throat, bronchitis, asthma, thirst, biliousness, dysentery, blood purifier in ulcer treatment. In Unani system of medicine EJ Leaf ash is used to strengthen teeth gums, EJ seeds are used as astringent, diuretic and also used to stop urinary discharges. The bark of EJ having strong antidiabetic properties. The siddha system of Indian medicine utilizes Jambolana seeds for hematinic, thermo-regulate, the traditional medicine of Madagascar's the Jambolana seeds are utilized to regenerate the β-cells of pancreas and leaves are used by women to contract vagina after delivery, reduce mucus and odors [20].

5. Comparative pharmacological properties

The uniform resemblances of pharmacological application both the species have been extensively analyzed with regardless of time, and tabulated in **Table 1**, the aim of the study, to put the researcher to focus on the beneficiary effect of bioactive constituents present in both the medicinal plants.

6. Conclusions

In a nutshell, both the species having identical pharmacological properties, bearing with different and rich source of phytoconstituents, currently, todays era getting conscious about the utilization of herbal medicaments, hence it was the preliminary choice of consumer world-wide. Otherwise, the traditional medicines

DOI: http://dx.doi.org/10.5772/intechopen.99225

S.N	*Nigella sativa* (black seed)		Uniform resemblances of both species		*Eugenia jambolana* (black plum)	
	Parts of BS	**Composition of constituent**	**Activity**	**Chechanism**	**Parts of BP**	**Composition of constitutent**
1.	Seeds	α-Hedrin, Steryl-glucosides, Acetylsteryl-glucoside	Anti-inflammatory	Anti-inflammatory activity is attributed to inhibition of cytokine, eicosanoids generation and measure lipid peroxidation through inhibition of cyclo-oxygenaseand 5-lipoxygenase pathway of archidonate metabolism. In addition, T cell- and natural killer cell-mediated immune responses are also accountable to its immune-modulatory activity.	Leaves	Ellagic acid, gallotannin betullinic acid, β sitosterol, eugenin, kaempferol triterpenoids, saponins and tannins phenolic compounds and flavonoids
2.	Oil	Nigellicimine, Nigellidine, Nigellimine-N-oxide	Cardiovascular actions	Cardiovascular depressant effects are mediated centrally via indirect and direct mechanisms that involved both 5-hydroxytryptaminergic and muscarinic mechanisms. Direct mechanism is virtue of volatile oild (TQ) which processes potent antihypertensive potential.	Seeds	Flavonoids, phenolic content-caffeic acid, ellagic acid, ferulic acid, tannins, terpenes
3.	Seeds	Arginine, Glutamic acid, Leucine, Lysine, Methionine, Tyrosine, Proline And Threonine	Anti-hyperlipidemic	Anti-hyperlipdemic effect is owing to significant reduction in hepatic HMG-COA reductase activity. In addition, this effect is attributed to blockage of the ex-vivo basal and in-vitro maximal formation of conjugated diene and malondialdehyde, and lengthened the lag times of low density lipoprotein, small dense low density lipoprotein and large buoyant low density lipoprotein. Methanolic extract possessing ω-6 linoleic acid along with palmitic acid is more effective that volatile extract containing thymol and isothymol phenolic antioxidant compounds. Thymoquinone has anti1hyperlipidemic as well as antioxidant activity	Plant pulp Seed	Triton X-100 induced hyperlipidemia
4.	Seeds	Palmitic acid (12.5%), Stearic and Myristic acid (30%).	Hypoglycemic effects	N. sativa and *Eugenia jambolana* has non-insulin-mediated mechanism for the demonstration of hypoglycemic activity. However, petroleum ether extract exerts an insulin1sensitizing action by enhancing the activity of the two major intracellular signal transduction pathways of the hormones receptor	Leave	Vit. C, gallic acid, tannins, anthocyanins including cyanidin, petunidin, Lupeol, β-sitosterol

S.N	*Nigella sativa* (black seed)		Uniform resemblances of both species		*Eugenia jambolana* (black plum)	
	Parts of BS	**Composition of constituent**	**Activity**	**Chechanism**	**Parts of BP**	**Composition of constitutent**
5.	Seeds	Esters Of Linoleic1 5a Caindd, N Tiann Ngilny,C	Antinociceptive effects	Antinociceptive effects of *N. sativa* oil and *Eugenia jambolana* having Flavonoids, phenolic and thymoquinone *N. sativa* of are mediated by indirect activation of the supraspinal µ1- and k-opioid receptor subtypes.	Seeds	Flavonoids, alkaloids, steroids
6.	Seeds	Enoate, Stigma-5, 22-Dien- 3-B-D-Gluco.	Anti-oxytocic potential	The volatile oil of *Nigella sativa* seeds inhibits the spontaneous uterine smooth muscle contractions induced by oxytocin stimulation. These effects are concentration-dependent and reversible by tissue washing.	Roots	Flavonoids, alkaloids, steroids
7.	Seeds	6-Methoxy-Coumarin, Hydroxy-Coumarin, 7-Oxy-Coumarin	Gastro-protective effects	*N. sativa* cause significant reduction in acidity and glutathione level while it produced a significant increase in mucosal histamine content	Leaves	Amylase
8.	Seeds	Cycloeucalenol, Cycloartenol, Sterol Esters	Neuroprotective action	Neuro-protective action of NSO is correlated to its ability to inhibit not only excessive reactive oxygen species (ROS) formation but also seizure generation	Seeds	Anthocyanins, volatile oils, terpenes
9.	Seeds	Arginine, Glutamic Lysine, Methionine, Nephro-protective effect	NSO acts in the kidney as a potent scavenger of free radicals	Crude extract	Flavonoids, glycosides	
10.	Seeds	Almitoleic acid, β-Sitosterol, α1Sitosterols (44–54%),	Anti-schistosomiasis	TQ were considered as protective agents against the chromosomal aberrations induced as a result of schistosomiasis	Crude extract of pulp	phenolic content and acetylated flavonol glycosides
11.	Seeds	Tyrosine, Proline and Threonine	Anxiolytic effect	*N. Sativa* oil increased brain levels of 5-HT but the levels of brain 5-HIAA decreased significantly. Brain and plasma levels of tryptophan also increased significantly following oral repeated administration of N. sativa oil. Based on this, it may be suggested that N. sativa oil is a useful choice for the treatment of anxiety.	Seeds	Flavonoids, alkaloids, steroids

S.N	*Nigella sativa* (black seed)		Uniform resemblances of both species		*Eugenia jambolana* (black plum)	
	Parts of BS	**Composition of constituent**	**Activity**	**Chechanism**	**Parts of BP**	**Composition of constitutent**
12.	Seeds	Almitoleic acid, β-Sitosterol, α1Sitosterols (44–54%), Cycloartenol, Sterol	Anti-malarial Effects	N. sativa oil can possibly be utilized as both supplements and as adjuvant. It has great importance when combine with chloroquine because the rate of loss and failure becomes less that's why it is safer for utilization. This will lessen the side effects of CQ. Total charge of treatment of malaria through chloroquine being the least expensive and mostly accessible	Methanolic extract of leaves	Polyphenols including Flavonoids, alkaloids, glycosides & phenolic compound, fatty oils
13.	Seeds	Almitoleic acid, β-Sitosterol, α1Sitosterols (44–54%), Cycloeucalenol,	Anti-parastic Effects	*Nigella sativa* oil serves to counter infection by tapeworms and also used in the treatment or control of nematode infestations. It was demonstrated that oil have the ability to lessen the quantity of *Schistosoma mansoni* worms and ova that are produced in both the liver and in the intestinal tract. It has ability to expel parasitic worms such as nodular worms, tapeworms, hookworms, earthworms and nodular worms. Displayed great properties to attack the tapeworms and earthworms.	Leaves	glycosides & phenolic compound, fatty oils
14.	Seeds	Cycloartenol, Sterol Esters and Sterol Glucosides	Influence on blood	In an ongoing report it was seen that menthol dissolvable parts of *Nigella sativa* oil Counting thymol and carvacol Had extremely solid inhibitory impact on aggregated platelets that are induced by arachidonic acid	Seeds	glycosides & phenolic compound, fatty oils
15.	Seeds	Cycloeucalenol, Cycloartenol, Sterol Esters and Sterol Glucosides	Treatment of Acne	The *Nigella sativa* oil moisturizer has demonstrated its adequacy as an effective treatment for skin break out by acne vulgaris A new common plant extricates, which does not have any consequences. One of its constituents α-pipene had in vitro impact against *Propionibacterium acnes*, That is one of the main considerations involve in the advancement of skin inflammation.	Leaves and fruit pulp extract	Triterpenoids, Resin, Resin, Phytosterol

S.N	*Nigella sativa* (black seed)		Uniform resemblances of both species		*Eugenia jambolana* (black plum)	
	Parts of BS	**Composition of constituent**	**Activity**	**Chechanism**	**Parts of BP**	**Composition of constitutent**
17.	Seeds and oil	Almitoleic acid β-Sitosterol, α1Sitosterols (44–54%)	Effect on reproductive system	The uptake of 1 ml/kg/day of black cumin oil enhances the release of sexual hormones that stimulated the increase protein production of liver enzymes, platelets number and in the blood it diminishing the level of cholesterol present in serum. *Nigella sativa* oil possess anti-oxidative activities to neutralize the damage in the epididymal sperm characters brought about by hydrogen peroxide (H2 02) treatment. Crude extract	Flavonoids, phenolic content – caffeic acid, ellagic acid, ferulic acid, tannins, terpenes	
18.	Seeds	Almitoleic acid, β-Sitosterol, α1Sitosterols (44–54%)	Effect on respiratory system	In Saudi Arab and neighboring nations Kalonji seeds and oils are commonly utilized for the cure o asthma. Carbonyl polymer of thymoquinone (nigellone) ends up being an incredible preventive agent for both bronchial asthma and asthmatic bronchitis. Essential oil can be utilized as probable respiratory energizer if thymoquinone is eliminated	Seeds	glycosides & phenolic compound, fatty oils
19.	Seeds	Sterol Esters and Sterol Glucosides	Anti-bacterial Activity	*Nigella sativa* oil have shown great properties against bacterial specie that are producing wound infections. The oil provided great preventing impacts on *Staphylococcus Aureus* and Streptococcus species. Thymohydroquinone was separated from the essential oil known to possess higher actions against gram+ive bacteria.	Crude extract of leaves and bark	Phenols and flavonoids
20.	Seeds and oil	Cycloartenol	Anti-fungal Effects	The essential oil of Kalnoji of various backgrounds has accounted for to have adequate inhibitory activity against disease causing strains of: yeasts, dermatophytes and Non-dermatophytic filamentous parasites alongside aflatoxin-creating organisms.	Roots	Flavonoids, phenolic content – caffeic acid, ellagic acid, ferulic acid, tannins, terpenes
21.	Seeds and oil	Cycloeucalenol, Cycloartenol Sterol	Antiallergic effect	Act on H1 and H2 receptors	Crude Extract	Flavonoids, alkaloids, steroids

DOI: http://dx.doi.org/10.5772/intechopen.99225

S.N	*Nigella sativa* (black seed)		Uniform resemblances of both species		*Eugenia jambolana* (black plum)	
	Parts of BS	**Composition of constituent**	**Activity**	**Chechanism**	**Parts of BP**	**Composition of constitutent**
22.	Seeds and oil	Thymoquinone, dithmoquinone, thymohydroquinone, nigellone, thymol	Anti-cancer	Act to dissolve the unwanted cells in the body by dissolving them and have significant cytotoxic effect against the majority of tumor cell lines	Crude extracts of roots	Phenols and flavonoids
23.	*Seeds*	*Thymoquinone, dithmoquinone, thymohydroquinone nigellone,*	*COVID-19 pandemic*	*Both the species exhibit to act on respiratory illness associated with type-II cells and secondary pathway of epithelial regeneration will be triggered*	*Water extract of roots*	*Flavonoids, phenolic content-caffeic acid, ellagic acid, tannins, terpenes Anthocyanins, volatile oils, terpenes*

Table 1.
Glimpse of phytochemical and pharmacological endorsement of both the species.

are still occupying remedy-kingdom in particular area of research. Inherent and varied activities with meticulously indorsed phytoconstituents from both the species is triggering zone to the drug research, whereas this chapter is entirely dedicated to bring out the best from research crafted by different scholars. NS is one of the most important medicinal herbs with considerable commercial value, the valuable Phytoconstituents bearing by these herbs is commendable and also the gap in research to fucose on, merely the principal constituents responsible for activity are the derivatives of thymoquinone (TQ), as evident by various scientific studies support its safe use for the long-term traditional food and medicinal purposes.

To date, number of studies showed that, EJ is evergreen tree, having food value, which provide remarkably diversified therapeutic application, to treat different disease and its disorder associated with physiological system. The studies suggested that the major constituents responsible for the activity are flavonoids, anthocyanins, carotenoids, essential oil, terpenes, tannins and phenolic compounds.

To jot down, NS and EJ having wider safety margin and praiseworthy therapeutic activity, against sustainably cure to different bacteria and virus, this era of treatment require the molecules isolated from natural sources, whereas the worldwide ban of antibiotic, steroidal hormones and outbreak of covid-19, this candidate will prove its effectiveness.

Acknowledgements

Author immensely grateful to the management of AIKTC and the book publishing family for giving me the opportunity to become a part of this novelty work. Last but not least my heartfelt thanks to Librarian of AIKTC for guidance support. I never deny the support and love of my children and family for providing me the quality time to draft this chapter.

Conflict of interest

The author declared no conflict of interest.

Notes/Thanks/Other declarations

Thanks to publishing house for giving me the opportunity to contribute.

Acronyms and abbreviations

NS	*Nigella sativa*
EJ	*Eugenia jambolana*
TQ	Thymoquinone
NSO	*Nigella sativa* oil
DPPH	2,2-diphenyl- 1-1picryhydrazyl hydrate
LOO	lipid peroxyl radicals
FRAP	Ferric reducing antioxidant power
GAE	Gallic acid equivalent
CE	Catechin equivalent
TAE	Tannic acid equivalent

AGEs	Acute gastroenteritis
CVD	Cardio Vascular Disease
AMD	Age Related Macular Degeneration

Author details

Nikhat Farhana[1,2]

1 Anjuman-I-Islam's Kalsekar Technical Campus, University of Mumbai, Mumbai, India

2 Department of Pharmaceutical Chemistry, AIKTC-SoP, Mumbai University, Mumbai, India

*Address all correspondence to: nik.nida13ada25@gmail.com

References

[1] Tapsell LC, Scientific TC, Sullivan DR. Health benefits of herbs and spices: the past, the present, the future. 2006;(September).

[2] Musharraf HM, Arman MSI. Prophetic medicine is the cheapest , safest and the best remedy in the prevention and treatment of hypertension (high blood pressure) – a mini review. 2018;3(5):245-50.

[3] Ayyanar M, Subash-Babu P. Syzygium cumini (L.) Skeels: A review of its phytochemical constituents and traditional uses. Asian Pac J Trop Biomed. 2012;2(3):240-246.

[4] Jhade D, Gupta S. Medicinal and Phamacological Potential of *Nigella sativa* : A Review. 2016;(December).

[5] Eid AM, Elmarzugi NA, Ayyash LMA, Sawafta MN, Daana HI. A Review on the Cosmeceutical and External Applications of *Nigella sativa*. 2017;2017.

[6] Datta AK, Saha A, Mandal A, Behar C. Black cumin (*Nigella sativa* L.) – a review. 2012;(January).

[7] Wu S. An efficient RNA-cleaving DNA enzyme can specifically target the 5-untranslated region of severe acute respiratory syndrome associated coronavirus (SARS-CoV). 2007;(November 2006):1080-6.

[8] Sallehuddin N, Nordin A, Bt R, Idrus H, Fauzi MB. Nigella sativa and Its Active Compound, Thymoquinone, Accelerate Wound Healing in an In Vivo Animal Model : A Comprehensive Review. 2020;

[9] Sharma D. Chapter -3 Health Benefits of *Syzygium cumini* (Jamun) Seeds Chapter -3 Health Benefits of *Syzygium cumini* (Jamun .... Chapter - 3 Health Benefits of *Syzygium cumini* (Jamun) Seeds Authors Master' s Student, Department of Food , Nutrition and Dieteti. 2020;(December).

[10] Ayyanar M, Subash-Babu P. Syzygium cumini (L.) Skeels: A review of its phytochemical constituents and traditional uses. Asian Pac J Trop Biomed. 2012;2(3):240-246.

[11] Bijauliya RK, Alok S, Sabharwal M, Chanchal DK. Syzygium Cumini (Linn.) - an Overview on Morphology, Cultivation, Traditional Uses and Pharmacology. Int J Pharm Sci Res. 2018;9(9):3608-3620.

[12] Ayyanar M, Subash-Babu P, Ignacimuthu S. Syzygium cumini (L.) Skeels., a novel therapeutic agent for diabetes: Folk medicinal and pharmacological evidences. Complement Ther Med. 2013;21(3): 232-243.

[13] Ramya S, Neethirajan K, Jayakumararaj R. Profile of bioactive compounds in Syzygium cumini-a review. Artic J Pharm Res. 2013;5(8):4548-4553.

[14] Baliga MS, Bhat HP, Baliga BRV, Wilson R, Palatty PL. Phytochemistry, traditional uses and pharmacology of Eugenia jambolana Lam. (black plum): A review. Food Res Int [Internet]. 2011;44(7):1776-1789. Available from: http://dx.doi.org/10.1016/j.foodres.2011.02.007

[15] Ijaz H, Tulain UR, Qureshi J, Danish Z, Musayab S, Zaman M, et al. *Nigella sativa* (Prophetic Medicine): A Review. 2016;(November).

[16] Islam MT, Guha B, Hosen S, Riaz TA. Nigellalogy : A Review on *Nigella Sativa* Nigellalogy : A Review on *Nigella Sativa*. 2017;(September).

[17] Khan Z, Hasan N, Ahmad N, Khalid M. Pharmacological Activity of *Nigella Sativa* : A Review Pharmacological Activity of *Nigella Sativa* : A Review. 2016;(April).

[18] Nesrain F, Nadia S, Jumat S. Physiochemical properties of Saudi *Nigella sativa* L. ('Black cumin') seed oil. 2021;1-9.

[19] Oliveira ACP, Endringer DC, Amorim LAS, Brandão MDGL, Coelho MM. Effect of the extracts and fractions of Baccharis trimera and Syzygium cumini on glycaemia of diabetic and non-diabetic mice. J Ethnopharmacol. 2005;102(3):465-469.

[20] Rao SS, Najam R. Efficacy of combination herbal product (Curcuma longa and Eugenia jambolana) used for diabetes mellitus. Pak J Pharm Sci. 2016;29(1):201-204.

Chapter 11

Garlic in Traditional Indian Medicine (Ayurveda) for Health and Healing

Vinod Kumar Joshi and Apurva Joshi

Abstract

Traditional Indian Medicine (TIM)- Ayurveda is a Sanskrit Language word, which signifies "true knowledge of life". It is recognized as one of the oldest Traditional health care systems of the World by World Health Organization. In fact, it was a main stream health care system till the introduction of convention medicine in India. Plant, animal and mineral origin natural substances are used in Ayurveda for health and healing. Of them, Garlic is one of the plant origin substances. Garlic is known as *Lasuna*, which signifies, destroyer of diseases. The fresh plants of Garlic are used as edible food substance and also the dried cloves are on ripening to alleviate the disorders rationally in TIM. Garlic is recommended as physical strength promoting, intellect promoting and as aphrodisiac to maintain healthy state of life. Its properties like- unctuous, hot, pungent, heavy has been described to alleviates skin diseases, intra abdominal tumor, chronic rhinitis, hemicranias, epilepsy, fainting etc. Its continuous use causes internal hemorrhage. The medicated milk, medicated oil preparation are used orally as well topically. A number of pharmaceutical forms are seen in more than 3000 years old original scriptures of Ayurveda and also in later works as it was in use by successive generation in India. A comprehensive review on Garlic is highlighted here, including original references with scientific evidences.

Keywords: Ayurveda, Traditional Indian Medicine, Plant, Animal, Mineral, Lasuna, Rasona, Garlic, Health, Healing

1. Introduction

According to World Health Organization (WHO), Traditional Medicine (TM) is a comprehensive term used to refer both to Traditional Medicine such as traditional Chinese Medicine, Indian Ayurvedic and Arabic Unani Medicine and Various forms of Indigenous medicine. Traditional medicine therapies include medication therapies-if they involve use of herbal medicines, animal parts and minerals-and non-medication therapies- if they are carried out primarily without the use of the medications, as in the case of acupuncture, manual therapies and the spiritual therapies. In countries where dominant health care system is based on allopathic medicine, or where TM has not been incorporated into the national health care system, TM is often termed, "complementary", alternative or non-conventional medicine (WHO, 2002) [1].

Across the world, TM is either as the mainstay of health care delivery or serves as a complement to it. The World Health Assembly (WHA) resolution on TM (WHA 62.13), adopted in 2009, requested the Director-General of World Health Organization (WHO) to update the WHO Traditional medicine strategy 2002–2005, based on countries' progress and current new challenges in the field of traditional medicine. The WHO Traditional Medicine Strategy 2014–2023 thus reappraises and builds on the WHO Traditional Medicine Strategy 2002–2005, and sets out the course for TM and CM (T&CM) in the next decade (WHO, 2013) [2].

Since ancient times, the Traditional Indian Medicine- Ayurveda is a main stream in health care system since ancient times based on use of natural origin substances available on earth. In Charaka Samhita three origins of medicinal substances has been defined- **तत् पुनस्त्रविधिं प्रोक्तं जङ्गमौद्भदिपार्थविम्** which are as follows [3–5];

Sthavara **(immobile)**, which includes- (i) *Vanaspati* (those with fruits and invisible flowers), (ii) *Vraksha* (those having both flower and fruits), (iii) *Virudh* (weak plant and shrub) and (iv) *Osadhi* (which perishes on maturing of fruits). Further, the vegetable parts used as drug are also described in both the texts, which constitutes; *mula* (root), *tvak* (bark), *niryasa* (exudate), *nala* (hollow stalk), *svarasa* (juice), *pallava* (young leaf), *kshara* (alkali) *kshira* (latex), *phala* (fruit), *pushpa* (flower), *bhasma* (ash), *taila* (oil), *kantaka* (thorn), *patra* (leaf), *sung* (flowering bud), *kanda* (rhizome/tuber/corm), *praroha* (aerial shoots) etc.

Jangama **(mobile)**, which includes- (i) *Jarayuja* (all placental bearing- animals, human beings etc.), (ii) *Andaja* (all egg bearing- birds, snakes, reptiles etc.), (iii) *Svedaja* (origin from sweating/humidity/dampness- microorganism, insects, worms etc.) and (iv) *Udbhija* (emerge out from earth- *Indragopa*, *manduka* (frog) etc. Further, danta (tooth/tusk), *asthi* (bone), *mutra* (urine), *purisa* (faeces), *khura* (hoof), *tunda* (beak), *loma* (hair), *nakha* (nail), *charma* (skin), *paksha* (wings), *pitta* (bile), *vrsana* (testicles), *antra* (intestine), *rakta* (blood), *yakrita* (Liver), *sringa* (horn), *mamsa* (flesh) etc.

Parthiva **(Earth origin),** which includes- *suvarna* (gold), *rajata* (silver), *mani* (gems), *mukta* (pearls), *manahshila* (realgar), *mritakapala* (earthen piece) *anjana* (galena), *kanchanagairika* (red ochre), *kasisa* (ferrous sulphate), *kamksi* (alum), *Kamsya* (bronze), *ayas* (iron), *tamra* (copper), *tuttha* (copper sulphate), *puspakasya* (purified ferrous sulphate), *riti* (brass), *lohamala* (iron by-product), *vajra* (diamond), *vaidurya* (Cat's eye), *vida* (ammonium chloride), *silajatu* (black bitumen), *sisa* (lead), *sudha* (lime), *suvarnamakshika* (Copper pyrite), *suvarchika*, *sphatika* (Rock-crystal), *harital/ala* (Orpiment) etc. under this group.

Those substances are actually used rationally in Ayurveda not empirically. The Principle and Practice of Ayurveda has its emergence from ancient Vedic period i.e. 3000–1500 before Christ Era (BCE). The Indian seers of ancient age observe the nature and their surroundings and evolved certain basic principles in accordance with the prevailing Laws of the nature- *Soma* (Lunar), *Surya* (Solar) and *Anal* (Air), which influences life of every individual in the universe. According to them, the creation of Ayurveda is for the wellness of all living being. They further emphasize on two objective of the Ayurveda- (i) *svasthasya svastha rakshanam* (protection of health of a healthy individual and (ii) *aturasya vikaraprasamanam* (alleviation of disorder in a diseased person). It is worthy to mention here that the definition of Health is told in one of original scriptures of Ayurveda- Sushruta Samhita(SS) coincide with WHO definition of Health as follows; "a state of physical, mental and social well-being and not merely the absence of disease or infirmity [6]. In SS the definition of Health is seen as follows:

समदोषः समाग्नश्चि समधातु मलःक्रयिः।.
प्रसन्नात्मेन्द्रयिमनः स्वस्थइतअिभधीयते॥.

One whose *doshas*, *agni* and function of *dhatu* and *malas* are in the state of equilibrium and who has cheerful mind, intellect and sense organs is treated as '*svastha*'(healthy) [7]. This definition is very near to definition of Health by WHO.

2. Evidence of use of similar vedic plants in original scriptures of tim

The evidence of use of natural substance as medicine in India has its foot-print in more than 5000 years old compendium i.e., *Rigveda* (3000 BCE) a compendium of knowledge (*Veda*) of ancient origin. The *Osadhi-sukta* (well saying on drug) of *Rigveda* is the foremost authoritative document of the knowledge about plants in that age. It says that plant came in existence much earlier from the Gods and has innumerable places of origin and habitat. They have potency like horse and they conquer diseases in the patient on circulating all over the body. Plants were used to make man (*dvipad*- two leg) and animals (*chatuspad*- four leg) free from disease. Atharvaveda (1500 BCE) mention quite a large number of the plants and other substances used as medicine [8].

On comprehensive review of the Vedic compendia, it is observed that a good numbers of plants with their similar name and uses are find places in CS and SS. A few of them are as follows; Asvattha (*Ficus religiosa* L.) is said king of trees in Aitareya Brahamana and its fruit popularly known as, '*Pippala*'. The versatile commentator of Vedic compendia- Sayana, interprets '*pippala*' as '*palaka phala*' (life sustaining fruit) [9]. In CS- *Asvattha* find place by the same name and its phala (fruit) and *patra* (leaf) are used. The *phala* (fruit) is enumerated among fruit group [10]. In SS also, *Asvattha-phalamulatvakasunga* (fruit-root-bark-terminal part of leaf) are used. Its fruit is said as *Vajikarana* (aphrodisiac) [11]. Another plant- *Sigru*, denotes a geographical region but in later text; Kausika Sutra, it has appeared as a plant and prescribed its application in worms [12]. In 27th chapter of CS, Sigru is enumerated with other drugs i.e., **yavani** (*Trachyspermum ammi* (L.) Sprague, **arjaka** (*Orthosiphon pallidus* Royle ex Benth) etc. are used freshly as adjuvant in the preparation of food items. Here, **Garlic** (*Lasuna*) is also find place in green vegetable group [13].

The observational experience on effect of plant initially on animals and thereafter in Human beings led to the genesis of science of Life- Ayurveda (Traditional Indian Medicine) during ancient India. The three natural origin substances i.e., *Audbhid* (plant), *Jangam* (animal), *Parthiva* (mineral) are used to prepare single and compounds drugs from them. On the other side former two are used as food substances. Ayurveda advocate that rational use of wholesome substance(s) by an individual in accordance with season and geographical region makes healthy long life, whereas unwholesome causes various disorders. Ayurveda is known as sub-division of Atharvaveda as honestly written in Charaka Samhita (CS) [14] and Sushruta Samhita (SS) the Original scriptures of Ayurveda- *Vedo hi Atharvanohya* [15]. It is worthy to mention here that many of the medicinal substances used in Vedic compendia are referred in original scriptures of Ayurveda with similar name and uses.

3. Ancient origin of ayurveda (aoa)

CS and SS are very well known as the original scriptures of TIM with their Vedic tradition, they are considered contemporary to each other as both were created during 1000 BCE. The available scriptures are written in Sanskrit language, which was the language of vocabulary, writing and teaching during that period. Thus, it is obvious that the complete writing is available in Sanskrit. The CS is the text of Internal Medicine and SS is Surgical Care of Disease a part from medical care. The entire work is presented in question-answer style by Master and Disciple. The contents of the text have been arranged in eight sections and 120 chapters in case of CS and the eight sections are comprising of; basic concepts, diagnosis, specific features, human body, fatal sign & symptoms, treatment, pharmaceutical and successful management [16]. Similarly, the SS, consisted of six chapters and 188 sections as follows; basic concepts, diagnosis, human body, treatment, pharmaceuticals and Uttartantra (deals with-diseases above the neck, pediatrics and internal medicine [16, 17].

On review, one can easily visualize the method of preparation of sizable number of compound formulations too, which are even purchased over the counter for health benefits. A few of the popular compound formulations, which are even today in common practice in Ayurveda are; *Triphala Rasayana churna, Trikatu Churna* and *Chyavanprasha Avaleha* [18].

4. Evidence of first use of Garlic-*Lasuna* in india

The use of Garlic in India dates back to more than 3000 years as evident from CS and SS the original available scriptures on Ayurveda in Sanskrita Language. In both the texts "Garlic" is known by the name of *Lasuna* and also by its synonym

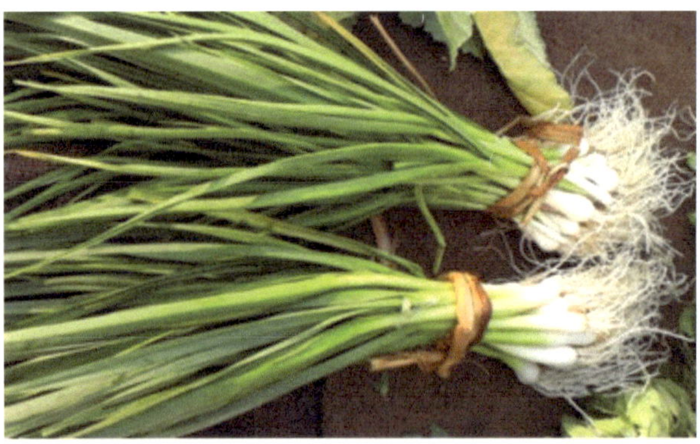

Figure 1.
Plant of Fresh Garlic.

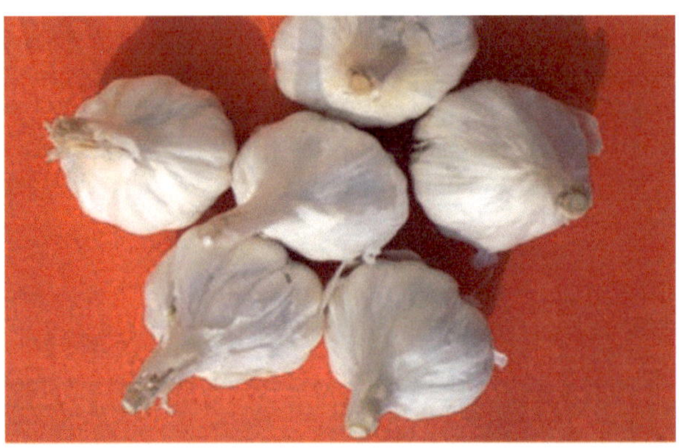

Figure 2.
Mature Garlic Bulb.

Rasona. On complete review of both the texts, it was observed in CS that the fresh garlic is placed in *harit varga* (green group) with other edible plant substances and consumed as food article [19, 20]. The green garlic is consumed while immature and still tender and a bulb not separated into cloves like a mature ones, whereas cloves are used when it is matured. Not only in Pan India but in the neighboring areas like; Nepal, Myanmar, Lao, Pakistan, Bangladesh, Bhutan, SriLanka (South-East Asian region) similar uses are reported. Thus, it is obvious that in Pan India, Garlic is in use since ancient times (**Figures 1** and **2**).

5. Use of Garlic-Lasuna for health and healing in CS and SS

5.1 Garlic-Lasuna for health in CS and SS

The Health benefits of Garlic- *Lasuna* are very much witness in ancient texts viz., CS and SS, which is based on the properties of the Lasuna (Garlic) like; *snigdha* (unctuous), *usna* (hot), *katu* (pungent), *guru* (heavy). and *snigdha* (unctuous), *usna* (hot), *tikshna* (sharp), katu (pungent), *picchila* (slimy), *guru* (heavy), *sara* (laxative), *svadurasa* (sweet) respectively. Of them, due to unctuous and slimy properties it has *vrisya* effect (promotion of 7th *Dhatu- sukra*), which is responsible for the quality formation of sperm cells and thereby *oja* (vital essence) with the result of that enhances body immunity to fight against disorders. Those properties are enhanced, if it is consumed either with milk, and/ or butter or clarified butter, thus in general it has health benefits. With clarified butter- it minimizes adverse effect owing to the properties like; hot, sharp and pungent. In SS it is considered beneficial to eye and advised for physical and mental strength promotion. It has *balya* (strengthening), *vrisya* (aphrodisiac) effects and promotes- *medha* (intellect), *svara* (voice), *varna* (complexion), *chakshu* (vision), and *bhagnasthi sandhana* (union of fractured bone) as recorded in SS [21, 22].

5.2 Garlic-Lasuna for healing in CS and SS

The Garlic-Lasuna has been prescribed to alleviates *krimi* (worms), *kustha* (dermatopathies), *kilasa* (leucoderma), *vata* (one of the three vitiated elements) and *gulma* (intra abdominal tumour), *Gaurava* (head in heaviness), *Siras sula* (headache), *Pinasa* (chronic rhinitis), *ardhavabhedaka* (hemicrania), *krimivyadhi* (helminthiasis), *apasmara* (epilepsy), *ghrananasa* (anosmia) and *pramoha* (fainting) through nasal route of administration.

In *Vimanasthana*, Lasuna is included among the drugs for non-unctuous medicated enema for intestinal worms. This medicated enema is said to be administered for three or five days continuously. In the next chapter Lasuna is enumerated in *katuskandha* (pungent-group) and medicated enema is prepared, which is prescribed along with *madhu* (honey), *taila* (oil) and *Lavana* (salt) in slesma (one of the three bio-elements) origin disorders. In the same chapter the useful part of *Lasuna-kanda* (garlic-tuber) for sirovirechana (head-evacuation- one of the procedures of Panchakarma (Five measures- *vamana-virechana-anuvasana-asthapana and sirovirechana*) has been included with other drugs in a group. The kshira-paka (medicated- milk) prepared of *suddha-suska Lasuna* (clean-dried garlic) in definite ratio of *lasuna* (garlic): *udaka* (water): *Kshira* (milk) cures *vatajagulma* (intra-abdominal tumor due to vata-vitiation), *udavarta* (upward movement of Vayu-), *gridhrasi* (sciatica), *visamajvara* (irregular-fever), *hridaroga* (cardiac-diseases), *vidradhi* (abscess) and *sotha* (inflammation). The Oral administration of *Rasona* (Garlic) paste with sesame oil before meals is prescribed to alleviate the intermittent fever.

Garlic is one of the ingredients of the *Kanakakshiri taila* (medicated oil preparation) prescribed as topical massage to alleviate worms and itching. In 9th chapter, two kinds of clarified butter based Garlic formulations are seen for *Unmada* (insanity) and *Apasmara* (epilepsy) and in both the preparations, Garlic is found as the major ingredient. Fumigation of Garlic with other plant drugs is recommended to alleviate *apasmara* (epilepsy) [23].

In SS Sutrasthana 39 chapter, *Lasuna-kanda* (garlic-bulb) is found with *alarka, ativisa, sringavera* for sirovirechana (head evacuation). It is included with other *katu* (pungent) drugs in *katu*-group (pungent group) and in *saka varga* (vegetable group) with other vegetables and its properties like; *snigdha* (unctuous), *usna* (hot), *tikshna* (sharp), *katu* (pungent), *picchala* (slimy), *guru* (heavy), *sara* (laxative), *svadurasa* (sweet) has been enumerated. It alleviates; *hridaroga* (cardiac disease), *jirna-jvara* (chronic fever), *kukshi-sula* (abdominal colic), *vibandha* (constipation), *gulma* (intra-abdominal tumour), *aruchi* (anorexia), *kasa* (cough), *sopha* (oedema), *durnama* (piles) *kustha* (dermatopathies), *analasada* (agni deficiency), *jantu* (worms), *samira* (vata), *svasa* (dyspnoea) and *kapha*. Here, the drug Lasuna and its synonym, "*Rasona*" is seen first time in SS. In case of insufficient milk production in lactating mother due to *krodha* (anger), *soka* (sorrow), *avatsalya* (loss of affection to baby) it is recommended as galactogogue. At the time of labor pain to remove the hardness of bowel, milk preparation of garlic with hingu, *sauvarchala* and *vacha* is recommended. In combination with other plant and mineral origin substances, it is recommended in eye diseases as *anjana* (anointment) and to pacify; *kandu* (itching), *timira* (diminished vision), *suklarma* (pterygium), *raktaraji* of the eye (redness of the eye). In ear diseases Garlic with other drugs in compound form of oil and clarified-butter preparations is recommended. The lukewarm oil, prepared with the juice of garlic is recommended as wholesome to earache, head evacuation and in intermittent fever in *ghrita* (clarified butter) form. At other place the milk preparation of Garlic (*Rasona*) is recommended to *Kshayaartha* (patient of tuberculosis). The juice of Garlic (Rasona) as major ingredient with other drugs in Clarified butter form is recommended to alleviate; *gulma* (intra-abdominal lump), *grahani* (duodenal disorder), *arsa* (hemorrhoids), *svasa* (dyspnoea), *unmada* (insanity), *kshaya* (tuberculosis), *Jvara* (fever), *kasa* (cough), *apasmara* (epilepsy), *mandagni* (loss of appetite), *pliha* (splenomegaly), *vatika-sula* (colic). In Uttaratantra of Sushruta Samhita, two compound formulations comprising of Garlic with other Drugs has been recommended as collyrium (externally) and oil in psychiatric disorders. In successive chapter, a compound of Garlic with other drugs in *apasmara* (epilepsy) [24].

6. Use of Garlic-*Lasuna* for health and healing in Astanga Hridaya (AH)

In AH (5th Cent.), which was popular text of the Ayurveda in Medieval times, the use of Garlic continued as evident from the similar name- *Lasuna* as referred in two previous original texts of Ayurveda. It is worthy to mention here that the similar verse line to line from Charaka Samhita has find place in AH gulma Chikitsa, which confirms the tradition continued during that period also. In 6th Chapter of Sutrasthana of AH, it is included in vegetable group. Its properties has been said as; *Bhristikshonah* (excessive sharp and hot), *katu* in *rasa* and *vipaka* (pungent-taste and also after digestion and metabolism), *sara* (laxative), *snigdha* (unctuous), *rochana* (stimulating the appetite), *guru* (heavy). It is one of the drugs which is having *vrisya* (aphrodisiac) in spite of *Katu* (pungent) *rasa* (taste) inclusively referred in *Rasabhediya* 10th chapter of Sutrasthana.

In this text a few new health benefits including earlier texts, like- *hridya* (beneficial to heart) *Kesya* (beneficial for hair), *vrisya* (aphrodisiac), *dipana* (enhancing digestive fire), *bhagnasandhanakrita* (union-promoting in fracture), *rasayana* (promotive therapy) are enumerated. In case of regaining mada (intoxication) *murcha* (fainting) and *sanyasa* (complete exhaustion) due to chronic alcoholism, the juice of Garlic is advised.

It alleviates intermittent fever, if consumed with oil in the morning. Also alleviates severe *Vatic* disorders (diseases caused by vitiation of Vata), *kilasa* (vitiligo), *kustha* (dermatopathies), *gulma* (intra-abdominal lump), *arsa* (hemorrhoides), *meha* (turbidity in urine), *krimi* (worm), *kapha* (one of the three bio-elements), *anil-vata* (one of the three bio-elements), *hidhma* (hiccough), *pinasa* (chronic Rhinitis), *svasa* (difficult breathing) and *kasa* (cough). At other place, the compound formulation of Garlic with other plant and mineral origin medicinal substances has been recommended to alleviate *apasmara* (epilepsy) [25]. Looking to the popularity of the AH, this treatise is included with two great treatise of ancient period i.e., CS and SS and all three are known together as *Brihattrayi* (greater treatise) of Ayurveda even today.

7. Carefulness on continuous use of Garlic-Lasuna

Its continuous use as food items causes vitiation of *pitta* (one of the elements among three *doshas*), which leads to raktapitta (internal hemorrhage). The prodromal symptoms of occurrence of internal hemorrhage has also been reported such as; *annannabhilasa* (aversion to food), *bhuktasyavidaha* (burning on immediate ingestion of food), *suktaamlagandharasa udgaara* (eructation having smell and taste of sour gruel), *charderbhikshanamaagamana* (nauseating and frequent urge for vomiting), *Charditasya vibhatsata* (disgusting vomitus-consisting blood), *svarabheda* (hoarseness of voice), *gatranam sadanam* (malaise), *paridaha* (burning around the body) etc. [26]. Similar caution has been found in AH as follows; continuous use of Garlic-*Lasuna* causes *raktapittapradusana* (vitiation of *rakta-pitta* causes internal-hemorrhage) [27].

8. Healing benefits of Garlic- Lasuna in later works of

8.1 TIM

Another noted- treatise on Principles and Practices of Ayurvedic Medicine i.e., Cakradatta of 11th Cent. also having single and compound preparations prescribed in number of disorders like; *Lasunadi yoga* (a compound formulation) having *Pippali mula* (root of *Piper longum* L.) and *Abhaya* (*Terminalia chebula* Retz.) has been prescribed to alleviate spleenomegaly. At other place, the Lasunadya ghrita (a compound preparation with clarified butter) is prescribed to alleviates *sula* (abdominal colic), *gulma* (abdominal lump), *arsa* (hemorrhoids), *udara-roga* (abdominal disorders), *pandu* (anemia), *pliha* (spleenomegaly), *yonidosha* (uterine disorders), *krimi* (worms), *jvara* (fever), *vata* and *kapha* disorders and *unmada* (insanity). In this text also its synonym *Rasona* is find place and *Rasona kshira* (Garlic-milk), *Rasona-taila* (Garlic-oil), *Rasona-pinda* (Garlic-bolus), *Rasona-sura* (Garlic-liquor), *Rasonadya-kalka* (Garlic-paste) and *Rasonadya ghrita* (Garlic-clarified butter) are some of the compound formulations advised in various ailments. It is interesting to mention here that the Rasona kshira is the same preparation of CS with little change in verse and the indications are the same as of *Lasuna-kshiram* of CS. i.e., The *kshira-paka* (medicated- milk) prepared of *suddha-suska Lasuna* (clean-dried garlic) in definite ratio of *lasuna* (garlic): *udaka* (water): *Kshira* (milk) cures *vatajagulma* (intra-abdominal tumor due to vata-vitiation), *udavarta* (upward movement of vayu), *gridhrasi* (sciatica), *visamajvara* (irregular-fever), *hridaroga* (cardiac-diseases), *vidradhi* (abscess) and *sotha* (inflammation) [28].

In popular manuscripts of 12th Cent.- Vangasena Samhita, single as well as compound formulations of Garlic-Lasuna has been prescribed. The fine paste of Garlic bulb with clarified butter with consumption of clarified butter in diet alleviates all kinds of Vatic disorders (diseases caused due to vitiation of vata-dosha in body). At other place, a compound preparation- *Rasonapinda* (bolus of Garlic), either with *jala* (water) or *madya* (alcohol) is praised to alleviate- *amavata* (vitiated vata with endotoxin), vitiated *vata* in particular location and entire body, *apasmara* (epilepsy), *svasa* (dysponea), *kasa* (cough), *gara* (poisoning),*unmada* (insanity), *vatabhagna* (fracture due to vitiated vata), *sula* (colic) and *jantu* (worm infestation). The oil prepared from the paste and juice of Garlic alleviates all types of pain due to vitiated *vata dosha* [29].

In the most popular work of Srangadharacharya- Srangadharasamhita of 13th Cent., single and compound from of Garlic- *Lasuna* are included. The *kalka* (paste) Of *Rasona-Lasuna* mixed with the oil of sesame is prescribed in *visamjvara* (inter-mittent- fever) and vatic diseases. In continuation to that a compound formulation prepared with matured Garlic-*Lasuna* is recommended to alleviate *akangavata* (vitiated *vata* in particular location), *sarvanga vata* (vitiated *vata* inentire body, *apasmara* (epilepsy), *unmada* (insanity), *gridhrisi* (sciatica), *sula* (colic) and *krimi* (worm infestation) etc. [30].

The author Sodhal has composed the text during 14th Cent. and named it Gadanigrah in which disorders along with their treatment are lucidly described. Amongst the vegetable origin drugs Garlic-*Lasuna* is also find place in many diseases as single and compound formulations. The compound formulation- *Lasunaddya ghritam* (Clarified butter preparation of Garlic with other drugs) with honey and sugar alleviates- *raktapitta* (internal hemorrhage), *kasa* (cough), *gulma* (intra abdominal tumor) etc. At other place with other vegetable drugs, clarified butter preparation of Garlic- *Lasuna* is prescribed in *kasa* (cough), *svasa* (dyspo-nea), *jvara* (fever), *hridaroga* (cardiac disease)etc. An exclusive clarified prepara-tion is made to overcome the *gulma* (intra abdominal tumor) and vatic disorders has been prescribed. The *Rasonapinda* (bolus of Garlic), either with *jala* (water) or *madya* (alcohol) is praised to alleviate- *amavata* (vitiated vata with endotoxin), vitiated *vata* in particular location and entire body, *apasmara* (epilepsy), *svasa* (dys-ponea), *kasa* (cough), *gara* (poisoning),*unmada* (insanity), *vatabhagna* (fracture due to vitiated vata), *sula* (colic) and *jantu* (worm infestation). The oil preparation of *Kalka* (paste) and svarasa (juice) of *Rasona*- Garlic cures all vatic disorders [31].

During 15th Cent. Kaiyadeva *Nighantu* (Materia.Medica) came into existence, which was created by Kaiyadeva. In fact, initially it was known as *Pathyaapathya vibodhaka* (knowledge on wholesome and unwholesome). In this Materia Medica, Garlic-*Lasuna* its synonyms, properties, action and therapeutic uses as an indi-vidual drug has been described. Here the similar properties as found in CS and SS are described. It is worthwhile to mention here that the therapeutic uses are also the same as found in original texts [32].

The noted author of 16th Cent.-Bhavamishra created Bhavaprakasa in which single and compound formulations are prescribed. In this text, the compound formulation consisting of *Lasuna* and other vegetable drugs prepared in mustard oil is poured in ear to alleviates- *karnasula* (earache) and *karna-nada* (tinnitus). The paste of Garlic mixed with sesame oil and rock salt cures *visamjvara* (intermittent fever) and all vatic disorders if consumed in the morning and Garlic paste in oil removes *apasmara* (epilepsy). In case of wound with maggots the paste of Garlic is applied to kill them. Administration of the paste of Garlic with sesame oil cures *ardit* (facial paralysis). *Rasonapinda* (bolus of Garlic), a compound formulation is advised to alleviate- *amavata* (vitiated vata with endotoxin), vitiated *vata* in particular location and entire body, *apasmara* (epilepsy), *svasa* (dysponea), *kasa* (cough), *gara* (poisoning),*unmada* (insanity), *vatabhagna* (fracture due to vitiated vata), *sula* (colic) and *jantu* (worm infestation) [33, 34]. He also created Bhavaprakasa *Nighantu* (Materia - Medica) in which Garlic-*Lasuna,* its synonyms, properties, action and therapeutic uses as single drug has been described. Almost similar properties, action and therapeutic uses are seen as found in CS & SS. Here, it is stressed that a person should not do exercise, exposure to Sunlight, anger, excessive water drinking while consuming Garlic- Lasuna, because of hot in potency [35].

Pandit Narhari in 17th Cent. created Raja- *Nighantu* (Materia Medica) in which Garlic –Lasuna along with synonyms are described. Further, its properties like- *Usna* (hot), *katu* (pungent), *picchala* (slimy) *snigdha* (unctuous), *guru* (heavy), *tikshna* (sharp), *svadurasa* (sweet) has been enumerated. By virtue of its properties it has health promotive effects viz- *atibalya* (excess strengthening), *vrisya* (aphrodisiac), medha (mental strengthening), *varnya* (improve complexion) etc. A part from that it also alleviates- *hridaroga* (cardiac disorder), *bhagnasthisandhankara* (union promoter of the fractured bone), *jvara* (fever), *gulma* (intra-abdominal tumor), *sula* (colic), *sopha* (inflammation) etc. [36].

During 18th Cent. Kaviraj Govind Das Sen compiled a manuscript and named it Bhaisajyaratnawali, which consist of 2600 formulations. In this work number of single and compound formulations of Garlic are included, which are as follows; *Lasuna- Kshira* (milk preparation of Garlic), *Lasunadi- ghrita* (clarified preparation of Garlic, *Rasona-kalka* (garlic-paste), *Rasona-taila* (garlic-oil), *Rasona- sura* (garlic- liquor), *Rasonadi-kvatha* (decoction of Garlic with other drugs) etc. They are recommended in *apasmara* (epilepsy), *svasa* (dysponea), *kasa* (cough), *gara* (poisoning), *unmada* (insanity), *vatabhagna* (fracture due to vitiated vata), *sula* (colic) and *jantu* (worm infestation) etc. Most of the preparations contains in Bhaisajyaratnawali are still in practice and prepared by the Ayurvedic Pharmaceutical industries [37].

In 19th Cent. Shaligram Nighantu- Bhusanam was created by Lala Shaligramji Vaisya, which is considered the last Nighantu of that time written in ancient style. In this Nighantu, Garlic-Lasuna has been placed under the heading of *kandasaka* of *sakavarga* (vegetable group). Here also, its synonyms like-*Rasona, suklakanda* etc. as referred in previous works are included. Similarly, properties, action, therapeutic uses find in CS, SS and later works are incorporated, which shows continuation of the TIM of ancient origin even during that period. The botanical name *Allium sativum* L. Is included here [38].

A good number of *Nighantu's* were come into existence during 20th Cent. Of them, the famous is Adarsha *Nighantu*, created by Vaidya Bapalal. In this *Nighantu*; Garlic- *Lasuna* is included in *Lasunadivarga* (Garlic group) and its names in various regional languages of India and, Latin scientific name *Allium sativum* L. has been included. Its properties like- *katu* (pungent), *madhura* (sweet) in taste, *usna* (hot) in potency, katu-vipaka (transformed state after digestion and metabolism) and *kapha* and *vata doshaghna* (pacifying *kapha* and *vata dosha*) is written in a way to make it more clear to the seekers of Ayurvedic based knowledge on Garlic. It is worthwhile to mention here that the author has give original textual references on Garlic-*Lasuna* compiled from CS, SS, AH, popular *Nighantu* of different period viz., Dhanvantari, Raja, Bhavaprakasa etc. Thus, it shows that the author has brought forward diversified knowledge at one place on Garlic-Lasuna. This Nighantu is included in the graduate course of Ayurveda taught in Ayurvedic institution in India [39].

9. Etymology of *Lasuna*- Garlic and binominal nomenclature based on usna (hot) potency

It is obvious that the Garlic by the name of Lasuna was much more earlier in use in India i.e., since ancient period and even one of the properties hot (usna) is referred in original scriptures of Ayurveda (1000 BCE). The etymology of the Lasuna is defined by Dalhana as follows; *Lasati bhinatti roganiti lasunam* means, which destroy diseases [40].

The binominal nomenclature / botanical name of the Garlic was confirmed by Linnaeus as *Allium sativum* L. in 16th Cent. It is interesting to note here that the genus *Allium*, Linn. was derived from the Celtic all (relating to the Celts or their languages-a branch of Indo-European family of Languages), signifies "hot", or "burning". Thus it seems that the genus- *Allium* L. has its base from the most prominent "hot" potency". It is worthwhile to mention here that a good number of binominal nomenclatures have its basis on Sanskrit names of the vegetable drugs as evident from William Roxburgh's, "Flora Indica" where he has mentioned that he has picked up names of the various drugs from the works of Amarkosa, Rajanighantu and Bhava-prakasha, which helped him to ascertain their Botanical nomenclature [41]. It is quite possible that the usna (hot) potency, which has included in almost all the works of Ayurveda have attracted Linnaeus and coined the genus Allium [42]. Ayurveda advocates that alleviation of any disorders is always due to the properties which exist in a Drug. In fact, any substance of natural origin qualifies a Drug if used rationally in accordance with the Basic Principles of Dravya-guna-karma (substance-properties-action).

10. Rationale use of natural substance and Garlic-Lasuna for health and healing

The natural origin-food substance(s) of plant and animal origin are predominance in *bhautika / saririka* gunas (physical / bodily attributes) in accordance with the geographical region. They are 20 in numbers and grouped in 10 pairs because relative to each other. They are as follows; *guru-laghu* (heavy-light), *sita-usna* (cold-hot), *snigdha-ruksha* (unctuous-non-unctous), *manda-tikshna* (dull-sharp), *sthira-sara* (stable-moving), *mrdu-kathina* (soft-hard), *visada-picchila* (non-slimy-slimy), *slakshna-khara* (smooth-rough), *sthula-sukshma* (massive/gross-fine), and *Sandra-drava* (thick-liquid). Because of relative to each other, they produce visible changes in the bodily substances. The judicious use of the food substances in accordance with the beneficial to the *prakriti* (natural body constitution) of a person keeps healthy all along the life, whereas contrary to that use of un-wholesome food leads to diseased state of the body. In diseased state apart from administration of wholesome food to alleviate the disorder drug potency is kept in mind before writing a prescription.

This potency in a drug is known as *Virya* in Ayurveda. In fact, out of aforesaid twenty(20) *gunas* eight(8) i.e., *guru-laghu* (heavy-light), *sita-usna* (cold-hot), *snigdha-ruksha* (unctuous-non-unctous) and *mridu-tikshna* (dull-sharp) are designated as *virya* (potency) because of excellent allowance of gunas acquired naturally in a medicinal substance. Considering the potency of a drug, it is prescribed in definite dose as compare to food substance consumed in large quantity. Thus food (having gunas) as well as drug (having *virya*) play important role in the alleviation of the disorders to bring back equilibrium of the three doshas and therefore in Ayurveda wholesome food (pathya) is the integral part of the prescription along with potential drug [43, 44]. The properties like- *snigdha* (unctuous), *picchala* (slimy) in Garlic- Lasuna have health benefits, which is enhanced when consumed with milk, butter or clarified butter based preparations, whereas- *guru* (heavy), *usna* (hot), *tikshna* (sharp), katu (pungent), *sara* (laxative), *svadurasa* (sweet) has healing effect in a diseased person with hot water, honey, sesame oil etc.

11. Lasuna- Garlic in the ayurvedic pharmacopoeia of india

In the Ayurvedic Pharmacopoeia of India Part-I, Vol.III, Garlic-Lasuna (bulb) is defined as follows; Lasuna consists of *Allium sativum* Linn.(Fam.Liliaceae);a perennial bulbus plant, cultivated as an important condiment crop in the country. *Rasona* and *Yavanesta* two synonyms with names in Indian regional languages are find place here. The macroscopic and microscopic description of a clove of the bulb is described. Following this; identity, purity and strength, thin layer chromatography, constituents, properties, action, important formulations- *Lasunadi* vati, *Lasunadi ghrita* and *Vacha-lasunadi* tail are included here. The therapeutic uses and prescribed dose; 3–6 g. of the Drug shows its importance in Ayurveda [45].

12. Scientific evidence of efficacy of *Allium sativum*- Lasuna (Garlic)

The pre-clinical study of Garlic extract (50–500 mg/ kg,) has been found anti-hypertensive response as reported by Sanfilippo and Ottaviano [46], Petkov [47], Chanderkar and Jain [48]; antiarrhythmic by Martin et al., [49], Isensee et. Al., [50]; cardioprotective effects on rodents by Saxena et al., [51], Kojima et al., [51] Ashraf et al.,[52], Sarvanan & Prakash [53], Cheng et al., [54]. The dietary intake of garlic powder (1.0 per cent) for 10- weeks significantly prohibited the incidence of ventricular arrythemias after ischaemia and reperfusion in the isolated rat heart (Langendrorff) preparation Martin et al., [55]. Cardioprotective effect of Garlic was observed against doxorubicin and hypocholesterolamic diet induced cardiac injuries and pulmonary hypertension- induced cardiac hypertrophy in laboratory- animals, Kojima et al., [56], Cheng et al., [57]. Fibrinolytic activity of garlic was observed in animals, Singh & Chaturvedi, 1974 [58]. The Garlic and its Phytoconstituents were reported to inhibit platelet aggregation and to increase the bleeding time and clotting time of experimental animals, Jain et al., [59], Allison et al., 2012 [60].

Garlic have been found other bioactivities viz., antidiabetic, Brahmchari and Augusti [61], Jain et al., [62], Padiya & Banerjee [63]; nephroprotective, Rafieian et al., [64]; chemopreventive /anticancer, Belman [65], Rao et al., [66], Ariga et al., [67]; antibacterial Rao et al., [68], Jezowa et al., [69]; anti-Helicobacter Pylori, Sivam [70]; antifungal, Tansey & Appleton [71]; antiviral, Tsai et al. [72]; anthelmintic, Abdel- Rahman et al. [73], antispasmodic, Gaffen et al., [74], Aquel et al., [75] anti-oxidant, Popov et al., [76], Dong et al., [77] anti-toxic, Bhatia & Ahujari [78], Senapati et al.,[79], immunomodulatory, Tabari & Ebrahimpour [80] in pre-clinical experimental animals.

On clinical study also, Garlic were seen effective in the patients of- hypertension in which significant lowering of systolic and diasystolic blood pressure was recorded, Sobenin et al. [81], Ashraf et al., [82]; coronary artery disease, Bordia et al., [83], Williams et.al, [84]; peripheral arterial occlusive disease, Kiessewetter et al., [85]; atherosclerosis, Rapp et al., [86], Budoff et al., [87]; hyperlipedemia, Bordia et al., [88], Bhusan et/al., [89], Mahanta et al., [90], Vorberg & Schinder [91], Jung et al., [92]; type-2 diabetes, Soebinin et al., [93], Ashraf et al., [94], Kumar et al., [95]; systemic sclerosis, Rapp et al., [96]; Common cold, Josling [97]; cold and flu, Nantz et al., [98]; Rheumatoid arthritis, Denisov et al., [99].

13. Conclusion

The use fresh plant as well as mature and dried cloves of Garlic is in use in Traditional Indian Medicine since ancient times as per the documented evidence in original scriptures of Ayurveda. The original works are written in Sanskrit Language, therefore, Garlic is seen by the name of *Lasuna* along with its popular synonym *Rasona*. The traditional Indian Medicine has its foot print in Vedic Compendia (3000 1500 BCE) as the similar named plants are find place in Charaka Samhita and Sushruta Samhita, thus the use of vegetable origin substances can be visualized more than 5ooo years in practice and in case of **Lasuna**, it is more than 3000 years. The etymology of the word Lasuna signifies- destroyer of diseases. The properties based action and therapeutic uses itself speaks about the rational use of Garlic- Lasuna in Ayurveda. The genus *Allium* seems to be based on one of the predominant properties 'hot' found in *Lasuna* as referred in both the original scriptures of Ayurveda. The bilingual name *Allium sativum* was coined by Linneaus in 16th Century, which was included later on in successive works.

As per the evidence, the varies uses of *Lasuna*-Garlic (*Allium sativum* L.) as food substance as well drug substances is well established in Indian Traditional Medicine, which is known as one of the traditional Medicines of the World by World Health Organization. The traditional continued since then and documented by successive generation in different period of times, and even tradition prevail in today's India. For Health; it is recommended as; strengthening, aphrodisiac, promoting- intellect, galactogogue in mother,, vision and complexion, beneficial to hairs etc. and for the alleviation of disorders it is prescribed in cardiac diseases, chronic and intermittent fever, abdominal colic, intra-abdominal tumor, piles, dermal disorders, worm infestation, diminished vision, pterygeum, difficult breathing, tuberculosis, insanity, epilepsy etc. Single and compound formulae like Garlic- juice, paste, bolus, clarified butter, oil, milk, liquor and oil, clarified butter, tablets etc., respectively. In fact, the rational use as well formulae are prepared on the basis of properties like; unctuous, hot, pungent, slimy, heavy etc.

It is worthwhile to mention here that the health benefits of Garlic-Lasuna as envision by ancient scholars of TIM- Ayurveda now proved scientifically by the various scholars working on *Allium sativum* L. like- hridaroga (antiarrhythmic, cardioprotective effects, ventricular arrythemias after ischaemia), *raktapitta*-internal hemorrhage (increase the bleeding time and clotting time), *jantughna* (antibacterial), kustha (dermatopathies- antifungal), krimighna (anthelmintic), sula (antispasmodic), *balya*–strengthening(immunemodulatory), vata-kapha disorders (common cold, cold and flu) etc., which corroborate the uses of Lasuna- Garlic in TIM- Ayurveda.

Thus, it is obvious that Lasuna- *Garlic (Allium sativum* L.) is one of the vegetable origin substances in India has its evidence of uses traditionally more than 3000 years for the protection of Health as well as Healing (alleviation of disorders rationally).

DOI: http://dx.doi.org/10.5772/intechopen.97495

Author details

Vinod Kumar Joshi[1]* and Apurva Joshi[2]

1 Faculty of Ayurveda, Department of Dravyaguna, Institute of Medical Sciences, Banaras Hindu University, Varanasi, India

2 Ozone Pharmaceutical Ltd., New Delhi, India

*Address all correspondence to: joshivkvns@gmail.com

References

[1] Anonyms, Key points; WHO traditional Medicine Strategy: 2002-2005, p.1-2, World Health Organization Geneva-27, Switzerland, (2002).

[2] Anonyms, WHO traditional Medicine Strategy: 2014-2023, p. 7, World Health Organization Geneva-27, Switzerland (2013).

[3] Agnivesa, Charaka Samhita, revised by Charaka and Dridhabala with the Ayurveda-Dipika Commentary of Chakrapanidatta, Edited by Vaidya Jadavji Trikamji Acharya, published by Chaukhambha Sanskrit Sansthan, Varanasi, p. 20 (1992).

[4] Susruta, Sushruta Samhita with the Nibandhasangraha Commentary of Sri Dlhanacharya, Edited by Vaidya Jadavji Trikamji Acharya, Published by Chaukhambha Orientalia, Varanasi, p.7-8 (1992).

[5] Joshi VK, Joshi A, Dhiman KS. The Ayurvedic Pharmacopoeia of India, development and perspectives. Journal of Ethnopharmacology. 2017; 197: 32-38. DOI: 10.1016/j.jep.2016.07.030

[6] https://en.wikipedia.org/wiki/World_Health_Organization

[7] Susruta, Sushruta Samhita with the Nibandhasangraha Commentary of Sri Dlhanacharya, Edited by Vaidya Jadavji Trikamji Acharya, Published by Chaukhambha Orientalia, Varanasi, p.2 (1992).

[8] Anonymous, edited by Sharma, P.V. History of Medicine in India, the Indian National Scienc Academy, Bahadur Shah Jafar Shah Zafar Marg, New Delhi-110002. p. 16 (1992).

[9] Anonymous, edited by Sharma, P.V. History of Medicine in India, the Indian National Scienc Academy, Bahadur Shah Jafar Shah Zafar Marg, New Delhi-110002. p. 40 (1992).

[10] Agnivesa, Charaka Samhita, revised by Charaka and Dridhabala with the Ayurveda-Dipika Commentary of Chakrapanidatta, Edited by Vaidya Jadavji Trikamji Acharya, published by Chaukhambha Sanskrit Sansthan, Varanasi, p. 159 (1992).

[11] Susruta, Sushruta Samhita with the Nibandhasangraha Commentary of Sri Dlhanacharya, Edited by Vaidya Jadavji Trikamji Acharya, Published by Chaukhambha Orientalia, Varanasi, p.7-8 (1992).

[12] Anonymous, edited by Sharma, P.V. History of Medicine in India, the Indian National Scienc Academy, Bahadur Shah Jafar Shah Zafar Marg, New Delhi-110002. p. 52 (1992).

[13] Agnivesa, Charaka Samhita, revised by Charaka and Dridhabala with the Ayurveda-Dipika Commentary of Chakrapanidatta, Edited by Vaidya Jadavji Trikamji Acharya, published by Chaukhambha Sanskrit Sansthan, Varanasi, p. 162 (1992).

[14] Agnivesa, Charaka Samhita, revised by Charaka and Dridhabala with the Ayurveda-Dipika Commentary of Chakrapanidatta, Edited by Vaidya Jadavji Trikamji Acharya, published by Chaukhambha Sanskrit Sansthan, Varanasi, p. 186 (1992).

[15] Susruta, Sushruta Samhita with the Nibandhasangraha Commentary of Sri Dlhanacharya, Edited by Vaidya Jadavji Trikamji Acharya, Published by Chaukhambha Orientalia, Varanasi, p.2 (1992).

[16] Sharma P.V., Charaka Samhita (text with English translation), Vol. I (Sutrasthana to Indriyasthana),

Chaukhambha Orientalia, Varanasi-221001, p. i-xiii- (1981).

[17] Sharma P.V., Susruta Samhita with English translation of text and Dalhan's commentary along with critical notes, Vol. I, SutrasthanaChaukhambha Visvabharati, Varanasi-221001, p. iii-vi (1999).

[18] Anonymous, The Ayurvedic Formulary of India, Part I, (Second Revised Edition, Government of India, Ministry of Health and Family Welfare, s Department of Indian System of Medicine & Homeopathy, New Delhi –110001, p.110 & 37-38 (2003).

[19] Agnivesa, Charaka Samhita, revised by Charaka and Dridhabala with the Ayurveda-Dipika Commentary of Chakrapanidatta, Edited by Vaidya Jadavji Trikamji Acharya, published by Chaukhambha Sanskrit Sansthan, Varanasi, p. 24, 426 (1992).

[20] Susruta, Sushruta Samhita with the Nibandhasangraha Commentary of Sri Dlhanacharya, Edited by Vaidya Jadavji Trikamji Acharya, Published by Chaukhambha Orientalia, Varanasi, p.171, 232 (1992).

[21] Agnivesa, Charaka Samhita, revised by Charaka and Dridhabala with the Ayurveda-Dipika Commentary of Chakrapanidatta, Edited by Vaidya Jadavji Trikamji Acharya, published by Chaukhambha Sanskrit Sansthan, Varanasi, p. 162 (1992).

[22] Susruta, Sushruta Samhita with the Nibandhasangraha Commentary of Sri Dlhanacharya, Edited by Vaidya Jadavji Trikamji Acharya, Published by Chaukhambha Orientalia, Varanasi, p.232 (1992).

[23] Agnivesa, Charaka Samhita, revised by Charaka and Dridhabala with the Ayurveda-Dipika Commentary of Chakrapanidatta, Edited by Vaidya Jadavji Trikamji Acharya, published by Chaukhambha Sanskrit Sansthan, Varanasi, p. 24, 251, 284, 286, 426, 440, 472, 476 (1992).

[24] Susruta, Sushruta Samhita with the Nibandhasangraha Commentary of Sri Dlhanacharya, Edited by Vaidya Jadavji Trikamji Acharya, Published by Chaukhambha Orientalia, Varanasi, p.171,230,232, 391, 393, 614, 617, 640, 645, 646, 760, 798, 805 (1992).

[25] Vagbhata, Astanga Hridaya (A compendium of the Ayurveda System) Composed by Vagbhata, with the commentaries – Sarvanga Sundara of Arundatta and Ayurvedarasyana of Hemadri, Chaukhambha Orientalia, Varanasi, reprint 9th Edition. p 109, 178, 571, 638, 687, 688, 931, 944 (2005).

[26] Agnivesa, Charaka Samhita, revised by Charaka and Dridhabala with the Ayurveda-Dipika Commentary of Chakrapanidatta, Edited by Vaidya Jadavji Trikamji Acharya, published by Chaukhambha Sanskrit Sansthan, Varanasi, p. 205 (1992).

[27] Vagbhata, Astanga Hridaya (A compendium of the Ayurveda System) Composed by Vagbhata, with the commentaries – Sarvanga Sundara of Arundatta and Ayurvedarasyana of Hemadri, Chaukhambha Orientalia, Varanasi, reprint 9th Edition. p.109 (2005).

[28] Cakradatta (Text with English translation), A treatise on Principles and Practices of Ayurvedic Medicine, edited and translated by Priya Vrat Sharma, Chaukhambha Orientalia, Varanasi. p. 176, 245, 323, 386. (1994),

[29] Vangsen Samhita 'Hari'Hindi commentary by Pd. Hariprasad Tripathi, Chaukhambha Sanskrit Series Office, Varanasi, First Edition p. 663, 700, 737 (2009).

[30] Pd. Srangadharacharya, Srangadhara-Samhita, son of Pd.

Damodara with the commentary Adhamalla's Dipika and Kasirama's Gudhartha- Dipika, Chaukhambha Orientalia, Varanasi-221001, p.174-175 (2008).

[31] Sodhal, Gadanigraha with the Vidyotini Hindi commentary Part I and II by Sri Indradev Tripathi and edited by Sri Ganga Sahay Pandey, Chaukhambha Sanskrit Sansthana, Varanasi-221001. p.10, 40, 56, 262,512 (2011)

[32] Kaiyadeva –Nighantuh (Pathyapathya-Vibodhaka) edited and translated by Prof. Priyavrat Sharma and Dr. Guru Prasad Sharma, Chaukhambha Orientalia, Varanasi-221001, p.225 (1979).

[33] Bhavamishra, Bhavaprakasa edited with Vidyotini commentary by Bhisagratna Pandit Sri Brahma Shankar Mishra (Part II), Chaukhambha Sanskrit Bhawan, Varanasi- 221001 p. 75, 156, 225, 235, 290, 471 (2010).

[34] K.C.Chunekar and N.P.Hota, Plants of Bhavaprakasa editor, S.K.Sharma, National Academy of Ayurveda, Dhanwantari Bhawan Road No. 66, Punjabi Bagh (West), New Delhi-110026 , p.185,271, 272 (1999).

[35] Bhavaprakasa Nighantu (Indian Materia Medica) of Bhavamisra, commentary by Prof. K.C. Chunekar, edited by Late Dr. G. S. pandey, Chaukhambha Bharati Academy, Varanasi-221001 p. 126-127 (2010).

[36] Pandit Narahari, Rajanighantu edied with Dravyagunaprakashika Hindi Commentary by Dr. Indradeva Tripathi, Chowkhambha Krisnadas Academy, Vranasi-221001,p 198 (2010).

[37] Bhaisajyaratnāvali of Sri Govind Das Edited with 'Siddhaprada' Hindi Commentary by Prof. Siddhi Nandan Mishra, Chaukhambha Surbharati Prakashan, Varanasi, p. 121,526, 540, 597, 612, 650, 970 (2005).

[38] Lala Shaligram Vaisya, Shaligram Nighantu- Bhusanam,Khemraj Shrikrishnadas Prakashana, Bombay-400004, p. 693-694 (2011).

[39] Shri Bapalal G. Vd. Nighantu Adarsha (Uttararardha), Chaukhambha Bharati Academy, Varanasi-221001, p.617-626 (1984).

[40] Sushruta Samhita of Susruta, with the Nibandhasangraha Commentary of Sri Dalhanacharya, Edited by Vaidya Jadavji Trikamji Acharya, Published by Chaukhambha Orientalia, Varanasi, p. 798 (1992).

[41] Joshi VK[1], Joshi A[2], Dhiman KS[3].The Ayurvedic Pharmacopoeia of India, development and perspectives. J Ethnopharmacol. 2017 Feb 2;197:32-38. doi: 10.1016/j.jep.2016.07.030. Epub 2016 Jul 9.

[42] Paxton's Botanical Dictionary comprising the names, history and culture of all Plants known in Britain with a full explanation of Technical Terms, revised and corrected by Samuel Hereman, Periodical Express Book Agency, Delhi, p.21-22 (1988).

[43] Charaka Samhita by Agnivesa revised by Charaka and Dridhabala with the Ayurveda-Dipika Commentary of Chakrapanidatta, Edited by Vaidya Jadavji Trikamji Acharya, published by Chaukhambha Sanskrit Sansthan, Varanasi, p. 12,13, 141, 135-150, (1992).

[44] Sushruta Samhita of Susruta, with the Nibandhasangraha Commentary of Sri Dlhanacharya, Edited by Vaidya Jadavji Trikamji Acharya, Published by Chaukhambha Orientalia, Varanasi, 173-186 (1992).

[45] Anonyms; The Ayurvedic Pharmacopoeia of India, Part-I, Vol.-III (First Edition), Government of India,Ministry of Health and Family Welfare, Department of Indian Systems

of Medicine & Homeopathy, New Delhi .p. 108-109 (2001).

[46] Sanfilippo, G. and Ottaviano, G. 1944. Pharmacological investigations on *Allium sativum* L., General action II. Action on arterial pressure and on respiration. Boll Soc Ital Biol Sper 19. 156-158.

[47] Petkov,V. 1966.Pharmacological and Clinical studies of garlic. Deut Zeit 106, 1861-1867.

[48] Chanderkar, A.G. & Jain, P.K. 1973. Analysis of hypotensive action of *Allium sativum* L. (garlic).Indian Journal Physiol Pharmacol 17, 132-133.

[49] Martin, N., Bardisa, L., pantoja, C., Vargas, M., Quezada, P. and Valenzuela, J. 1994. Anti-arrythmic profile of a garlic dilysate assayed in dogs and isolated atrial preporations. J Ethnopharmacol 43,1-8.

[50] Isensee, H., Rietz, B. and Jcob, R. 1993. Cardio protective actions of garlic (Allium sativum),Arzneimittel Forschung 43,94-98.

[51] Saxena, K.K., Gupta, B. Kulshrestha, V.K., Srivastava, R.K. and Prasad, D.N.1980. Effect of garlic pretreatment onisoprenaline-induced myocardial necrosis in albino rats. Indian J Physiol Pharmacol 24, 233-236.

[52] Ashraf, M.Z. Hussain,M. and Fahim, M. 2000. Endothelium mediated vasorelaxant effect of garlic is not mediated through nitric oxide. Indian J. Pharmacol 32.160.

[53] Sarvanan, G. & Prakash, J. 2004. (*Allium sativum*) on lipid peroxidation in experimental myocardial infarction in rats. J Ethnopharmacol 94, 155-158.

[54] Cheng, Y.C., Chang, M.H., Tsai, C.C., Chen T.S.,Fan, C.C., Lin, C.C., Lai, C.H., Tsai, F.J., Lin, J.A. and Huang, C.Y. 2013. Garlic oil atinuates the cardiac apoptosis in hamster fed with hypercholesterol diet. Food Chem 136, 1296-1302.

[55] Martin, N., Bardisa, L., pantoja, C., Vargas, M., Quezada, P. and Valenzuela, J. 1994. Anti-arrythmic profile of a garlic dilysate assayed in dogs and isolated atrial preporations. J Ethnopharmacol 43,1-8.

[56] Kojima, R., Toyama, Y and Ohnishi, S.T. 1994. Protective effects of an aged garlic extract on doxorubicin- induced cardiotoxicity in the mouse. Nutr Cancer 22, 163-173.

[57] Cheng, Y.C., Chang, M.H., Tsai, C.C., Chen T.S.,Fan, C.C., Lin, C.C., Lai, C.H., Tsai, F.J., Lin, J.A. and Huang, C.Y. 2013. Garlic oil atinuates the cardiac apoptosis in hamster fed with hypercholesterol diet. Food Chem 136, 1296-1302.

[58] Singh,G. & Chaturvedi,G.N. 1974. Anticogulant and fibrinolytic effect of Garlic (*Allium sativum* and *Allium ascalonicum*), an experimental study. J Res Indian Med 9 (4), 1-7.

[59] Jain P.K., Chandarkar, A.G.., Bulakh, P.M., Reddy, B.V., Ranade,S.M. and Mathur, V.P. 1977. Observation on effect of *Allium sativum* on some haematological values in rabbits & human volunteers. J. Shivaji Uni 17, 121-123.

[60] Allison, G.L., Lowe, G.M. and Rahman, K. 2012. Aged garlic extract inhibits platelet activation by increasing intracellular cAMP and reducing the interaction of GPIIB / IIIa receptor with fibrinogen. Life Sci 91, 1275-1280.

[61] Brahmchari, H.D. and Augusti., K.T. 1962. Orally effective hypoglycemic agents from plants. J Pharm Pharmacol 14. 254-255.

[62] Jain, R.C., Vyas, C.H. and Mahatma, O.P.1973. Hypoglycemic action of onion and garlic. Lancet 2,1491.

[63] Padiya, R. & Banerje e, S.K. 2013. Garlic as anti-diabetic agent:Recent progress and patent reviews. Recent Pat FoodNutr Agric 5,105-127.

[64] Rafieian-Kopaei, M., Baradaran, A., Merrikhi, A., Nematbakhs, M., Madihi, Y. and Nasri, H. 2013. Efficacy of co- administration of garlic extract and metformin for prevention of gentamicin-renal toxicity in wister rats: A Biochemical study. Int J Prev Med 4, 258-264.

[65] Belman, S. 1983. Onion and Garlic oils inhibit tumour promotion. Carcinogenesis 4, 1063-1065.

[66] Rao, A.R., Sadhana, A.S. and Goel, H.C. 1990. Inhibition of skin tumour in DMBA- induced complete carcinogenesis system in mice by garlic (*Allium sativum*). Indian J Exp Biol 28, 405-408.

[67] Ariga, T., Tsuji, K., Saki, T. Moritomo, T. and Yamamoto, J.I. 2000. Antithrombotic and antineoplastic effects of phyto-granulosulphur compounds. Biofactors 13. 251-255.

[68] Rao, R.R., Rao, S.S. and Venkatraman, P.R. 1946. Investigation on plant antibiotics. Part I. Studies on allicin, the antibacterial principle of *Allium sativum* (garlic). J. Sci Ind Res. 5,31.

[69] Jezowa, L., Rafinski, T. and Wrocinski, T. 1966. Investigations on the antibiotic activity of *Allium sativum* L. Herba Pol 12, 3-13.

[70] Sivam, G.P. 2001. Protection against Helicobacter Pylori and other bacterial infections by garlic. J. Nutr 131, 1106-1108.

[71] Tansey, M.R. & Appleton, J.A. 1975. Inhibition of fungal growth by garlic extract. Mycologia 67.409-413.

[72] Tsai, Y., Cole, L., Davis, L.E., Lockwood, S.J. Simmons, V. and Wild, G.C. 1985. Antiviral properties of garlic: *In vitro* effects on influenza B, herpes simplex and coxsackie virus. Planta Med 5, 460-461.

[73] Abdel- Rahman, , E.H., Kandil, O.M. and Abdel Megeed, K.N. 1998. Comperative studies of lethal effects of *Bacillus thuringiensis*, *Allium sativum* and *Nerium oleander* on *Trichostrangylide* parasites. Egypt J Zool 30, 193, 134-141.

[74] Gaffen, J.D. Taveres, I.A. and Bennett, A. 1984. The effect of garlic extracts on contractions of rat gastric fundus and human platelet aggregation.J Pharm Pharmavol 36, 272-274.

[75] Aquel, M.B., Gharaibah, M.N. and Salhab, A. S.1991. Direct relaxant effects of garlic juice on smmoth and cardiac muscles. J. Ethnopharmacol, 33,13-19.

[76] Popov, I., Blumestein, A. and Lewin, G. 1994. Antioxidant effects of aquous garlic extract. 1st Communication: Direct determination using the photochemluminescence. Arzneim Forsch 44, 602-604.

[77] Dong, R., Duan, Y.Q., Wang, X.Y., Liu, Y. and Gao, G.L. 2000. Effect of garlic on peroxidation in rats with diabetes. China J Public Hygeine 16, 205-206.

[78] Bhatiua,B., Ahuja, P.L. 1984.Cold tolerance of CCI4 treated mice and its modification by administration of garlic oil and glucose. Int J Biometerol 28, 93-99.

[79] Senapati, S.K., Dey, S., Dwivedi, S.K. and Swarup D. 2001. Effect of garlic (*Allium sativum*) extract on tissue lead levels in rats. J ethnopharmacol 16, 229-232.

[80] Tabari, M.A. and Fbrahimpour, S. 2014. Effect of aged garlic extract on immune response to experimental fibrosarcoma tumor in BALB/ c mice. Indian J Cancer 51, 609-613.

[81] Sobenin, I.A., , Andrianova, I.V., Gorchakova, T.V. and Orekhov, A.N. 2009. Time released gastric powder tablets lower systolic and diastolic blood pressure in men with mild and moderate arterial hypertension.Hypertens Res 32, 433-437.

[82] Ashraf, R., Khan, R. A., Ashraf, I and Qureshi, A.A. 2013. Effects of *Allium sativum* (garlic) on systolic and diastolic blood pressure with essential hypertension. Pak J Pharm Sci 26,859-863.

[83] Bordia, A. Verma, S.K. and Srivastava, K.C., 1998. Effect of garlic (*Allium sativum*) on blood lipids, blood sugar, fibrinogen and fibrinolytic activity in patients with coronary artery disease. Prostaglandins Leukot Essent Fatty Acids 58, 257-263.

[84] Williams, M.J., Sutherland, W.H., McCormick, M.P., Yeoman, D.J. and de Jong, S.A., 2005. Aged garlic extract improves endothelial function in men with coronary artery disease Phytother Res 19,314-319.

[85] Kiessewetter, H., Jung, F., Jung, E.M., Blume, J., Mrowietz, C., Birk, A., Koscielny, J. and Wenzel, E. 1993. Effects of garlic coated tablets in peripheral arterial occlusive disease. Clin Investig 71, 383-386.

[86] Rapp, A. Grohmann, G.,Oelzner, P. Uehleke, B. and Uhlemann, C. 2006. Does garlic influence rheologic properties and blood flow in progressive systemic sclerosis? J Forsch Komplement Med 13 (3), 141-146.

[87] Budoff, M.J., Ahmadi, N., Gul K.M., Liu, S.T., Flores, F.R., Tiano, J., Takasu, J. Miller, E. and Tsimikas, S. 2009. Aged garlic extract supplement with B vitamins, folic acid and L-arginine retards the progression of subclinical atherosclerosis: A randomized clinical trial. Prev Med 49, 101-107.

[88] Bordia, A., Bansal, H.C., Arora, S.K. and Singh, S.V. 1975b. Effect of essential oil of garlic and onion on alimentary hyperlipedemia. Atherosclerosis 21, 15-19.

[89] Bhushan, S., Sharma, S.P., Singh S.P., Agrawal, S., Indrayan, A. and Seth, P. 1979. Effect of garlic on normalblood cholesterol level. Indian J Physiol Pharmacol 23, 211-214.

[90] Mahanta, R.K., Goswami, R.K., Kumar, D. and Goswami, P. 1980. Effect of *Allium sativum* (Garlic) on blood lipids. Indian Med Gaz 114,157-160.

[91] Vorberg, G. and Schneider, B. 1990. Therapy with garlic: Results of a placebo-controlled double- blind study. Br J Clin Pract 69 (8),7-11.

[92] Jung, E.s., Park, S.H., Choi, E.K., Ryu, B.H.., Kim, D.s., Kim, Y.G. and Chae, S.w. 2014. Reduction of blood lipid parameters by a 12-wk supplementation of aged black garlic:A randomized controlled trial. Nutrition 30, 1034-1039.

[93] Sobein, I.A., Nedosugova, L.V., Filatova, L.V., Balabolkin, M.I., Gorchakova, T.V. and Orekhov, A.N. 2008b. Metabolic effects of time-released garlic powder tablets in Type 2 diabetes mellitus: The result of double-blinded placebo-controlled study. Acta Diabetol 45, 1-6.

[94] Ashraf, R., Khan,R.A. and Ashraf, A. 2011. Garlic (*Allium sativum*) supplementationwit standard antidiabetic agent provides better diabetic control in type 2 diabetes mellitus. Park J pharm Sci 24,565-570.

[95] Kumar, R. Chhatwal, S. Arora, S. Sharma, S., Singh, J. Singh, N. Bhandari, V. and Khurana, A. 2013. Antihyperglycemic, anti-inflammatory and adenosine deaminase- lowering effects of garlic in patients with type 2 diabetes mellitus wih obesity. Diabetes Metab Syndr Obes 6, 49-56.

[96] Rapp, A. Grohmann, G.,Oelzner, P. Uehleke, B. and Uhlemann, C. 2006. Does garlic influence rheologic properties and blood flow in progressive systemic sclerosis? J Forsch Komplement Med 13 (3), 141-146.

[97] Josling, P. 2001. Preventing the common cold with a garlic supplement: A double-blind , placebo- controlled survey. Adv Therapy 18,189-193.

[98] Nantz, M.P., Rowe,C.a., Muller, C.E., Creasy, R.a. Stanilka, J.A. andPercival, S.s.2012. Supplementation with aged garlic extract improves both NK and YS-T cell function and reduces the severity of cold and Flu symptoms:A randomized double-blind, placebo-controlled nutrition intervention. Clin Nutr 31, 337-344.

[99] Denisov, L.N., Andrianova, I. V. and Timofeeva, S.S. 1999. Garlic effectiveness in rheumatoid arthritis. Ter arkh 71 (8),55-58.

Chapter 12

Pinaceae Species: Spruce, Pine and Fir as a New Culinary Herb and Spice

Nabila Rodríguez Valerón, Diego Prado Vásquez and Rasmus Munk

Abstract

The Pinaceae family has traditionally been used as medicine, resorted to as a famine food and for ornamental purposes as Christmas trees. In the last few years numerous restaurants have been using different species of *Pinaceae* family as a garnish or an aromatic spice, using them in different culinary applications like oils and infusions to flavor dressings and broths. *Abies grandis* (Grand fir), *Pseudotsuga menziesii* (Douglas fir), *Pinus sylvestris* (Scots pine) and *Picea abies* (Norway spruce) were researched on taxonomy, habitats and non-edible uses, culinary traditions, health and nutritional properties, aroma profile. The main compounds in Pinaceae family are monoterpenes, oxygenated monoterpenes, sesquiterpenes, oxygenate sesquiterpenes, diterpenes and hydrocarbons, especially α-β-pinene, limonene, α-terpinene, and even bornyl acetate, responsible for aroma compounds such as citrusy-, woody-, herbal-, or piney aromas. Modern gastronomy uses, sensory analysis and culinary applications were applied for demonstrating the possibilities on modern culinary application in this novel yet traditional spice.

Keywords: Spruce, Fir, Pine, Pinaceae, Spice, Herbs, Culinary

1. Introduction

The Pinaceae family species has been used for many years as an edible food source, especially the genera Abies, Pseudotsuga, Pinus and Picea. Among *Abies grandis* (Grand fir), *Pseudotsuga menziesii* (Douglas fir), *Pinus sylvestris* (Scots pine) and *Picea abies* (Norway spruce) are the most common in contemporary and traditional gastronomy [1] (**Figures 1-4**).

1.1 Taxonomy, habitats and non-edible uses

All the species mentioned above have a long history of supplying pitch, turpentine, wood, tar and resin for construction, but also as medicine (**Table 1**). People used to chew the hard amber colored resin of pine as toothpaste. It was rubbed on the teeth to whiten them, and in spring the fresh resin could be applied to wounds to encourage healing [7].

Abies grandis (Grand fir) is most common in lowland coastal areas. It grows from near the sea level to ca. 1,800 m a.s.l., on a variety of soils derived from granitic

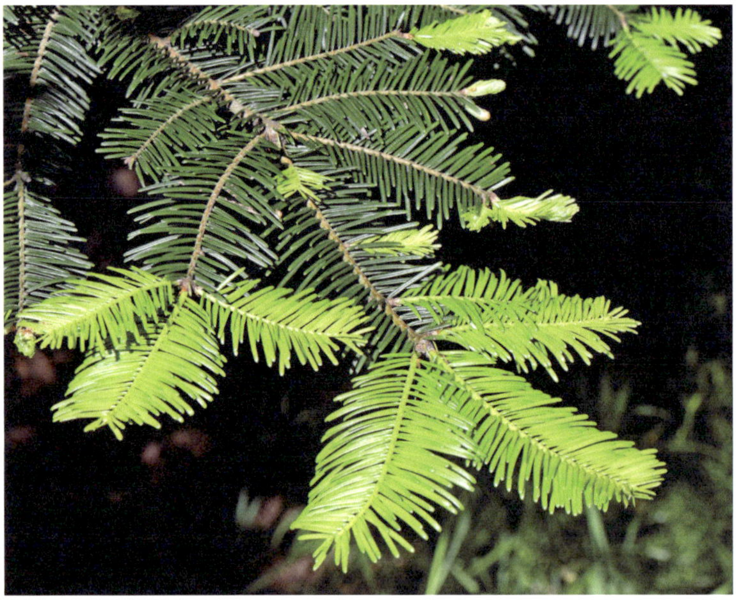

Figure 1.
Abies grandis *(Grand fir) [2].*

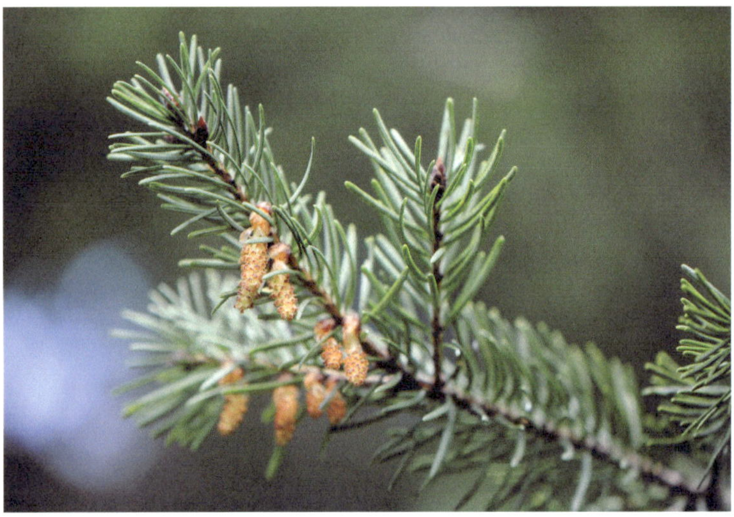

Figure 2.
Pseudotsuga menziesii *(Douglas fir) [3].*

or basaltic rock. It grows best on alluvial soils with a relatively high ground water table. Rapid growth and great size make this species an important tree for producing timber. The wood is soft and white and an excellent source of pulpwood. Young trees are valued as Christmas trees because they tend to grow very symmetrically and have glossy green foliage. Grand fir is a common sight in large gardens and city parks and it was planted in nearly all landscape gardens laid out in the nineteenth century in Europe [8].

Pseudotsuga menziesii (Douglas fir) is common in a variety of climatic zones, landscapes and habitats. It benefits from high rainfall, yet also grows well on better drained sites, commonly on slopes or elevated, no longer flooded river terraces. Giant trees can measure up to 100 metres, Somewhat further inland the species also grows

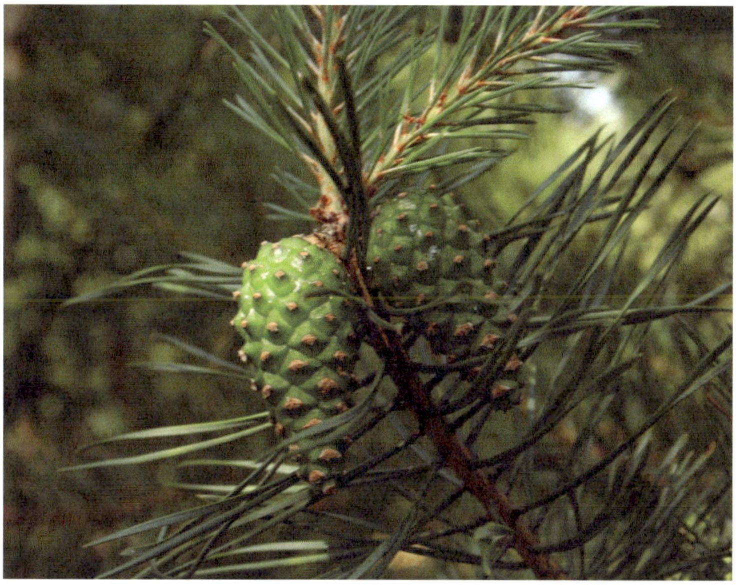

Figure 3.
Pinus sylvestris *(Scots pine) [4].*

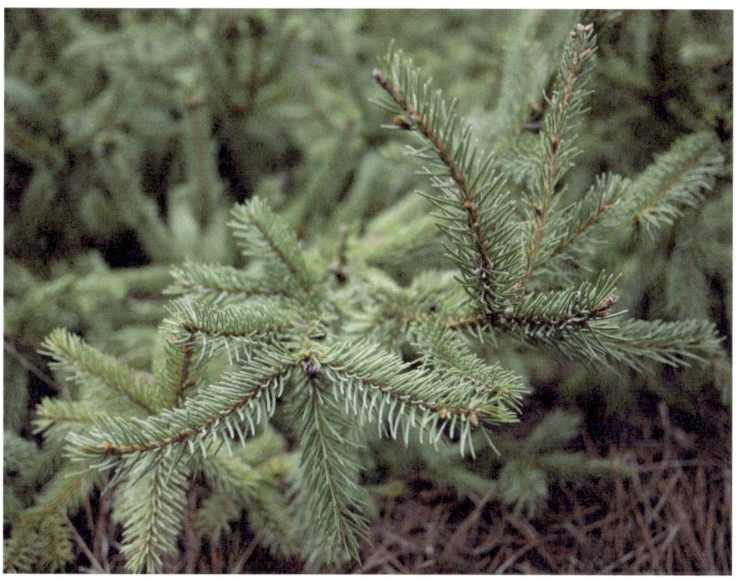

Figure 4.
Picea abies *(Norway spruce) [5].*

in valley bottoms near streams, still reaching great height and living up to 800–1,000 years. These coniferous forests are of similar composition as those on the coast. Var. glauca is a smaller, but still quite large tree that grows in the Rocky Mountains [9].

Douglas fir is one of the world's most important timber trees. The huge size, especially of the coastal variety, as well as the excellent wood properties make it the preferred tree for knot-free sawn timber of great length. However, the more continental variety *P. menziesii var. glauca* grows much slower and to a more moderate size, thus yielding denser, heavier wood, excellent for cooperage for vats and tanks for breweries and distilleries. Douglas fir has been introduced to many countries in

Specie	*Abies grandis* (Douglas ex D.Don) Lindl.	*Pseudotsuga menziesii* (Mirb.) Franco	*Pinus sylvestris* L.	*Picea abies* (L.) H. Karst
Kingdom	*Plantae*	*Plantae*	*Plantae*	*Plantae*
Phylum	*Tracheophyta*	*Tracheophyta*	*Tracheophyta*	*Tracheophyta*
Class	*Pinopsida*	*Pinopsida*	*Pinopsida*	*Pinopsida*
Order	*Pinales*	*Pinales*	*Pinales*	*Pinales*
Family	*Pinaceae*	*Pinaceae*	*Pinaceae*	*Pinaceae*
Genus	*Abies*	*Pseudotsuga*	*Pinus*	*Picea*

Table 1.
Taxonomy of the most widely used species [6].

plantation forestry as well as an ornamental tree and a good number of cultivars are known and used in horticulture. In the NW USA and W Canada it is also grown as a Christmas tree [9].

Pinus sylvestris (Scots pine) grows naturally in a variety of habitats, the common denominator of which is deficiency of nutrients in the soil. Thus, on the Atlantic seaboard with high levels of precipitation it grows on ancient igneous or metamorphic rocks with little or no soil – in Scotland and Norway up to 70o N, while south of the Baltic Sea it grows on podzolized glacial sands left after the Ice Age. In the central Alps it is restricted to the drier slopes and valleys below other conifers like Picea, while in the Caucasus it ascends to 2,600 m on rocky outcrops and scree. In much of Siberia, it occupies the drier sites, but in Scandinavia and NE Europe it often borders acidic peat bogs. In the steppes of Russia and Mongolia it only grows along stream courses [10].

Pinus sylvestris is an important timber tree, but most of the production goes to the paper industry. Most of the 'pine' used for furniture in W Europe is in fact spruce (*Picea abies*). In Russia and Scandinavia resin is extracted by "destructive distillation" from the stumps and roots of felled trees to produce "Stockholm tar" which is used as a wood preservative. In much of western Europe, it is a widely planted forestry tree for timber; it was introduced in the USA for similar purposes and for use as Christmas trees [10].

Picea abies (Norway spruce) is widespread and dominant in Boreal conifer forests of northern and northeastern Europe, the natural distribution shows continental tendencies but in the western mountains of Central Europe an ecotype has evolved that is adapted to sub-Atlantic weather conditions with heavy 'wet' snowfall in early winter. Although it can grow on most substrates, it is most common on acid soils [6].

Norway spruce is an important timber tree in Europe. Outside the Boreal Forest zone most commercial timber is now harvested from plantations or from managed forests in which other trees are suppressed. The wood is used for pulpwood as well as construction, furniture (most of the popular 'pine' furniture is made with wood from Norway spruce), and for special purposes like the sound boards of pianos and the bodies of guitars and violins. The famous Stradivarius violins were made with wood of Norway Spruce from the Alps. In Europe this species is the most popular Christmas tree [6].

2. Culinary traditions

As for culinary uses, the *Pinaceae* family has mainly been used as a famine, emergency, or survival food in different traditional communities in Finland, Sweden and Norway, for example the indigenous Sámi people. It is also consumed in northwestern North America and Russia for the same purposes [7].

Considered as a famine or emergency/survival type of food, the inner bark (cambium) of *Abies grandis* (Grand fir), *Picea abies* (Norway spruce) and *Pinus sylvestris* (Scots pine) has been eaten cooked, usually dried, and then ground into a powder. It is then used as a thickening in soups or mixed with cereals to make bread [11]. Large sheets of bark of *Pinus sylvestris* are taken from trees in spring and early summer by the Sami people in northern Sweden and Finland and either dried and ground into a flour (as *Abies grandies*) or eaten directly (fresh) "as delicacies". The flour can be stored for a long period of time and can be mixed with reindeer milk, fat from boiled milk, blood or fish and meat soups. Pine inner bark has probably also been used as a seasoning, added to meats instead of salt. It has also been used to make flat bread chips where the main ingredient was Scots pine inner bark, it is seasoned with brown sugar and roasted over fire [7].

Young pine cones from different Pinus spp., like *Pinus kochiana* and *Pinus sylvestris,* have been used in Armenia, Eastern Europe, Russia and Georgia to make jam, syrup and confiture. Immature female cones from Picea abies have also been used this way [12]. *Abies spp.* have also been used for making chewing gum from needles, branches and cones [13]. *Picea abies* and *Abies grandis* resin has been consumed as chewing gum in Sweden and North [11, 14], also sap of several Pinus spp. has been used for drinks and reduced to make syrups [13].

There are approximately 29 *Pinus spp.* that produce seeds that have been used as food items [15]. The most valuable one is *Pinus pinea*, that is traditionally used to produce pine nuts in Mediterranean countries like Italy, Turkey, Spain and Portugal [16]. In Turkey it is commonly eaten as a snack or for making sweets like "halva" and cold drinks [17]. Native North Americans used to make them into a butter or grinded them to make balls as delicacies [14].

Young twigs and leaves from *Pseudotsuga spp.* and *Abies spp.* have been used as a substitute for coffee, spruce beer from *Picea spp.* has been made from the shoots and an infusion of the leaves has been used as a beverage [13] young shoot tips are also used as a tea substitute [14, 18]. *Picea abies* and *Pinus sylvestris* shoots and catkins have been eaten raw or cooked as snacks and added to other recipes as a flavoring (**Table 2**) [11, 12].

Specie	Parts used	Use	Source
Abies grandis (Douglas ex D.Don) Lindl.	Inner bark Resin, gum Shoots	Bread, stews Candy, drink Infusion, drink, Snack	[11, 13, 14]
Pseudotsuga menziesii (Mirb.) Franco	Inner bark Resin Sap Shoots Branches, leaves	Bread Snack, drink Candy, drink, sweetener Infusion, drink, candy Spice	[13, 14, 18]
Pinus sylvestris L.	Inner bark Seed Shoots Catkins Pinecones	Bread Nuts Snack, flavoring Snack, flavoring Jam, candy	[6, 11, 12]
Picea abies (L.) H. Karst	Inner bark Shoots Catkins Pinecones	Bread Snack, flavoring, drink Snack, flavoring Jam, candy	[12, 13]

Table 2.
Traditional common uses of Pinaceae spp.

3. Health and nutritional properties

In the past few years nutraceutical products that claim to counteract human diseases have received increasing attention. The products are enriched with natural extracts such as ginger, onion, garlic, turmeric, etc.

The use of pine (*Pinus sylvestris*) was an important nutritional factor that historically helped prevent scurvy (from Vitamin C deficiency). The high nutritional value of inner bark when peeled in spring is well known today. Important nutrients from inner bark include carbohydrates, vitamin C, and fiber to balance the consumption of protein and fatty meat, fish and reindeer milk from which the bulk of calories, protein, minerals and vitamins were derived [19] (**Table 3**).

Pinaceae species have been investigated by scientific communities because of their potential properties in food, medicine, and cosmetics. *Picea abies* has recently been studied for its potential antimicrobial activity in which the main bioactive compounds are aldehydes, ketones, alcohols, esters, and hydrocarbons [21].

One study proved the antibacterial activity of *Picea abies* extract on the growth of *E. coli* interfering with the metabolic activity of the microorganism [21]. Furthermore, other studies have identified that compounds responsible for antimicrobial activity are present in the *Picea abies* species. Specifically, monoterpenes such as α-terpineol, α-3-carene, α and β-pinene, limonene, γ and β- terpinene, linalool, borneol as well as sesquiterpenes such as cadinene, γ-muurolene, α-humulene, all of them are responsible for its aroma profile [21].

Essential oil from various *Pinaceae spp.* trees is often associated with a positive impact on health. It has been noted to have relaxing effects when inhaled or and to counteract certain mental health issues, for instance sleep disorders. Other results reported are that some molecules making up the aromas, such as α-pinene, can relieve stress [22]. In addition, the atmosphere in forests impacts the cerebral activity. Based on all these observations compounds present in *Pinaceae spp.* can be related to relaxation of the human body [23].

Pine nuts are well-known around the world because of their nutritional value, and widely eaten in Turkey and Spain among other countries. They are high in vitamin E and K, minerals such as iron, magnesium, phosphorus, zinc, copper, potassium, and manganese. Moreover, they are a source of fiber, niacin, and riboflavin, and high in polyunsaturated fats [24].

Pseudotsuga menziesii cones among other species of *Pinaceae spp.* have been studied for their antioxidant activity. In one study on the possible bioactive effects in humans, the samples gave a positive result for anti-viral and anti-bacterial properties [25]. This study analyzed the total phenol content (TPC), the ferric reducing

Part used	Energy (kcal)	Water	Protein	Fat	Carbohydrates	Starch	Total Sugars	Ash
Inner bark (Summer)	107,6	62,2	0,8	2,0	9,9	6,7	3,2	0,64
Inner bark (Autumn)		62,4	2,33		4,3	0,65	3,3	
Inner bark Flour (Summer)			1,5	2,3	6,0			

Table 3.
*Comparisons between nutritional content of Scots Pine (*Pinus sylvestris L.*) inner bark harvested in summer and autumn [7, 20].*

ability of plasma (FRAP), and 2,2-diphenyl-1-picrylhydrazyl, in three different stages of cones, green, matured and opened, resulting in high scores in the first, green, stage for all the species [25].

The terpenes such as pinene, limonene (both enantiomers), 1,8-cineole, and borneol were studied as anti-bacterial agents to counteract *Listeria monocytogenes*. Pinene was the most active component and 1,8 cineole and borneol less, therefore they might be considered to Listeria or to prevent its growth. These kinds of molecules are present in fir, pine, and spruces, and they are considerably cheaper than essential oils from spices and herbs, because most of the antimicrobial activity comes from phenolic compounds [26].

4. Aroma profile

Pinaceae spp. represents the largest genus of the conifers, with many different species spread over the world, especially in North America, Europe and Asia. There are also a few in south-east Asia and even some in South America. It is the most common tree in the world and a popular material for the manufacture of wood products, and due to its characteristic smell it is commonly used as a natural and pleasant aroma [26].

Furthermore, the species produces oleoresin, the mix of monoterpene (C10), sesquiterpene (C15) and diterpenes (C20) commonly called resin acids and phenolic compounds. Conifers use them as a form of chemical defense in needles and wood to deter insect attacks and to inhibit the growth of fungi [22, 27].

The organoleptic profile of *Pseudotsuga menziesii* is mainly created by monoterpenes such as (Z) and (E)-β-ocimene (green, woody, tropical), β-pinene (piney, woody, terpy), sabinene, α-terpinolene (woody, terpy, citrus), α-terpineol (woody, earthy, cooling), γ-terpinene (citrus, terpenic), limonene (citrus, herbal, terpenic) or geranyl acetate (fruity, floral, rose) and cintronellyl acetate. On the other hand, *Picea abies* contains different concentrations of monoterpenes, oxygenated monoterpenes, sesquiterpenes, oxygenate sesquiterpenes, diterpenes and hydrocarbons. Volatile compounds such as α-β-pinene, limonene, ρ-cymene (woody, terpy, harsh), (E)- caryophyllene (woody, camphoric, peppery), δ-cadinene (woody), bornyl acetate (camphor, woody, pine), β-phellandrene (green and terpy) or δ-3-carene (citrus) are responsible for the characteristic aromas of this species of pines [28].

Abies grandis contains a complex mixture of monoterpenes, sesquiterpenes and diterpenoid acids, used to deter insect pests and their symbiotic fungal pathogens [29]. In previous research, it was shown that the leaf oil of *Abies grandis* is dominated by β-pinene (20.3–31%), responsible for piney, woody flavor; bornyl acetate (12.7–26.2%), for balsamic odor and camphoreous flavor; β-phellandrene (13.7–25.2%), responsible for minty odor; and camphene (8.3–11.5%), giving a woody, fir needle odor and camphereous, minty, green, spicy flavor, with moderate amounts of α-pinene (4.4–7.4%), responsible for herbal, pine, fresh odor and woody, tropical flavors; α-terpinene (1.1–2.2%), responsible for woody, citrus odor and terpenic, citrus, lemon and lime flavor; terpinolene (1.3–2.9%), giving a herbal, pine, citrus odor and woody, lemon, lime and floral flavor; and α-terpineol (1.1–3.6%), responsible for terpenic, pine, citrus and floral odor, lemon, lime and woody flavors [21, 28].

According to a study performed by the department of botany and genetics at Vilnius University in Lithuania, the composition in needle essential oil for Pinus sylvestris L. is principally formed by α-pinene [30] that contributes aromas to pine, cypress, citrus fruits, herbs, spices, and mastic [28]. *Pinus sylvestris L.* is mainly composed of α-pinene (22.48%) which aromas are piney, woody [28]; σ-3-carene responsible for citrus and terpenic aroma [31]; muurolol (4.42%) responsible for herbal and honey [32]; camphene (3.39%) or germacrene (2.97%), giving woody aroma, and minty-cooling flavor [28]; β- caryophyllene (3.32%) responsible for spicy-peppery- notes [32]; β-elemene (1.79%) responsible for herbal aroma, myrene (1.57%), β-pinene (1.52%), bornyl acetate (1.79%) and β-ocimene (1.12%) all of them are responsible for woody, green, citrus, or camphor aroma. In lower concentration are β-phellandrene (0.86%) responsible for green, terpy; α-humulene (0.84%), γ-muurolene (0.82%), α-copaene (0.73%), or sabinene (0.45%) responsible for woody [28].

Also, other compounds are present in the aroma profile of this species, such as (E)-2-hexenal (0.32%) responsible of fruity aroma; terpinolene (0.30%) giving citrus (lime peel) and woody aroma; 2-undecanone (0.27%) and undecanone (0.05%) giving fruity aroma; terpinolene (0.30%) responsible for citrus; α-terpineol or terpinyl acetate (0.08%) giving floral notes such as lavender or citrus notes such as lime [28, 30].

A study performed by Friedrich-Alexander-Universität Erlangen-Nürnberg detected the presence of 44 odor-active compounds in wood from Pinus sylvestris L. Among the main compounds identified were fatty acid degradation products, and some terpenoic substances [22] The majority of the molecules identified were (E,E)-nona-2,4-dienal, vanillin, phenylacetic acid, 3-phenylpropanoic acid, δ-octalactone and α-pinene. Also 11 compounds were identified for the first time as odor substances in wood, among them the heptanoic acid, γ-octalactone, δ-nonalactone and (E,Z,Z)-trideca-2,4,7-trienal [22].

According to the results of the study in wood, the presence of α-Pinene is high, which is to be expected since it is long known to be an aroma component in Pinus sylvestris. The fatty notes come from mono- and di-alkenals, such as (E,E)-Nona-2,4-dienal and (E,E)-Deca-2,4-dienal – for the first time reported in wood. The cheesy aroma can be assumed to result from pentanoic acid, butanoic acid as well as 3-methylbutanoic acid. The phenylacetic acid can be related to the honey-like notes, and vanillin to the vanilla-like aroma. Furthermore, the citrusy notes can come from octanal, linalool or nonanal whereas green and grassy aromas from pentanal and hexanal compounds. The pencil-like smell can be assumed to result from

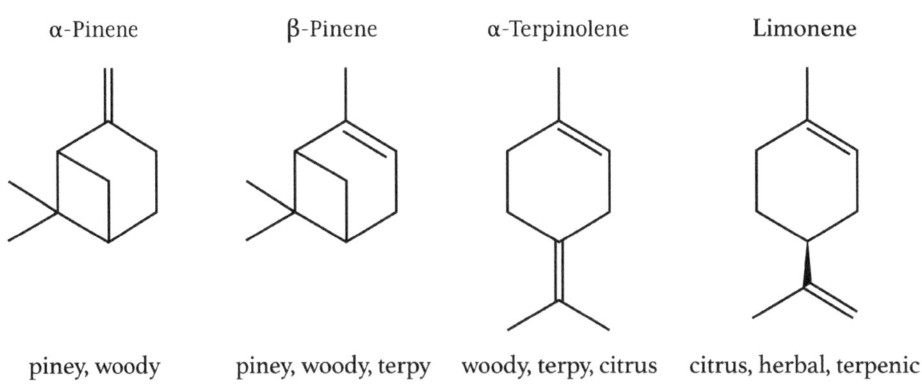

Figure 5.
Principal aroma components in Pinaceae spp. [33, 34].

thymoquinone, whereas peppery and plastic like aromas from α-bisabolol. There have also been found vomit-like notes that can be associated with 3-phenylpropanoic acid or blood-like and metallic aromas can be trace back to (E,Z,Z)-trideca-2,4,7-trienal molecules [22]; – these are of course less pleasant in gastronomic applications (**Figure 5**).

5. Modern gastronomy uses

In more recent research modern contemporary restaurants have been using to use several *Pinaceas spp.* often in combination with new culinary techniques.

Shoots from *Pseudotsuga menziesii* (Douglas fir), *Abies grandis* (Grand fir) and *Picea abies* (Norway spruce) are used in contemporary cuisine. They are served raw or cooked as garnish in different preparations like fish, meats and salads [35, 36]. Shoots and leaves are used as a spice in creams and chocolate ganache [37]. Branches and shoots are being used to make "gin" and sodas [38, 39]. Also, flavored salt is use blending salt and leaves [40].

Oils and flavored butters can be made from different *Pinaceas spp.* with different techniques like blending or infusing with neutral oils. *Pinus spp.* shoots can be used to infuse oil (neutral sunflower oil) to make "pine shoot oil" as seasoning for a fish dish [41]. Green pines cones can be cold infused to make green pine cone oil as a seasoning [42]. Or mixed leaves with butter infused in a vacuum bag and cooked at 80°C for 10 hours [43].

Other techniques are used for the leaves, like blending and sous vide-cooking to improve the flavor, and extracts mixed with flour has been used to make udon noodles [44]. Emulsions like mayonnaise can be made with the blended and strained oil [35, 45]. Pickles and vinegar from young shoots of Abies grandies, Pseudotsuga menziesii and Picea abies can be made by adding vinegar [40].

Green pine cones have been used as a flavoring for infusions to make granités, dehydrated merengues and gelatins [46], also for making jams and syrups. The leaves can be blended with simple syrup [47].

Wild yeast from Pinus spp. has been used to make fermented drinks, both alcoholic beverages and low alcoholic "sodas", using leaves, cones and branches [48].

Specie	Parts used	Technique/use	Source
Abies grandis (Douglas ex D.Don) Lindl.	Shoots Leaves	Spice, herb, pickle, beverage Spice, beverage, oil, syrup	[45]
Pseudotsuga menziesii (Mirb.) Franco	Shoots Leaves	Spice, herb, pickle, beverage Spice, beverage, oil, syrup	[35, 36]
Pinus sylvestris L.	Leaves Flowers Cones	Spice, beverage, oil, syrup Pickle, herb Jam, syrup, pickle	[42, 46]
Picea abies (L.) H. Karst	Shoots Leaves	Spice, herb, pickle, beverage Spice, beverage, oil, syrup	[35]

Table 4.
Modern contemporary uses of Pinaceaes spp.

Pinus spp. species pollen has been used as thickening agent, and mixed with flour to make bread and pastries [48] (**Table 4**).

6. Sensory analysis

A study carried out by restaurant Alchemist in Copenhagen, Denmark, showed that three different species of *Pinaceae*, *Abies grandis*, *Picea abies* and *Pseudotsuga menziesii* have completely different aroma profiles [1].

In the sensory analysis study *Abies grandis* was related to different attributes, such as citric, present in young needles for this specie, as it is shown in **Table 5**. Other attributes such as intense flavor, grapefruit flavor or "not woody" were found. These attributes might be related to the concentration of different terpenes such as limonene, β-pinene, sabinene or camphene. Despite that the concentration of bornyl acetate is a compound highly related to woody attribute, "not woody" was the most selected attribute [1].

According to the same study *Pseudotsuga menziesii* was related to natural, dark color, not astringent and bitterness [1]. These attributes might be related to the terpenes concentration such as α-pinene, phellandrene, or sabinene [49].

Abies grandis is related to *Pseudotsuga menziesii* citric attribute is common in both samples but is perceived with more intensity in *Abies grandis* [50].

On the other hand, the Picea abies attributes are in complete contrast to the other species (**Table 5**). This result is what was expected, since the aroma profile is different, as demonstrated in a research conducted by Nabil Haman at Piazza University [21].

Astringent is one of the molecules in major concentration (typical in this species), and directly related with astringency in this samples. Besides, the concentration of cinnamon acid (responsible for cinnamon aroma) or ferulic acid (responsible for vanilla aroma) [51] might be closely related to sweetness.

Abies grandis	*Pseudotsuga menziesii*	*Picea abies*
Citrusy	Natural	Astringent
Grapefruit flavor	Dark color	Sweet
Intense flavor	Not astringent	Earthy
Not woody	Bitterness	Woody
Fruity flavor	Citrusy	Crunchy

Table 5.
Summary of the most characteristic attributes used to describe each sample.

Pinaceae	Ice cream	Mean	Spruce tonic	Mean
Picea abies	109	4.687	230	4.855
Pseudotsuga menziesii	612	4.072	851	4.506
Abies grandis	534	4.759	467	5.048
	p- value	0.366		0.102

Table 6.
Averages liking of scale 1–9 in ice cream and gin tonic per each sample of spruces and p-value.

Furthermore, in the same study two different culinary applications were performed, according to the attributes for each species. One of the applications was an ice cream, according to Angelo Corvitto's recipe [52] with some modifications according to another research [1]. The second application was an alcoholic cocktail, spruce tonic, prepared according to Difford's guide [53] with Pinaceae spirit (40%) and tonic water [1].

Table 6 shows the averages for liking for each sample. Abies grandis has the highest score for both recipes, 5.048 for the spruce tonic, followed by *Picea abies* and *Pseudotsuga menziesii*. For the ice cream the average liking is 4.759 for Abies grandis followed by *Picea abies* and *Pseudotsuga menziesii* as is shown in **Table 6**. The reason that *Pseudotsuga menziesii* was less accepted by consumers might be related by bitterness. Also, the consumers acceptability of *Abies grandis* for both recipes might be related to citric flavor [49].

6.1 Culinary applications

According to the results from the sensory analysis of the *Pinaceae spp.* Article [1] two recipes were developed in the Alchemist restaurant development kitchen.

6.1.1 Abies grandis ice cream and spruce complements

Abies grandis ice cream, blueberry jam, pickled Pinus spp. shoots and *pinus sylvestris* inner bark crumble (**Figure 6**).

6.1.2 Spruce tonic

Douglas fir spirit was used to make a version of a gin tonic, replacing the gin with the Douglas fir spirit and drops of Douglas fir syrup (**Figure 7**).

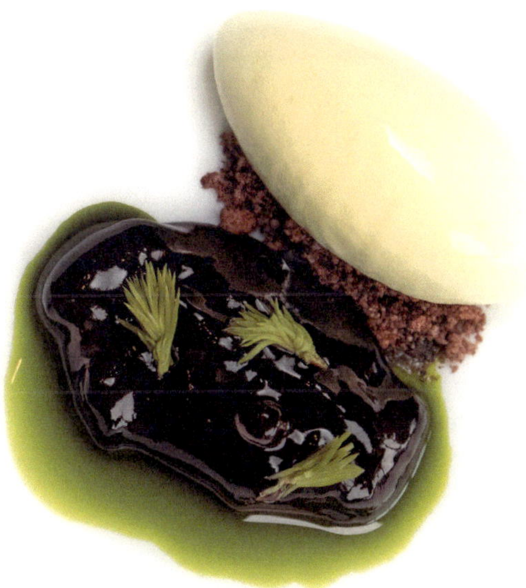

Figure 6.
Dessert: Abies grandis *ice cream and spruce garnishes.*

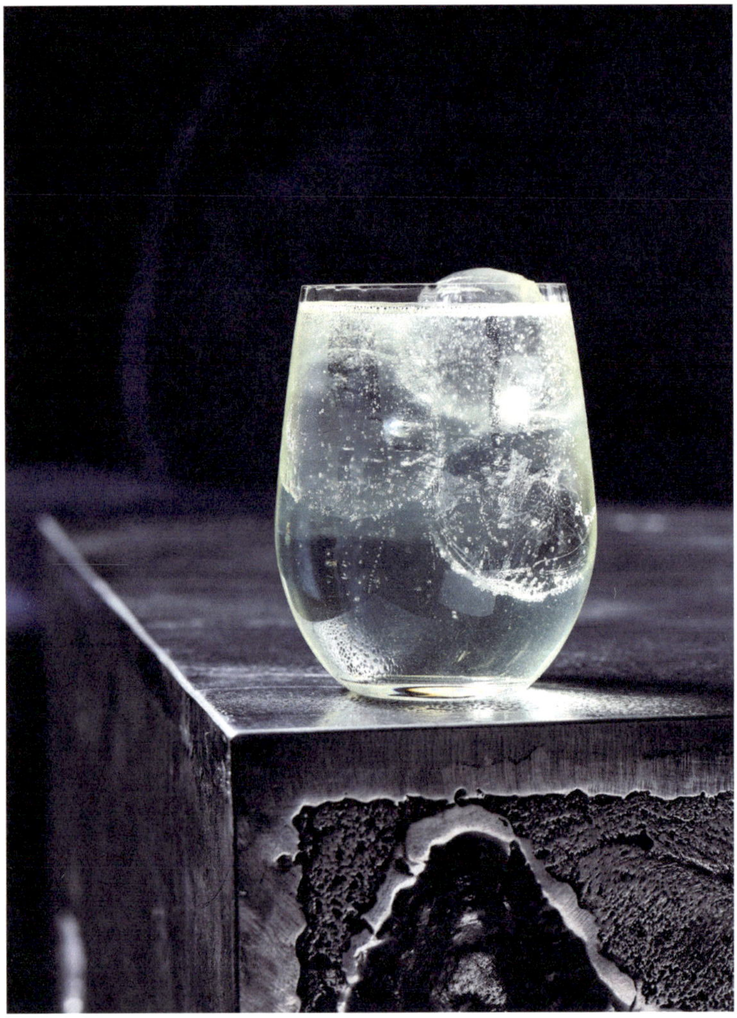

Figure 7.
Cocktail: Spruce tonic.

7. Conclusions

In the past, Pinaceae spp. has been considered as emergency or survival food during years of famine, and even as something shameful to eat [7]. But in the last years the consumption of *Pineaceae spp.* as a herb and spice has increased thanks to fine dining restaurants like elBulli in Spain or Noma in Denmark. Here the leaves, shoots, branches, pine cones and female flowers are used as a regular ingredient showcasing the potential of this species as a herb and spice [36, 42].

Until now, *Pinaceae spp.* has been considered as one flavor or generic aroma profile called "pine" or "spruce", without taking into consideration the large differences between each species [1].

Pinaceae spp. has the same potential as many commonly used spices like cinnamon or vanilla, in many different levels of gastronomy from fine dining to home cooking. It can be added to almost any type of preparation as shown in the "Modern gastronomy uses" chapter.

Author details

Nabila Rodríguez Valerón, Diego Prado Vásquez* and Rasmus Munk
Alchemist Explore, Research and Development, Alchemist Aps,
København, Denmark

*Address all correspondence to: dp@alchemist.dk

References

[1] Valerón, N. R., Vásquez, D. P., & Munk, R. (2021). The Pinaceae species, flavor attributes for new culinary spices. International Journal of Gastronomy and Food Science, 23(January). https://doi.org/10.1016/j.ijgfs.2021.100306

[2] "File:Abies grandis 001.jpg" by Krzysztof Golik is licensed with CC BY-SA 4.0. To view a copy of this license, visit https://creativecommons.org/licenses/by-sa/4.0

[3] "Pseudotsuga menziesii - Douglas Fir 2" by A_Nautilus is licensed with CC BY-NC-SA 2.0. To view a copy of this license, visit https://creativecommons.org/licenses/by-nc-sa/2.0/

[4] "Pinus_sylvestris_cones_pl.jpg" by Pleple2000 is licensed with CC BY-SA 4.0. To view a copy of this license, visit https://creativecommons.org/licenses/by-sa/4.0y Jebulon, CC0, via Wikimedia commons

[5] "Picea abies 'Frohburg'" by F. D. Richards is licensed with CC BY-SA 2.0. To view a copy of this license, visit https://creativecommons.org/licenses/by-sa/2.0/

[6] Farjon, A. (2010). A handbook of the world's conifers Volume II. The Oxford handbook of compositionality. Retrieved from http://www.ruhr-uni-bochum.de/mam/phil-lang/content/werning_oup_2012_offprint.pdf

[7] Bogdanova, S. (2016). Bark Food. The Continuity and Change of the Pine Inner Bark Use for Food by Sámi People in Northern Fennoscandia. The Arctic University of Norway. Retrieved from http://munin.uit.no/handle/10037/9295

[8] Farjon, A. (2013). Abies grandis. The IUCN Rd List of Threatened Species 2013 (Vol. 8235).

[9] Farjon, A. (2013). Pseudotsuga menziesii, The IUCN Red List of Threatened Species (Vol. 8235).

[10] Gardner, M. (2013). Pinus sylvestris. The IUCN Red List of Threatened Species 2013 (Vol. 8235).

[11] Svanberg, I. (2012). The use of wild plants as food in pre-industrial Sweden. Acta Societatis Botanicorum Poloniae, 81(4), 317-327. https://doi.org/10.5586/asbp.2012.039

[12] Schofield, J. J., & Tyler, R. W. (1989). Discovering Wild Plants: Alaska, Western Canada, the Northwest. (Alaska Northwest, Ed.).

[13] Elias Yanovsky. (1936). Food Plants of the North American Indians. Miscellaneous publication no 237 (Vol. 23). Washington, D.c. https://doi.org/10.2307/2478422

[14] Moerman, D. E. (1998). Native American Ethnobotany. (I. Timber Press, Ed.). Oregon.

[15] Ciesla, W. (1998). Non-Wood Products From Conifers. Non Wood Forest Products (Vol. 12). Rome.

[16] United Nations. (2013). Unece Standard Ddp-24 2013 Edition.

[17] Dogan, Y., Baslar, S., Ay, G., & Mert, H. H. (2004). The use of wild edible plants in western and central Anatolia (Turkey).

[18] Facciola, S. (1990). Cornucopia: A source Book of Edible Plants. (Kampong Publications, Ed.). California.

[19] Zackrisson, O., Östlund, L., Korhonen, O., & Bergman, I. (2000). The ancient use of Pinus sylvestris L. (Scots pine) inner bark by Sami people in northern Sweden, related to cultural and ecological factors. Vegetation

History and Archaeobotany, 9(2), 99-109. https://doi.org/10.1007/BF01300060

[20] Rautio, A., Norstedt, G., & Östlund, L. (2013). Nutritional Content of Scots Pine Inner Bark in Northern Fennoscandia. Economic Botany, 67(4), 363-377. https://doi.org/10.1007/s12231-013-9254-3

[21] Haman, N., Morozova, K., Tonon, G., Scampicchio, M., & Ferrentino, G. (2019). Antimicrobial effect of picea abies extracts on *E. coli* growth. Molecules, 24(22). https://doi.org/10.3390/molecules24224053

[22] Schreiner, L., Bauer, P., & Buettner, A. (2018). Resolving the smell of wood - Identification of odour-active compounds in Scots pine (Pinus sylvestris L.). Scientific Reports, 8(1), 1-9. https://doi.org/10.1038/s41598-018-26626-8

[23] Park, B. J., Tsunetsugu, Y., Kasetani, T., Hirano, H., Kagawa, T., Sato, M., & Miyazaki, Y. (2007). Physiological effects of Shinrin-yoku (taking in the atmosphere of the forest) - Using salivary cortisol and cerebral activity as indicators-. Journal of Physiological Anthropology, 26(2), 123-128. https://doi.org/10.2114/jpa2.26.123

[24] Geisler, M., & Romero, C. (2019, October). Pine Nuts. Technical Information. International Nut and Dried Fruit Council, 13. Retrieved from http://www.agmrc.org/commodities-products/nuts/pine-nuts/

[25] Hofmann, T., Visi-Rajczi, E., & Albert, L. (2020). Antioxidant properties assessment of the cones of conifers through the combined evaluation of multiple antioxidant assays. Industrial Crops and Products, 145(November), 111935. https://doi.org/10.1016/j.indcrop.2019.111935

[26] Mourey, A., & Canillac, N. (2002). Anti-*Listeria monocytogenes* activity of essential oils components of conifers. Food Control, 13(4-5), 289-292. https://doi.org/10.1016/S0956-7135(02)00026-9

[27] Steele, C. L., Crock, J., Bohlmann, J., & Croteau, R. (1998). Sesquiterpene Synthases from Grand Fir (Abies grandis). Journal of Biological Chemistry, 273(4), 2078-2089. https://doi.org/10.1074/jbc.273.4.2078

[28] McGee, H. (2020). Nose Dive. A field guide to the world's smells. (P. Press, Ed.) (1o). New York.

[29] Phillips, M. A., & Croteau, R. B. (1999). Resin-based defenses in conifers. Trends in Plant Science, 4(5), 184-190. https://doi.org/10.1016/S1360-1385(99)01401-6

[30] Lazutka, J. R. (2001). Genotoxicity of dill (*Anethum graveolens* L.), peppermint (Mentha×piperita L.) and pine (Pinus sylvestris L.) essential oils in human lymphocytes and *Drosophila melanogaster*. Food and Chemical Toxicology, 39(5), 485-492. https://doi.org/10.1016/S0278-6915(00)00157-5

[31] The Good Scents. (1980). The Good Scents Company Information System.

[32] Semiz, G., Heijari, J., Isik, K., & Holopainen, J. K. (2007). Variation in needle terpenoids among Pinus sylvestris L. (Pinaceae) provenances from Turkey. Biochemical Systematics and Ecology, 35(10), 652-661. https://doi.org/10.1016/j.bse.2007.05.013

[33] Trapp, S., & Croteau, R. (2001). Defensive resin biosynthesis in conifers. Annu. Rev. Plant Physiol. Plant Mol. Biol.

[34] Yoo, S. K., Day, D. F., & Cadwallader, K. R. (2001). Bioconversion of α- and β-pinene by Pseudomonas sp. strain PIN. Process Biochemistry, 36(10), 925-932. https://

doi.org/10.1016/S0032-9592(00)00248-X

[35] Gestalten, N., & Borderless Co. (2018). Nordic By Nature: Nordic Cuisine and Culinary Excursions. gestalten.

[36] Redzepi, R. (2010). Noma: Time and Place in Nordic Cuisine. (Phaidon Press., Ed.). Copenhagen.

[37] Bøttger, M. (2010). Dragsholm Slot - Fra fjord til jord - til bord. Politikens.

[38] Laursen, T. (2018). Wildfooding. Retrieved May 18, 2021, from https://wildfooding.com/gin/

[39] Mosca, Valeria; Tosoni, Stephano; Lanthier, C. (n.d.). Selvatiq. Retrieved May 18, 2021, from https://www.selvatiq.com/

[40] Emborg, R. (2014). Th Wizards Cookbook. Ronny Emborg.

[41] Luis Aduriz, A. (2004). Clorofilia. (Imagen Mab, Ed.). Errenteria.

[42] Ferran, J. A., & Soler. (2005). elBulli2003. Barcelona.

[43] Holmboe Bang, E. (2017). Maaemo. Cappelen Damm.

[44] Dufresne, W., & Meehan, P. (2017). WD-50, The Cookbook. (A. Bourdain/Ecco, Ed.).

[45] Laursen, T., & Boerlum, J. (2021). Den lille vilde. (P. Forlag, Ed.). Copenhagen.

[46] Ferran, J. A., & Soler. (2008). A Day at elBulli. (P. Press, Ed.). New York.

[47] Wetzel, B. (2020). Lummi: Island Cooking. Prestel.

[48] Baudar, P. (2018). The Wildcrafting Brewer: Creating Unique Drinks and Boozy Concoctions from Nature's Ingredients. Chelsea Green Publishing.

[49] Beauchamp, G. K., & Jiang, P. (2015). Comparative biology of taste: Insights into mechanism and function. Flavour, 4(1), 1-3. https://doi.org/10.1186/2044-7248-4-9

[50] Adams, R. P., Kauffmann, M., & Callahan, F. (2015). The leaf essential oil of Abies grandis. Phytologia, 97(January).

[51] Pérez-Rodríguez, N., Pinheiro de Souza Oliveira, R., Torrado Agrasar, A. M., & Domínguez, J. M. (2016). Ferulic acid transformation into the main vanilla aroma compounds by Amycolatopsis sp. ATCC 39116. Applied Microbiology and Biotechnology, 100(4), 1677-1689. https://doi.org/10.1007/s00253-015-7005-3

[52] Corvitto, A. (2011). The secrets of ice cream, ice cream without secrets (2o edition). Barcelona: Sant Cugat del Valles: Vilbo. Spain.

[53] Simon Difford. (2013). Diffordsguide Cocktails : The Bartender's Bible. (F. B. LTD, Ed.) (11th ed.). Ontorio, Canada.

Chapter 13

Genetic Resources of The Universal Flavor, Vanilla

Minoo Divakaran and N.T. Fathima Rafieah

Abstract

Commercially cultivated vanilla (*V. planifolia*) is native to Mexico and its cultivation and breeding programmes face major bottlenecks. This study reports presence of important agronomic characters in two important and endangered species of Vanilla, *V. aphylla* and *V. pilifera*, indigenous to India. *V. aphylla* was tolerant to Fusarium wilt and had longer flower life than the cultivated vanilla. *V. pilifera* flowers were fragrant, showed signs of insect pollination and had large fruit size. The species were amenable to interspecific hybridization and successful reciprocal crosses were done. Sequence similarity studies indicated the clustering of leafy and leafless species separately.

Keywords: interspecific hybridization, *V. apylla*, *V. pilifera*, sequence similarity

1. Introduction

The genus Vanilla includes about 110 species and the species have been treated in various monographic works [1, 2] including the life history of *V. planifolia* [3]. *Vanilla planifolia* (Salisb.) Ames (syn. *V. fragrans* Andrews.), is a tropical climbing orchid known for yielding the delicate popular flavor, vanilla [4] and is the second most expensive spice traded in the world market [5] (Spices Board 2000). The major vanilla producing countries are Madagascar, Comoro, Indonesia, Mexico and the Reunion, of which, Madagascar holds the prominent position.

Vanilla was introduced to Europe from Mexico, in about 1500 and its reputation of being an aphrodisiac followed it to countries where it was introduced. The importance of vanilla since early times in Mexico, is evident by the mention of offering vanilla as a medicinal beverage as part of a tribute during reign of Itzcóatl (Aztec Emperor) in 1427 and citing vanilla as a remedy for fatigue in Badianus manuscript in 1552 [6]. *Vanilla planifolia*, which yields the vanilla of commerce, is native to Mexico and parts of Central America and the history of origin of cultivated vanilla suggests that the entire stock outside Mexico may be from a single genetic source. For the last 400 years, humans have been playing important role in the dispersal and spread of vanilla in the New World.

2. Species of Vanilla

Studies of divergence among species of agronomic importance have been receiving greater attention. Genomics-based tools are efficient to characterize and

IntechOpen

identify genetic diversity in Vanilla and act as a significant tool for genomics-assisted plant breeding [7]. RAPD polymorphism was used to estimate the level of genetic diversity and interrelationships among few related species *Vanilla planifolia*, including both leafy and leafless types such as *V. tahitensis*, *V. andamanica*, *V. pilifera* and *V. aphylla*. Studies revealed that there is very limited variation within collections of *V. planifolia*, indicative of its narrow genetic base [8]. The British introduced *Vanilla planifolia* into India about 200 years ago whereas five other species are native viz., *V. pilifera* Holt., *V. andamanica* Rolfe., *V. aphylla* Blume., *V. walkeriae* Wight. and *V. wightiana* Lindl.

V. pilifera originally described from Malaya, recorded in Thailand is found in the Mikir hills of Northeast India. *V. aphylla*, an endangered species, previously known from Thailand is found in South India [9]. *V. andamanica* is endemic to Andaman group of Islands and is believed to be same as *V. albida* [10]. *V. tahitensis*, which is commonly exploited throughout the tropics, is indigenous to the Tahiti Islands. The presence and absence of leaves, and floral characters (colors of flower, lip, hairs on lip and ovary-pedicel etc.,), morphologically distinguish these species (**Table 1**).

A preliminary analysis of the various characters of Vanilla species including the above species, showed presence and absence of leaves formed an important part in the classification of the genus which in general had the basic chromosome number x = 16. Most of the Indian species were leafless, except *V. pilifera* which was intermediate in character, i.e., leafless in early stages and long narrow leaves at maturity and the chromosome number in *V. aphylla* is 2n = 64, whereas the cultivated vanilla and *V. tahitensis* had a somatic chromosome number of 2n = 32 [10, 11]. Differences in floral characters existed in flower color and lip characters (**Table 2**). In *V. pilifera* vines, leaves developed as the vine grew with flowers that were narrower (2.8 x 0.8 cm) with distinct pure white ovary-pedicel (**Figures 1** and **2**), pale green tepals, purplish violet and longer (6 mm approx.) hairs on white lip. *V. aphylla* is leafless (with scales-1.8 cm) and yellowish-cream flowers (petal size 3 x 1.2 cm approx.) having tuft of hairs that are cream near tip, deep reddish inside (2–3 mm) and light green ovary-pedicel (**Figures 3** and **4**).

Species	Leaf type		Internode	Median ridge
	Shape	Size		
V. aphylla	Scale leaves to leafless	2.1 cm in fresh shoots	6.5 cm	Absent in fresh shoots
V. pilifera	Narrow (intermediate to *V. planifolia* and *V. aphylla*)	L (8.5–16.5 cm) B (1.6–3.1 cm)	7 cm	Present all along the stem

Table 1.
Vegetative characters of Vanilla aphylla *and* V. pilifera.

Species	Petal color	Ovary-pedicel	Tuft of hair on the lip	Nature	Fruit size after pollination – 4 weeks
V. aphylla	Yellowish cream, L-3 cm, B-1.2 cm	Light green	Cream near tip, reddish brown inside (2–3 mm)	Longer life	14 cm (L) 3 cm (B)
V. pilifera	Pale green, narrower, L-2.8 cm, B-0.8 cm	White	Violet and longer (6 mm)	More brittle	11.5 cm (L) 3.3 cm (B)

L, Length; B, Breadth.

Table 2.
Variations in floral characters.

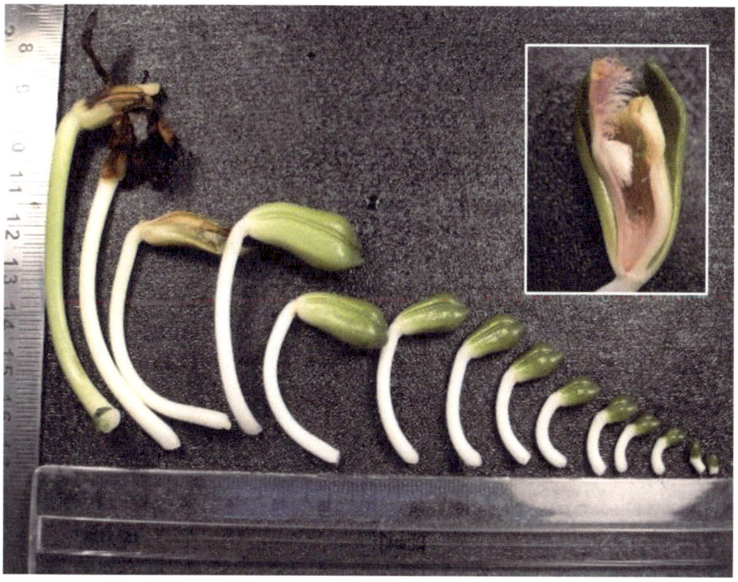

Figure 1.
Members of V. aphylla *inflorescence arranged sequentially (Inset: Close-up of an opened flower).*

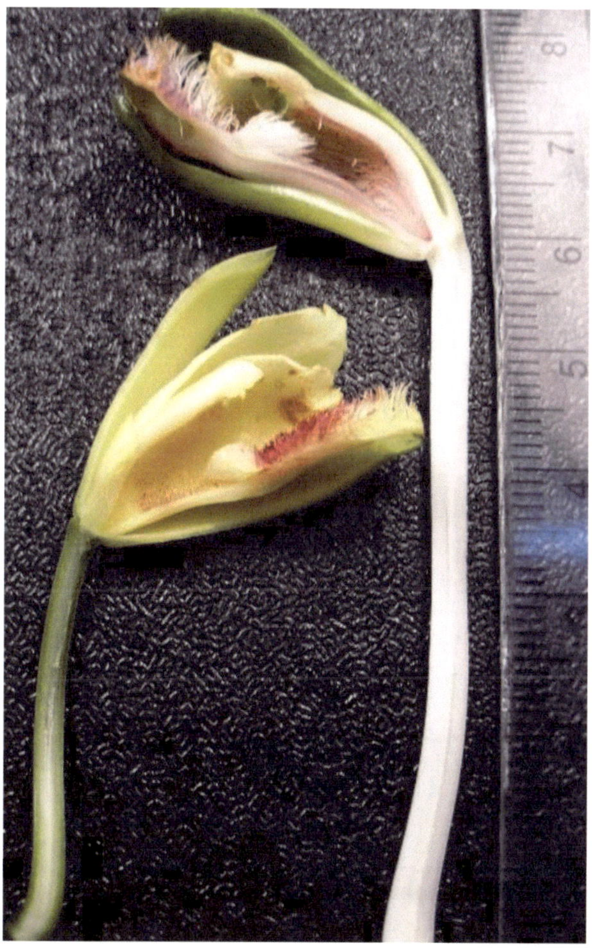

Figure 2.
Members of V. pilifera inflorescence arranged sequentially (Inset: Close-up of an opened flower).

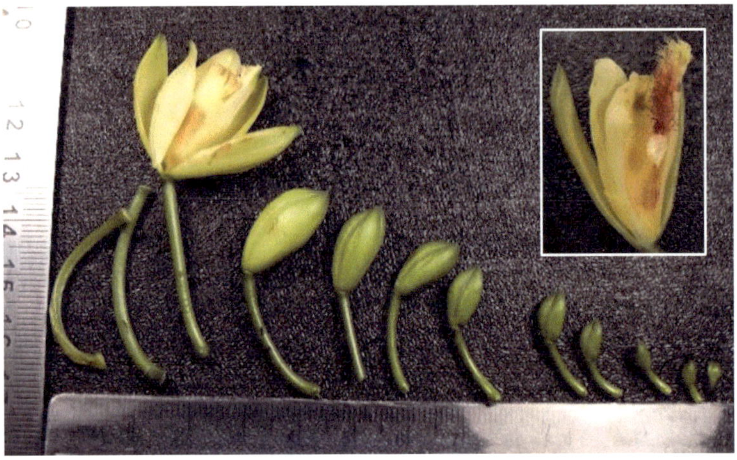

Figure 3.
L.S. of flowers of V. aphylla *(L) and* V. pilifera *(R).*

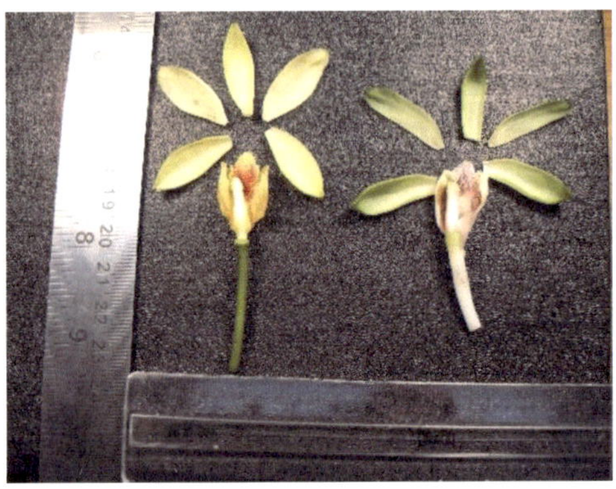

Figure 4.
Comparison of dissected out flowers of V. aphylla *(L) and* V. pilifera *(R).*

3. Biotechnological applications

Micropropagation and *in vitro* conservation techniques for the different species of Vanilla [12] and interspecific hybridization as a tool for gene flow of desirable characters from wild species into cultivated species, through pollen, have been reported [13]. Genetic interrelationships studies, using RAPD profiles [8], among different species revealed that the leafless forms of vanilla, *V. aphylla* and *V. pilifera* formed a separate sub-cluster. All the other leafy vanilla types formed a separate sub-cluster. *V. pilifera*, which showed an intermediate leaf character, showed only 50–56.1% similarity to *V. planifolia* but closely resembled *V. aphylla* (76.8%). Thus, the present study reveals the presence of important agronomic characters for introgression into cultivated vanilla and which can be utilized to overcome major bottlenecks in vanilla breeding. The presence of fragrance which attracts insects, coupled with signs of fruit set without hand pollination, holds *V. pilifera* as a potential candidate for breeding programmes, to overcome the problem of lack of natural seed set in vanilla. *V. aphylla* which was tolerant to *Fusarium oxysporum* [8] and its crossability to cultivated vanilla can be utilized as a bridging species and to help wipe out diseases arising out of monoculture. Interspecific hybridization has been reported and hence transfer of these desirable traits into cultivated vanilla,

V. planifolia, may not be hindered. The advent of biotechnological tools, offers techniques for transfer of these characters into *V. planifolia*, thus making the dream of transforming vanilla into a fragrant, natural seed setting, disease tolerant commercially important orchid can be turned into a reality.

The identification of a hydratase/lyase type enzyme as being a vanillin synthase offers new opportunities for the Vanilla pod-based industries. The accumulation of vanillin glucoside in the capsules of cultivated vines in response to environmental challenges may now be assessed at the molecular level. Likewise, the basis for development of genetic markers for the selection of vanilla orchid varieties with improved aromatic properties has now been laid down. Vanillin produced biologically is termed 'natural' vanillin and has a high economic value compared with chemically synthesized vanillin. Likewise, in the transition towards a bio-based economy, it is important to develop sustainable production systems to replace those currently based on fossil fuels. The demonstration that a single enzyme in the vanilla pod catalyzes the conversion of ferulic acid and ferulic acid glucoside into vanillin and vanillin glucoside provides several options for biotechnological applications [14].

4. Materials and methods

4.1 Genomic DNA isolation

Genomic DNA was isolated from approximately 100 mg fresh leaves by grinding in a pestle and mortar using liquid Nitrogen and following the procedure using DNeasy® Plant Mini Kit (Qiagen, USA). The ground sample powder (100 mg) was transferred to microfuge tubes. Followed by addition of 400 μl AP1 buffer and 4 μl RNase A and mixed by vortex. The tubes were incubated at 65°C for 10 min in a water bath with intermittent mixing 2–3 times by inverting the tubes. Added 130 μl buffer P3 to the tube, mixed and incubated for 5 min on ice. The lysate was centrifuged for 5 min at 14,000 rpm. The samples were then loaded onto the QIAshredder spin columns and centrifuged at 14,000 rmp for 2 min. The flow-through was transferred to a new tube without disturbing the pellet. Added 1.5 volume of buffer AW1 and mixed by pipetting. The contents were then loaded in 650 μl fractions onto the DNeasy mini spin column and centrifuged at 8000 rmp for 1 minute. The flow-through was discarded. The spin column was placed into a new 2 ml collection tube and added 500 μl buffer AW2, followed by centrifugation for 1 min at 8000 rpm. This last step with buffer AW2 step was repeated, with centrifugation at 14,000 rpm for 2 min. The spin columns were placed in fresh microfuge tubes and 100 μl AE buffer was added onto the membranes and incubated at room temperature for 5 min. The tubes were then centrifuged at 8000 rpm for 1 min. This step was repeated with another 100 μl of AE buffer. The eluted samples were stored at −20°C.

4.2 Measurement of purity and DNA concentration

Quality and quantity of genomic DNA was monitored by using UV/Vis. Spectrophotometry and quality was confirmed by using 0.8% Agarose Gel Electrophoresis. Each of the sample DNA was diluted to 5 ng/μL in double distilled water for use as a PCR template.

4.3 PCR amplification of DNA barcoding region and sequencing

PCR reactions were carried out using universal primers for the DNA barcode regions matK, nrDNA-ITS, rbcL and trnH-psbA. All the specific locus primers were purchased with universal M13 primer sequence at their 5′ ends, thus enabling the direct sequencing of the PCR products using the universal M13 primers. The PCR amplification was performed in a 20 μl reaction mixture, consisting of 1X PCR buffer (2 mM Mgcl2), 200 μM each of dATP, dCTP, dGTP, dTTP; 0.5 μM of each forward and reverse primers and 1 U of Taq polymerase (TakaRa-Taq), and (5–20 ng) DNA template. DNA amplification was performed in a thermal cycler (Eppendoff, Germany). When the reaction has finished, the tubes were stored at 4°C. PCR products were separated by agarose gel electrophoresis (1.8%). The list of primers, their nucleotide sequences, annealing temperature and the specific PCR cycling conditions are shown in **Table 3**. A large volume PCR reaction (100 μl) per sample loci was done and PCR purification was done using Nucleospin Gel and PCR Clean-up kit (Macherey-Nagel, Germany). The purified PCR products were sequenced using M13 universal primers (M13 forward and M13 reverse primers) on ABI 3730xl

S. No	DNA region	Primers Name	Sequence (5′-3′)	Reference	PCR reaction conditions
1	*matK*	390F	CGATCTATTCATTCAATATTTC	[15]	95°C for 4 min. 95°C for 45 sec. } 48°C for 30 sec } 35X 72°C for 50 sec. } 72°C for 8 min.
		1326R	TCTAGCACACGAAAGTCGAAGT		
3	ITS	ITS4	TCCTCCGCTTATTGATATGC	[16]	94°C for 4 min. 94°C for 40 sec. } 55 for 40 sec. } 36x 72°C for 1 min. } 72°C for 8 min.
		ITS5	GGAAGTAAAAGTCGTAACAAGG	[17]	
4	ITS	ITS-P5	CCTTATCAYTTAGAGGAAGGAG	[18]	94°C for 4 min. 94°C for 30 sec. } 55°C for 40 sec. } 34x 72°C for 1 min. } 72°C for 10 min.
		ITS-u4	RGTTTCTTTTCCTCCGCTTA		
5	*rbcL*	rbcL_1F	ATGTCACCACAAACAGAAAC	[19]	95°C for 4 min. 95°C for 45 sec. } 55°C for 30 sec. } 35x 72°C for 50 sec. } 72°C for 8 min.
		rbcL_724R	TCGCATGTACCTGCAGTAGC	[20]	
6	*rbcL*	rbcL_1F	ATGTCACCACAAACAGAAAC	[19]	95°C for 1 min. 95°C for 30 sec. } 51°C for 30 Section } 35x 72°C for 1 min. } 72°C for 5 min.
		rbcLa_r	CTTCTGCTACAAATAAGAATCGATCTC	[21]	
7	*rbcL*	rbcL_1F	ATGTCACCACAAACAGAAAC	[19]	95°C for 1 min. 95°C for 30 sec. } 51°C for 30 sec. } 35x 72°C for 1 min. } 72°C for 5 min.
		rbcLa_SI_Rev	GTAAAATCAAGTCCACCRCG	[22]	
8	*rbcL*	rbcL_1F	ATGTCACCACAAACAGAAAC	[19]	95°C for 1 min. 95°C for 30 sec. } 51°C for 30 sec. } 35x 72°C for 1 min. } 72°C for 5 min.
		rbcLaj634R	GAAACGGTCTCTCCAACGCAT	[23]	
9	trnH-psbA	psbA3_f	GTTATGCATGAACGTAATGCTC	[24]	92°C for 4 min. 94°C for 1 min. } 52°C for 1 min. } 35x 64°C for 1 min. } 64°C for 8 min.
		trnHf_05	CGCGCATGGTGGATTCACAATCC	[25]	

Table 3.
List of primers used for amplification of different loci and their PCR conditions.

DNA sequencer at AgriGenome labs facility, Kochi, India. Each DNA barcode region was sequenced.

The different universal primers used in this study for the amplification are shown in **Table 4** along with the amplified product size.

The final edited sequences are provided in FASTA format below for each of the successful sequencing reactions:

>Vanilla S matk.

TCTCACATTTAAATTATGTGTCAGATCTACTAATACCCTATCCCATACATC
TGGAAATCTTAGTTCAAATTCTTCAATGCTGGGTCAAAGATGTTCTTTCTTTG
CATTTATTGCGATTGTTTTTTCACGAATATCATAATTTGAATAGTCTCGTTAC
TTCAAAGAAATCTATTTATGTCTTTTCAAAAATAAATAAAAGATTTTTTTAT
TCCTACATAATTTTTATGTATATGAATCCGAATATCTATTCCTGTTTCTTCGT
AAACAGTCTTCTTATTTACGATCAACATCTTCTGGAGTGTTTCTTGAACAAA
CACATTTCTATGTAAAAATAGAACATATTCATCTTATAGTAGTAGTGTGTTG
TAATTCTTTCAAAAGGGACCTATGGTTTCTCGAAGATCCTTTCATGCATTAT
GTTCGATATCAAGGAAAAGCTATTCTGGGTTCAAAAGGAACTCTTATTCTGG
TGAATAAATGGAAATATTATCTTATTAATTTTTGGCAATCTTATTTTCACTTT
TGGTCTCAACCAGATAGGATCTATAGAAAGCAATTCTCCGACTATTCCTTTT
CTTTCCTGGGGTATTTTTCAAGTGTATTAAAAAATACTTTGGTAGTCAGAAA
TCAAATGCTAGAGAATTGCTTTCTCATAAATACTCCGACTCAGAAATTAGAT
ACCATAGCCCCGGTTATTTCTCTTATTGGATCCTTGTCGAAGGCAAAATTTT
GTACGTTAATGGGTCATCCCATTAGTAAACCGATCTGGACCGATTTATCGGA
TTCTGAGATTATTGATCGATTTTGTCGAATATGTAGAAATCTTTGTCGTTATC
ACAGTGGATCCTCAAAAAAACAGGTTT.

>VG matk.

TTCTCACATTTAAATTATGTGTCAGATCTACTAATACCCTATCCCATACAT
CTGGAAATCTTAGTTCAAATTCTTCAATGCTGGGTCAAAGATGTTCTTTCTTT
GCATTTATTGCGATTGTTTTTTCACGAATATCAGAATTTGAATAGTCTCGTTA
CTTCAAAGAAATCTATTTATGTCTTTTCAAAAAAAAATAAAAGATTCTTTTTA
TTCCTACATAATTTTTATGTATATGAATTCGAATATCTATTCATGTTTCTTCG
TAAACAGTCTTCTTATTTACGATCAACATCTTCTGGAGTGTTTCTTGAACAAA
CACATTTTTATGGAAAAATAGAACATATTCATCTTATAGTAGTAGTGTGTTT
TAATTCTTTAAAAAGCGACCTATGGTTTCTCGAAGATCCTTTCATGCATTAT
GTTCGATATCAAGGAAAAGCTATTCTGGGTTCAAAAGGAACTCTTATTCTGT
TGAATAAATGGAAATATTATATTATTTATTTTTTGCAATCTTATTTTCACTTT
TGGTCTCAACCAGATAGGATCTATAGAAAGCAATTCTCTGACTATTCCTTTT
CTTTCCTGGGGTATTTTTCAAGTGTATTAAAAAATACTTTGGTAGTCAGAAA
TCAAATGCTAGGGAATTGCTTTCTCATAAATATTCCGATTCAGAAATTAGAT
ACCACAGCCCCGGTGATTTCTCTTATTGGATCCTTGTCGAAGGCAAAATTTT
GTACGTTAATGGGTCATCCCATTAGTAAACCGATCTGGACTGATTTATCGGA
TTCTGAGATTATTGATCGATTTTGTCGAATATGTAGAAATCTTTGTCGTTATC
ACAGTGGA.

>VP matk.

TTCTCACATTTAAATTATGTGTCAGATCTACTAATACCCTATCCCATACAT
CTGGAAATCTTAGTTCAAATTCTTCAATGCTGGGTCAAAGATGTTCTTTCTTT
GCATTTATTGCGATTGTTTTTTCACGAATATCAGAATTTGAATAGTCTCGTTA
CTTCAAAGAAATCTATTTATGTCTTTTCAAAAAAAAATAAAAGATTCTTTTTA
TTCCTACATAATTTTTATGTATATGAATTCGAATATCTATTCATGTTTCTTCG
TAAACAGTCTTCTTATTTACGATCAACATCTTCTGGAGTGTTTCTTGAACAAA
CACATTTTTATGGAAAAATAGAACATATTCATCTTATAGTAGTAGTGTGTTT
TAATTCTTTAAAAAGCGACCTATGGTTTCTCGAAGATCCTTTCATGCATTAT
GTTCGATATCAAGGAAAAGCTATTCTGGGTTCAAAAGGAACTCTTATTCTGT
TGAATAAATGGAAATATTATATTATTTATTTTTTGCAATCTTATTTTCACTTT

S. No	Plant Name	Matk	ITS		rbcL Primers				trnH-psbA
		(product size)	(product size)	(product size)	(product size)	(product size)	(product size)	(product size)	(product size)
1	*V1*	390F/1326R (1000 bp)	ITS4/ITS5 (800 bp)	—	rbcL_1F/rbcL_724R (NA*)	rbcLa_f/rbcLa_r (700 bp)	rbcLa_f/rbcLa_SI_Rev (600 bp)	rbcLa_f/rbcLaj634R (650 bp)	psbA3_f/trnHf_05 (750 bp)
2	*VG*	390F/1326R (1000 bp)	ITS4/ITS5 (800 bp)	ITS-P5/ITS-u4 (800 bp)	rbcL_1F/rbcL_724R (NA*)	rbcLa_f/rbcLa_r (NA*)	rbcLa_f/rbcLa_SI_Rev (600 bp)	rbcLa_f/rbcLaj634R (650 bp)	psbA3_f/trnHf_05 (800 bp)
3	*VP*	390F/1326R (1000 bp)	ITS4/ITS5 (800 bp)	ITS-P5/ITS-u4 (800 bp)	rbcL_1F/rbcL_724R (NA*)	rbcLa_f/rbcLa_r (NA*)	rbcLa_f/rbcLa_SI_Rev (600 bp)	rbcLa_f/rbcLaj634R (650 bp)	psbA3_f/trnHf_05 (800 bp)

**NA, No amplification.*
The Bold text indicates successful sequencing was done for these samples.
The ITS region was very problematic while sequencing and only V1 was completed, while sequencing is pending for VG and VP samples.
Loci rbcL and trnH-psbA has been successfully amplified but has not yet been sent for sequencing.

Table 4.
List of primers pairs used for amplification of different barcode loci and its estimated product sizes in agarose gel, for the Vanilla *species under study.*

TGGTCTCAACCAGATAGGATCTATAGAAAGCAATTCTCTGACTATTCCTTTT
CTTTCCTGGGGTATTTTTCAAGTGTATTAAAAAATACTTTGGTAGTCAGAAA
TCAAATGCTAGGGAATTGCTTTCTCATAAATATTCCGATTCAGAAATTAGAT
ACCACAGCCCCGGTGATTTCTCTTATTGGATCCTTGTCGAAGGCAAAATTTT
GTACGTTAATGGGTCATCCCATTAGTAAACCGATCTGGACTGATTTATCGGA
TTCTGAGATTATTGATCGATTTTGTCGAATATGTAGAAATCTTTGTCGTTATC
ACAGTGGA.

>VS ITS.

AGTGGAAGTAAAAGTCGTAACAAGGTTTCCGTAGGTGAACCTGCGGAAG
GATCATTGACGAGAGCTATGACTGATCGAGTGATCTGTGCAACCTGTGGGG
GTGCGACGGCTGTTTGATGTCGCATTCTTCCATCGCAGAGCTCCTGCTTCCA
GGGGGAGCTCGATGCTGTGGGGGGATAAACAACAGCCTATGGGCGTGGTCA
TACGCCAAGGGAGAGCAAATGTTAAGCCGCCAACGGGTGTGTTGTGCGTCG
CCAGGCCCAGTGGGGTATGGCAAACGAACACTGAACGACTCTCGACAACGG
ATATCTTGGCTCTCGCATCGATGAAGAACGCAGCGAAATGCGATACGTGTTG
TGAATTGTAGAATCCCGTGAACCATCCATTTTTTGAACGCAAGTTGCGCCCG
AGGATGCAAGCCGAGGGCACTCCTGCATGGGTGTAATGCGTTCTGTCGCTC
CTCGCGCAGGCATGGAATCGTTGGTTTAGATCAGCGGCCCCTCGCCAGGAT
GCGATCGATGGCACCCTGTGCTACGGCATGGCGTGTTCAAGCGTTGGGCGA
TGGTCGGCTGTAGACACGGCAAGAGGTGGATGCCACCGAGTGTTGTGGTGT
TGGCCAGTAGGAACCGATGTTGCAGTGCGACAAGGTGATGCCCCTTGCAAA
TCCAACTCCATGCTCCATGGTGTGGAATCGTGACCCCATGTTAGGTGAGGCT
ACCCGCTGAGTTTAAGCATATCAATAAGCGGA.

5. Result and discussion

5.1 Presence of important agronomic characters

Among the different species of vanilla studied *Vanilla aphylla* Blume and *V. pilifera* Holtt., flowered synchronously (**Figure 5**). *V. aphylla* occurs naturally in South India (**Figure 6**) and *V. pilifera* (**Figure 7**) in Assam, Northeast India. Flowers of both the species opened sequentially and lasted for one day in *V. pilifera*, whereas it lasted for 2 days in *V. aphylla*. In the former, signs of fruit set were observed even without pollination (**Figures 1** and **8**) whereas *V. apylla* flowers did not set fruit (**Figure 3**), ruling out the possibility of natural fruit set in this species, which is thus similar to *V. planifolia* (**Table 5**).

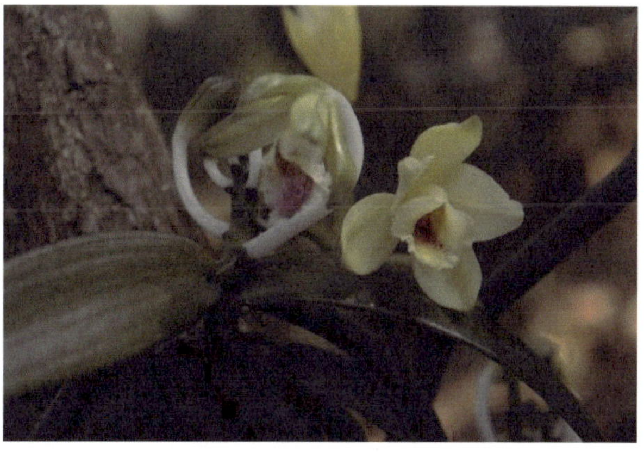

Figure 5.
V. pilifera *(T) inflorescence in comparison with that of* V. aphylla *(B). Arrow Indicates signs of natural fruit set without pollination in* V. pilifera.

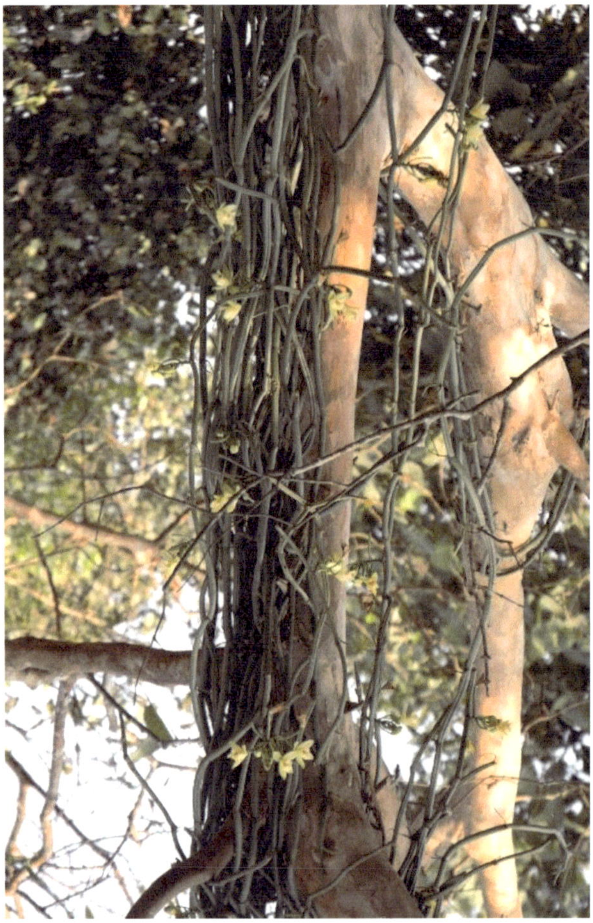

Figure 6.
V. pilifera *flower with a leaf (which develops at maturity).*

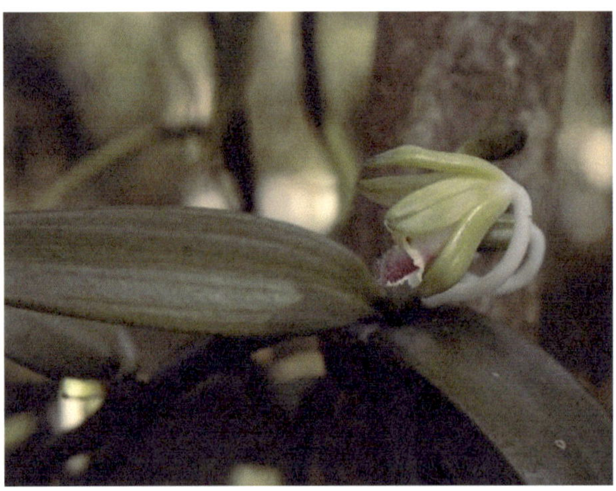

Figure 7.
Vine of V. aphylla *in bloom.*

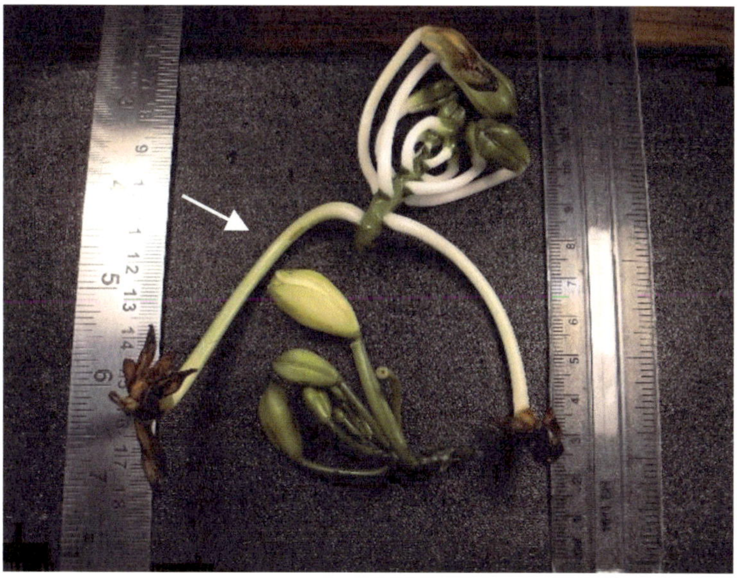

Figure 8.
Cross section of the ovary pedicel of V. aphylla *without pollination, and after 24 hrs.*

Species	Disease resistance	Fragrance	Natural seed set	Crossability	Fruit size	Flower life (hours)
V. aphylla	Tolerant to *Fusarium oxysporum*	—	Not seen	Crossable to *V. pilifera* and *V. planifolia*		> 36
V. pilifera	—	Highly fragrant	Symptoms seen	Crossable to *V. aphylla*	Larger	~24
V. planifolia	Susceptible		Not seen	Crossable to *V. aphylla*		< 24

Table 5.
Important agronomic characters.

Cross sections of the ovary pedicel were observed after closing of the flowers. Persistent perianth is characteristic to the genus and also indicative of effective pollination. In flowers where pollination is not effected, the perianth is shed after the flower closes. Perianth in *V. pilifera* were found to persist even without pollination and the cross sections indicated initiation of seed set (**Figures 9** and **10**), whereas *V. apyhlla* did not show any indications (**Figures 11** and **12**). Since rostellum is present in both the species, natural pollination without an aid is ruled out. It can be suspected, that the fragrance of the *V. pilifera* flowers attracts insects (which were found to frequent the flowers often) to visit them and bring about effective pollination.

Pollinations both self and interspecific hybridizations between the two species were done and fruits set was observed (**Figure 13**).

5.2 Sequence analysis

General observations from the experiment

1. The matK sequences of VG and VP are identical.

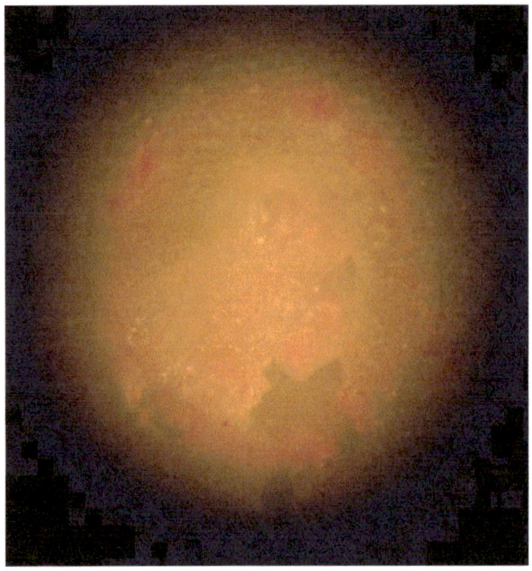

Figure 9.
Cross section of the ovary pedicel of V. aphylla *without pollination, and after 24 hrs.*

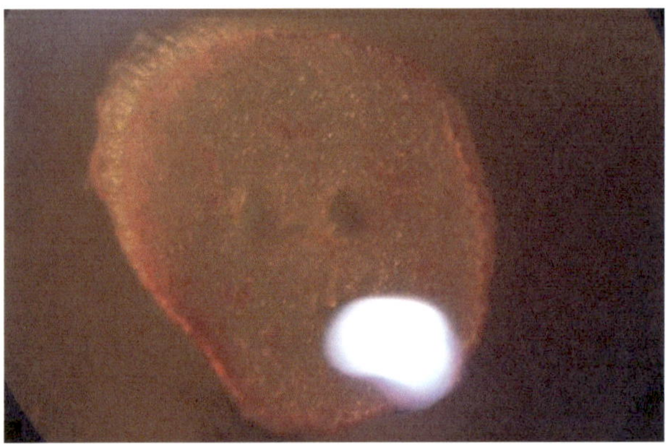

Figure 10.
C.S. of ovary-pedicel of V. pilifera *without pollination, showing indications of seed set.*

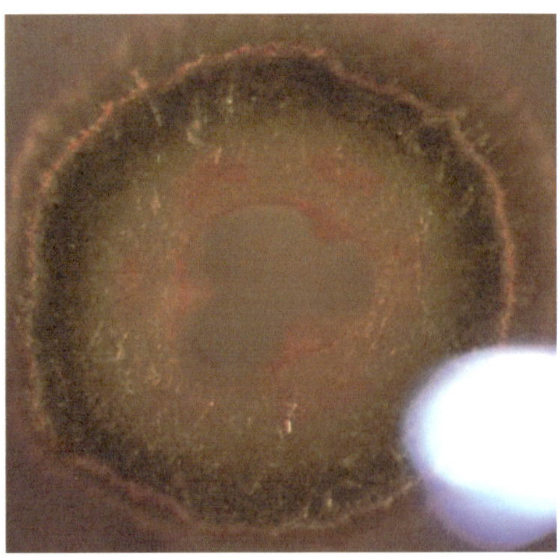

Figure 11.
C.S. of ovary-pedicel of V. pilifera *without pollination, showing indications of seed set.*

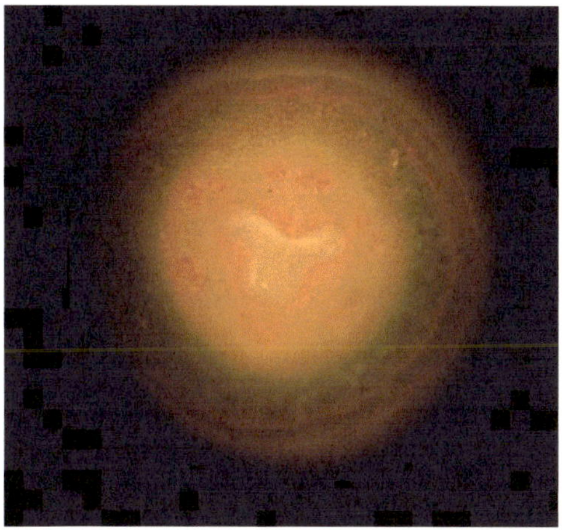

Figure 12.
Flowers of V. pilifera *in comparison with* V. aphylla.

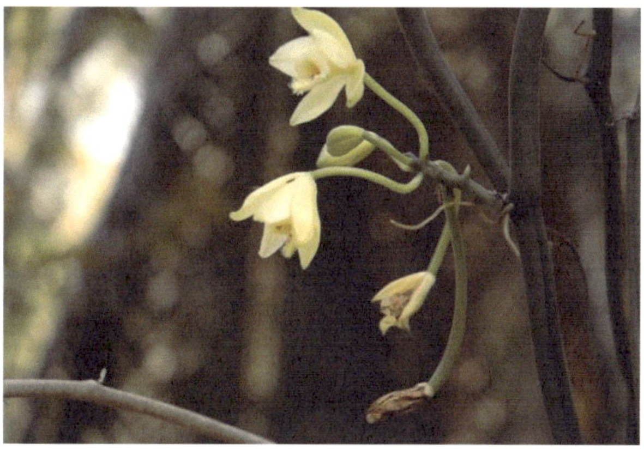

Figure 13.
V. aphylla *inflorescence with fruit set after interspecific hybridization.*

2. The matK sequence of V1 was different from VG/VP at 21 nucleotide positions as shown in **Table 6** below.

Nucleotide position	1	1	2	2	2	3	3	3	3	3	4	4	4	5	5	6	6	6	6	6	7
	3	9	0	3	5	2	2	6	7	8	7	9	9	0	6	4	6	6	8	9	7
	7	0	3	8	2	3	8	7	7	3	1	2	8	5	3	0	1	7	5	5	3
VS matk	T	T	T	C	C	C	T	G	C	G	G	C	A	G	C	A	C	C	T	T	C
VG matk	G	A	C	T	A	T	G	T	A	C	T	A	T	T	T	G	T	T	C	G	T
VP matk	G	A	C	T	A	T	G	T	A	C	T	A	T	T	T	G	T	T	C	G	T

Table 6.
Matk sequence analysis.

3. Blast search of the matk sequences of VG/VP in the NCBI blast search gave 100% match with *Vanilla planifolia* (Accession No. KJ566306.1), as in the NCBI search results shown below.

Description	Max score	Total score	Query cover	E value	Ident	Accession
Vanilla planifolia chloroplast, complete genome	1563	1563	100%	0.0	100.00%	KJ566306.1
Vanilla planifolia chloroplast, complete genome	1546	1546	100%	0,0	99.65%	MF197310.1
Vanilla planifolia tRNA-Lys (trnK) gene, partial sequence; and maturase K (matK) gene, compl	1524	1524	100%	0.0	99.17%	JN181462.1
Vanilla planifolia maturase K (matK) chloroplast pseudogene, partial sequence	1507	1507	100%	0.0	98.82%	AF263687.1
Vanilla planifolia chloroplast matK pseudogene	1507	1507	100%	0.0	98.82%	AJ310079.1
Vanilla planifolia plastid partial matK gene for maturase K, specimen voucher Chase O-199 K	1423	1423	95%	0.0	98.40%	AJ581443.1
Vanilla somae voucher KFBG290 maturase K (matK) gene, partial cds: plastid	1419	1419	100%	0.0	96.93%	KY966974.1
Vanilla aphylla chloroplast DNA, complete genome	1419	1419	99%	0.0	97.03%	LC085348.1
Vanilla pilifera voucher V5 maturase K (matK) gene, partial cds: chloroplast	1354	1354	99%	0,0	95.64%	FJ816099.1
Vanilla siamensis voucher V2 maturase K (matK) gene, partial cds: chloroplast	1315	1315	97%	0,0	95.23%	FJ816097.1
Vanilla planifolia voucher SBB-0324 maturase K (matK) gene, partial cds: chloroplast	1314	1314	84%	0.0	100.00%	JN004635.1
Vanilla planifolia isolate AD7LN25 maturase K (matK) qene. Partial cds: chloroplast	1284	1284	89%	0.0	97.11%	MF349972.1

4. Blast search of the matk sequences of VS in the NCBI blast search gave maximum identity with *Vanilla somae* (Accession No.KY966974.1). See the NCBI search results below.

Description	Max score	Total score	Query cover	E value	Ident	Accession
Vanilla somae voucher KFBG290 maturase K (matK) gene, partial cds: plastid	1570	1570	99%	0.0	99.54%	KY966974.1
Vanilla aphylla chloroplast DNA, complete genome	1570	1570	99%	0.0	99.54%	LC085348.1
Vanilla pilifera voucher V5 maturase K (matK) gene, partial cds: chloroplast	1489	1489	100%	0.0	97.81%	FJ816099.1

Description	Max score	Total score	Query cover	E value	Ident	Accession
Vanilla pompona chloroplast. Complete genome	1474	1474	100%	0,0	97.45%	MF197310.1
Vanilla planifolia chloroplast. Complete genome	1469	1469	100%	0.0	97.34%	KJ566306.1
Vanilla planifolia tRNA-Lys (trnK) gene, partial sequence: and maturase K (matK) gene, complel	1452	1452	100%	0.0	96.99%	JN181462.1
Vanilla siamensis voucher V2 maturase K (matK) gene, partial cds: chloroplast	1447	1447	98%	0.0	97.33%	FJ816097.1
Vanilla planifolia maturase K (matK) chloroplast pseudogene, partial sequence	1435	1435	100%	0.0	96.64%	AF263687.1
Vanilla planifolia chloroplast matK pseudogene	1435	1435	100%	0.0	96.64%	AJ310079.1
Vanilla planifolia isolate AD7LN25 maturase K (matK) gene, partial cds: chloroplast	1408	1408	90%	0.0	99.23%	MF349972.1
Vanilla roscheri voucher NMK:838.10216 maturase K (matK) gene, partial cds: chloroplast	1395	1395	93%	0.0	97.89%	KU748308.1
Vanilla aphylla voucher V1 maturase K (matK) gene, partial cds: chloroplast	1391	1391	96%	0.0	96.79%	FJ816096.1

5. Blast search of the ITS sequences of VS in the NCBI blast search gave maximum identity with Vanilla shenzhenica (Accession No. JF796930.1). See the NCBI search results below.

Description	Max score	Total score	Query cover	E value	Ident	Accession
Vanilla somae voucher KFBG290 maturase K (matK) gene, partial cds: plastid	1570	1570	99%	0.0	99.54%	KY966974.1
Vanilla aphylla chloroplast DNA, complete genome	1570	1570	99%	0.0	99.54%	LC085348.1
Vanilla pilifera voucher V5 maturase K (matK) gene, partial cds: chloroplast	1489	1489	100%	0.0	97.81%	FJ816099.1
Vanilla pompona chloroplast. Complete genome	1474	1474	100%	0,0	97.45%	MF197310.1
Vanilla planifolia chloroplast. Complete genome	1469	1469	100%	0.0	97.34%	KJ566306.1
Vanilla planifolia tRNA-Lys (trnK) gene, partial sequence: and maturase K (matK) gene, complel	1452	1452	100%	0.0	96.99%	JN181462.1
Vanilla siamensis voucher V2 maturase K (matK) gene, partial cds: chloroplast	1447	1447	98%	0.0	97.33%	FJ816097.1
Vanilla planifolia maturase K (matK) chloroplast pseudogene, partial sequence	1435	1435	100%	0.0	96.64%	AF263687.1
Vanilla planifolia chloroplast matK pseudogene	1435	1435	100%	0.0	96.64%	AJ310079.1

Description	Max score	Total score	Query cover	E value	Ident	Accession
Vanilla planifolia isolate AD7LN25 maturase K (matK) gene, partial cds: chloroplast	1408	1408	90%	0.0	99.23%	MF349972.1
Vanilla roscheri voucher NMK:838.10216 maturase K (matK) gene, partial cds: chloroplast	1395	1395	93%	0.0	97.89%	KU748308.1
Vanilla aphylla voucher V1 maturase K (matK) gene, partial cds: chloroplast	1391	1391	96%	0.0	96.79%	FJ816096.1

6. The ITS sequences matching with different Vanilla sp. were downloaded and subjected to analysis using MEGA7.0 software (**Table** 7).

	VS ITS	*JF796930.1_Vanilla_shenzhenica*	*KY966687.1_Vanilla_somae*	*AF151006.1_Vanilla_aphylla*	*JF825978.1_Vanilla_siamensis*	*FJ425830.1_Vanilla_imperialis*	*FJ425840.1_Vanilla_roscheri*	*FJ425835.1_Vanilla_barbellata*	*FJ425834.1_Vanilla_africana*	*EU498163.1_Vanilla_bahiana*	*GQ867241.1_Vanilla_planifolia*	*GQ867237.1_Vanilla_pompona*	*AF391785.1_Vanilla_hirsuta*	*EU498165.1_Vanilla_edwallii*
VS ITS	0													
JF796930.1_Vanilla_shenzhenica	20	0												
KY966687.1_Vanilla_somae	20	0	0											
AF151006.1_Vanilla_aphylla	27	19	19	0										
JF825978.1_Vanilla_siamensis	42	39	39	41	0									
FJ425830.1_Vanilla_imperialis	40	33	33	41	47	0								
FJ425840.1_Vanilla_roscheri	41	34	34	45	53	40	0							
FJ425835.1_Vanilla_barbellata	55	48	48	55	66	57	58	0						
FJ425834.1_Vanilla_africana	63	51	51	56	66	56	60	76	0					
EU498163.1_Vanilla_bahiana	96	89	89	96	101	97	99	107	100	0				
GQ867241.1_Vanilla_planifolia	107	100	100	107	119	106	113	110	110	45	0			
GQ867237.1_Vanilla_pompona	99	92	92	99	104	98	103	107	104	20	45	0		
AF391785.1_Vanilla_hirsuta	101	92	92	102	114	101	102	108	100	39	31	43	0	
EU498165.1_Vanilla_edwallii	132	133	133	136	143	136	143	141	146	139	150	136	146	0

Table 7.
Estimates of evolutionary divergence between sequences.

The number of base differences per sequence from between sequences are shown. The analysis involved 14 nucleotide sequences. All ambiguous positions were removed for each sequence pair. There was a total of 657 positions in the final dataset. Evolutionary analyses were conducted in MEGA7 (**Figure 14**).

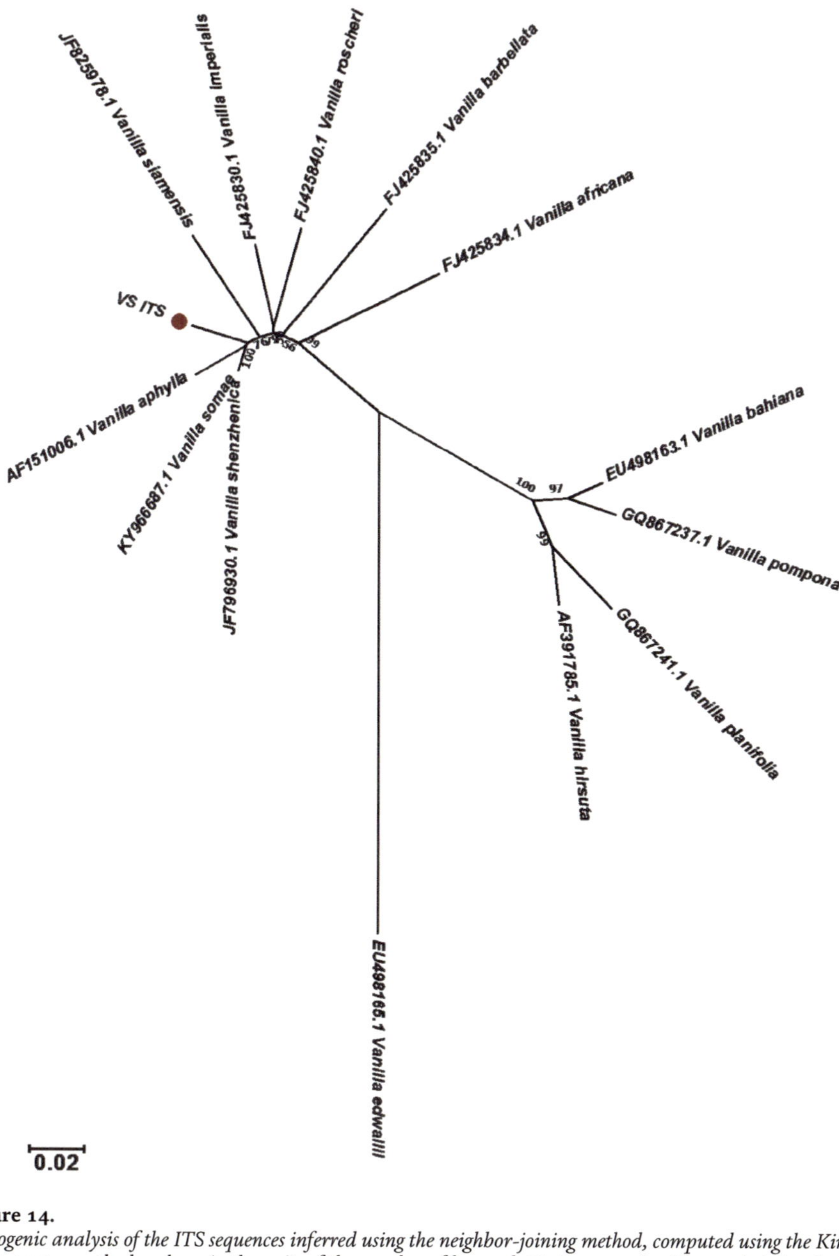

Figure 14.
Phylogenic analysis of the ITS sequences inferred using the neighbor-joining method, computed using the Kimura 2-parameter method and are in the units of the number of base substitutions per site. The analysis involved 14 nucleotide sequences. All ambiguous positions were removed for each sequence pair. There was a total of 657 positions in the final dataset. The analyses were conducted in MEGA7.

6. Conclusions

The analysis involved 14 nucleotide sequences. All ambiguous positions were removed for each sequence pair. There was a total of 657 positions in the final dataset. The analyses were conducted in MEGA7. The phylogeny analysis also revealed the separate clustering offer leafy and leafless species. *Vanilla siamensis*, a leafy species, indicating signs of self-pollination in its wild, in Thailand, clustered with leafless *V. aphylla* species.

The studies further reveal the complexity of the biosynthesis of the natural vanillin synthesis. However, it is to be further analyzed whether leafy character is associated with enhanced photosynthetic products that indirectly affect the vanillin synthesis too. This reiterates the need for conservation of the genetic resources [12] of Vanilla across the continents, for implementing meaningful breeding programs, to enhance vanillin productivity in addition to disease resistance and reproductive behavior.

Acknowledgements

The first author acknowledges the former Directors of Indian Institute of Spices Research, Kozhikode, Kerala from where she initiated these studies. The authors are thankful for the financial support rendered by University Grants Commission (MRP and CPE funds), DST-FIST funds, for taking up these research initiatives, in their laboratory and express gratitude to Scientists at Centre for Medicinal Plant Research, Kottakkal, Malappuram, for support in Sequencing work.

Author details

Minoo Divakaran* and N.T. Fathima Rafieah
Department of Botany, Providence Women's College, Kozhikode, Kerala, India

*Address all correspondence to: minoodivakaran@gmail.com

References

[1] Correll, D. S. (1953). Vanilla-its botany, history, cultivation and economic importance. Economic Botany, 7(4), 291–358. DOI:10.1007/bf02930810

[2] Bouriquet G (1954) Le vanillier et la vanille dans le monde. Encyclope'die Biologique XLVI. Lechevalier, Paris VI

[3] Swamy, B. G. L. (1947). On the life-history of Vanilla planifolia. Botanical Gazette, 108(3), 449–456. DOI:10.1086/335429

[4] Purseglove JW, Brown EG, Green CL, Robbins SRJ (eds.) 1981. Spices. Vol. 2. Longman Inc., New York, pp 644-735.

[5] Spices Board 2000. Vanilla Status paper. Spices Board, Cochin, India, pp. 33.

[6] Lubinsky P (2004) Vanilla diversity in Mexico. In: Bakto Fla-vors, Rutgers University (eds) Vanilla 2004 Europe, Second International Congress, Cannes, France, 30 Sept–01 Oct 2004.

[7] Hu, Y., Resende, M. F. R., Jr., Bombarely, A., Brym, M., Bassil, E., and Chambers, A. H. (2019). Genomics-based spanersity analysis of Vanilla species using a Vanilla planifolia draft genome and genotyping-by-sequencing. Scientific Reports, 9(1). DOI:10.1038/s41598-019-40144-1

[8] Minoo, D., Jayakumar, V. N., Veena, S. S., Vimala, J., Basha, A., Saji, K. V., Nirmal Babu, K., and Peter, K. V. (2007). Genetic variations and interrelationships in Vanilla planifolia and few related species as expressed by RAPD polymorphism. Genetic Resources and Crop Evolution, 55(3), 459–470. DOI:10.1007/s10722-007-9252-3

[9] Satish K and Manilal K.S. 1993. Vanilla aphylla Blume. Amer. Orch. Soc. Bull. 62, 394–397.

[10] Seidenfaden G. 1978. Orchid genera in Thailand VI Neottioideae. Dansk. Bot. Ark. 32, 138–146.

[11] Franklin, W.M., 1963. Chromosome number and behavior in a Vanilla hybrid and several Vanilla species. Bull. Torrey Bot. Club 90, 416–417

[12] Minoo, D., Nirmal Babu, K., and Peter, K. V. (2006). Conservation of Vanilla species, in vitro. Scientia Horticulturae, 110(2), 175–180. DOI:10.1016/j.scienta.2006.07.003

[13] Minoo, D., Nirmal Babu, K., Ravindran, P. N., and Peter, K. V. (2006). Interspecific hybridization in vanilla and molecular characterization of hybrids and selfed progenies using RAPD and AFLP markers. Scientia Horticulturae, 108(4), 414–422. DOI:10.1016/j.scienta.2006.02.018

[14] Gallage, N. J., Hansen, E. H., Kannangara, R., Olsen, C. E., Motawia, M. S., Jørgensen, K., Holme, I., Hebelstrup, K., Grisoni, M., and Møller, B. L. (2014). Vanillin formation from ferulic acid in Vanilla planifolia is catalysed by a single enzyme. Nature Communications, 5(1). DOI:10.1038/ncomms5037

[15] Cuenoud, P., Savolainen, V., Chatrou, L. W., Powell, M., Grayer, R. J., and Chase, M. W. (2002). Molecular phylogenetics of Caryophyllales based on nuclear 18S rDNA and plastid rbcL, atpB, and matK DNA sequences. American Journal of Botany, 89(1), 132–144. DOI:10.3732/ajb.89.1.132

[16] White, T. J., Bruns, T., Lee, S., and Taylor, J. (1990). AFmplification and direct sequencing of fungal ribosomal rna genes for phylogenetics. In PCR Protocols (pp. 315–322). Elsevier. doi:10.1016/b978-0-12-372180-8.50042-1

[17] Sang, T., Crawford, D. J., and Stuessy, T. F. (1995). Documentation of

reticulate evolution in peonies (Paeonia) using internal transcribed spacer sequences of nuclear ribosomal DNA: Implications for biogeography and concerted evolution. Proceedings of the National Academy of Sciences, 92(15), 6813–6817. DOI:10.1073/pnas.92.15.6813

[18] Cheng, T., Xu, C., Lei, L., Li, C., Zhang, Y., and Zhou, S. (2015). Barcoding the kingdom Plantae: New PCR primers for ITS regions of plants with improved universality and specificity. Molecular Ecology Resources, 16(1), 138–149. DOI:10.1111/1755-0998.12438

[19] Olmstead, R. G., Michaels, H. J., Scott, K. M., and Palmer, J. D. (1992). Monophyly of the Asteridae and identification of their major lineages inferred from DNA sequences of rbcL. Annals of the Missouri Botanical Garden, 79(2), 249. DOI:10.2307/2399768

[20] Fay, M. F., Swensen, S. M., and Chase, M. W. (1997). Taxonomic affinities of Medusagyne oppositifolia (Medusagynaceae). Kew Bulletin, 52(1), 111. DOI:10.2307/4117844

[21] Kress, W. J., and Erickson, D. L. (2007). A two-locus global DNA barcode for land plants: The coding rbcL gene complements the non-coding trnH-psbA spacer region. PLoS ONE, 2 (6), e508. DOI:10.1371/journal.pone.0000508

[22] Kress, W. J., Erickson, D. L., Jones, F. A., Swenson, N. G., Perez, R., Sanjur, O., and Bermingham, E. (2009a). Plant DNA barcodes and a community phylogeny of a tropical forest dynamics plot in Panama. Proceedings of the National Academy of Sciences, 106(44), 18621–18626. DOI:10.1073/pnas.0909820106

[23] Fazekas, A. J., Burgess, K. S., Kesanakurti, P. R., Graham, S. W., Newmaster, S. G., Husband, B. C., Percy, D. M., Hajibabaei, M., and Barrett, S. C. H. (2008). Multiple multilocus DNA barcodes from the plastid genome discriminate plant species equally well. PLoS ONE, 3(7), e2802. DOI:10.1371/journal.pone.0002802

[24] Sang, T., Crawford, D. J., and Stuessy, T. F. (1997). Chloroplast DNA phylogeny, reticulate evolution, and biogeography of Paeonia (Paeoniaceae). American Journal of Botany, 84(8), 1120–1136. DOI:10.2307/2446155

[25] Tate, J.A., Simpson, B.B. (2003). Paraphyly of Tarasa (Malvaceae) and diverse origins of the Polyploid species. Systematic Botany. 28. 723-737. DOI: 10.1043/02-64.1

Section 4

Functional Products

Chapter 14

Herbs and Spices Fortified Functional Dairy Products

Vinod Kumar Paswan, Hency Rose, Chandra Shekhar Singh, S. Yamini and Aman Rathaur

Abstract

Recently, an increased interest in exploiting the functional and medicinal health attributes of herbs and spices has been observed worldwide among the health conscious consumers to preserve and promote the health and nutrition and immunity particularly during the Covid-19 pandemic era. Fortification of dairy products with these herbs and spices so as to exploit the functional and medicinal attributes have also gained momentum. Herbs and spices are rich source of bioactive compounds such as anti-oxidants, vitamins, micro- and macro-minerals, phytochemicals like flavonoids, alkaloids, glycosides, tannins, essential oils, coumarin, organic acids, phenols and saponins. Milk and other dairy products have been popular compatible vehicles for delivering functional, nutritional and other health benefits of phytochemicals of herbs and spices among the consumers. This chapter explores the quality and functional attributes of herbs and spices fortified dairy products such as herbal spiked milk, curd and yoghurts, paneer, cheese and ice creams and other dairy products.

Keywords: bioactive compounds, herbs and spices, dairy products, functional foods, antioxidants, phytochemicals

1. Introduction

Food habits and disease prevention have a clear link; the effects of food on diseases including diabetes, obesity, osteoporosis, hypertension, and cardiovascular disease have been reported in the literature [1]. The indigenous knowledge of traditional medicinal plants are becoming more widely recognized around the world. Since it is the world's largest producer of traditional medicinal herbs, India is considered as the "Botanical Garden of the World" and "Land of spices" [2]. Herbs and their extracts have been used to fortify foods as preservatives, flavorings, medicinal agents, and food additives throughout history [3]. Consumer knowledge and interest in adding herbs to dairy and food products to enhance dietary strategy and balanced nutrition for achieving health benefits from foods beyond providing basic nutrition has increased worldwide as a result of the advent of functional foods, and consequently, the demand for value-added functional foods has grown worldwide [4]. Since India is the world's largest producer of milk, a significant amount of liquid milk is utilized for traditional dairy products. Incorporating herbal bioactives into conventional Indian dairy products facilitate to compete in the global functional food market, which is growing at a rapid pace [5].

2. Herbs and their classification

Herbs and spices are plants or parts of plants, mostly leaves and seeds, that are used for their taste, flavor, aroma, and imparting color in food products, or for medicinal and functional properties. These are cultivated primarily in temperate and tropical climates and harvested to be used as flavorings or seasonings [6]. The diverse phytochemicals and bioactive compounds present in herbs and spices give additional nutraceutical, medicinal and functional health benefits. In addition to leaves and seeds, spices may be derived from different other parts of the plant such as bark, buds and flowers, fruits and seeds, rhizomes and roots, or sometimes the complete whole plant tops [7]. Although, the term 'spice and 'herbs' are used interchangeably, 'herb' is considered as a subset of spice and refers to plants with aromatic leaves with medicinal and functional health benefits. In addition to taxonomic classification, herbs and spices have been classified according to seasonality and lifespan, based on usage and applications and on the basis active principles and functional and medicinal properties present in them. Classification of herbs based on their seasonality and lifespan, usage and bioactive phytochemicals present in them has been presented in **Table 1** [6, 8].

Classification	Properties	Examples
According to the usage		
Medicinal herbs	Curative and healing properties and used as pharmaceutical and therapeutical purposes.	Tulsi, sage, pepper mint, rosemary, thyme, asparagus, *Aloe vera*, garlic, cinnamon leaf, neem, brahmi, ashwagandha, amla, malabar nut, coriander, ginger, onion etc.
Culinary herbs	Have strong flavors and/or imparts color in food and thus used in cooking.	Borage, chives, mint, parsley, basil, dill, thyme, sage, oregano, chervil, paprika, turmeric, saffron etc.
Aromatic herbs	Have pleasant smelling flowers or foliage and used for aroma.	Lemon verbena, clove pink, lavender, bergamot, myrtle, scented geranium, sweet violet, rose etc.
Ornamental herbs	Used for decoration and Ornamental purposes.	Chives, lavender, chicory, yarrow, jewelweed, rosemary, chamomile, thyme, sage, feverfew etc.
According to the active constituents		
Aromatic herbs	Owing to the presence of volatile essential oils, they have a good odor and are widely used both therapeutically and as flavorings. These are of two types:	
	Stimulant Herbs: Increases the body's energy and movements, and most commonly affects the digestive, respiratory, and circulatory systems.	Capsicum, damiana, fennel, garlic, ginger, peppermint, sage, thyme, catnip, feverfew, lemon grass, penny royal etc.
	Nerving Herbs: These are used to relieve and heal the nervous system, but these also have an impact on the digestive, respiratory, and circulatory systems.	Chamomile, crampbark, dong quai, ginger, hops, lobelia, skullcap, valerian, catnip, lady's slipper, and sarsaparilla etc.
Astringent herbs	They have an impact on the digestive, circulatory, and urinary systems because of astringent components including tannins.	Bayberry, comfrey, eyebright, golden seal, peppermint, red raspberry, slippery elm, white oak, white willow, black walnut, crampbark, mullein, and penny royal etc.

Classification	Properties	Examples
Bitter herbs (phenolics, saponins, and alkaloids)	The presence of phenols and phenol glycosides, alkaloids, or saponins, and are classified into subcategories such as laxative herbs, diuretic herbs, digestive herbs etc.	Aloe vera, blessed thistle, yam root, cascara, licorice, pumpkin, senna, yellow dock, yucca, barberry, gentian, safflowers, and golden seal etc.
Mucilaginous herbs	Polysaccharides give mucilaginous herbs their properties, including a smooth, mild flavor that tastes sweet in water. They aid in the removal of toxins from the digestive system, as well as its regulation and the reduction of bowel transit time.	Althea, aloe vera, burdock, comfrey, dandelion, echinacea, fenugreek, kelp, psylium, slippery elm, dulse, konjak root, Irish moss, and mullein etc.
Nutritive herbs	Provide carbohydrates, and fats, as well as vitamins and minerals.	Banana, barley grass, bilberry, broccoli, grapefruit, hibiscus, lemon, oat straw, onion, red clover, apple, asparagus, banana, barley grass, bilberry, broccoli, cabbage, carrot, cauliflower, spirulina, stevia, wheat germ etc.
According to seasonality and lifespan		
Annuals	Complete their life cycle in one season within a year	Anise, basil, borage, calendula (pot marigold), chamomile, chervil, cilantro/ coriander, dill bouquet, dill dukat, fennel, smoky, marjoram, parsley, shiso, saffron, summer savory etc.
Biennials	Grow for more than one season	Caraway seeds, prime rose, bai zhi, mullein, teasel, viper's bugloss, angelica, caraway, clary, watercress, and parsley etc.
Perennials	Which live for two seasons and only bloom in the second.	Alfalfa, allspice, aloe vera, angelica, avens, bee balm, bay leaves, catnip, chamomile, common thyme, dill, echinacea, fennel, lavender, lemon balm, mint: spearmint/ peppermint/ applemint/ orangemint, marjoram sweet, mitsuba, oregano, rosemary, stevia, salad burnet, sage, tarragon, watercress, yarrow etc.

Table 1.
Classification of herbs based on their usage and applications, active principles in them and their seasonality and lifespan.

3. Functional properties of herbs

Herbs and their extracts have been shown to be beneficial to one's health. Flavonoids, polyphenols, phenolic acid, terpenoids, sulphides, carotenoids, coumarins, lignans, saponins, curcumins, phthalides, and plant sterols are only a few of the natural bioactive compounds found in it. These naturally occurring bioactive compounds shows several biological effects such as antimicrobial, anti-inflammatory, antioxidant, antiallergic and antihypertensive effects [9]. Herbs are very high in natural antioxidants. Antioxidants are substances that inhibit or prevent the oxidation process. Synthetic antioxidants, such as butyl hydroxy anisole or butylhydroxytoluene, are commonly used in the food industry to prevent the deterioration of food quality (including the degradation of lipids, carbohydrates and proteins). Such antioxidants, on the other hand, are volatile and easily decompose at high temperatures, and their ingestion may pose serious health risks. Herbal phytochemical based natural antioxidants are currently in high demand among consumers, owing

Common name	Scientific name	Bioactive components	Functional and medicinal properties
Basil	*Ocimum basilicum*	Phenolic acids (rosmarinic acid & caffiec acid), flavanol glycosides (quercetin & kaempferol), anthocyanins	Anti-asthmatic, anti-stress, gastric anti-ulcer activity, antioxidant, antibacterial, anti-fungal, antiviral, anti-mutagenic, antitumor and immuno-stimulant activities.
Aloe vera	*Aloe barbadensis miller*	Aloin, emodin, lupeol, auxins, gibberellin, Vitamins A, C & E (antioxidants)	Antibacterial, antiviral, antiseptic, analgesic wound healing, anti-inflammatory gastroprotective, antitumor.
Arjuna	*Terminalia arjuna*	Flavonoid and phenolic content, sitosterol	Antioxidant & free radical scavenger activities, heart tonic for healthy cardiovascular system, lowers blood cholesterol.
Sage	*Salvia triloba*	Phenolic acid, flavonoids	Anti-oxidative properties and anti-inflammatory activities.
Ashwagandha	*Withania somnifera*	Steroidal lactones, alkaloids and flavonoids	Antitumor, respiratory stimulant activities and immuo-stimulating effect.
Pudina leaf	*Mentha sp.*	Menthol, mint L-carvone, essential oils	Digestive health, natural coolant and mouth-freshener
Coriander leaf	*Coriandrum sativum*	Essential oils, linalool	Rich in antioxidant, help lower blood sugar, fight infections, and promote heart, brain, skin, and digestive health
Rosemary	*Salvia rosmarinus*	p-cymene, linalool, thymol	Rich source of antioxidants and anti-inflammatory compounds, help to boost the immune system and improve blood circulation.
Origanum	*Origanum vulgare*	carvacrol, β-fenchyl alcohol, thymol, rich in phenolic content	Antibacterial agent, reduction of asthma, cramping, diarrhea, and indigestion.

Table 2.
Some important herbs commonly used for development of functional dairy products, their bioactive components and functional and medicinal properties.

to concerns about the safety of synthetic antioxidants. Antioxidant properties are demonstrated by phenolic compounds found in herbs [10, 11]. Herbal bioactive compounds have also been shown to prevent or reduce the risk of degenerative diseases such as diabetes, cancer, obesity, and cardiovascular disease [12].

Polyphenols are plant secondary metabolites which work as antioxidants, scavenge free radicals and protects against cancer, cardiovascular disease, asthma, infection, and diabetes. Based on the number of phenol rings and the structural elements that hold these rings together, polyphenols are divided into 4 groups; phenolic acids, flavonoids, stilbenes and lignans. Acid fruits contain phenolic acids, which are further divided into hydroxyl benzoic and hydroxyl cinnamic acids [13]. Flavanoids are a form of polyphenol that is abundant in the human diet and is responsible for the attractive colors of flowers, fruits, and leaves [14]. Flavonoids are classified into six classes, as flavonols, flavones, flavanones, flavanols, anthocyanins, and isoflavones. Plant stilbenes are antifungal phytoalexins. Many studies confirms that supplementation of polyphenol-rich herbs with a healthy diet can help prevent coronary heart disease, reduce cancer cell growth, and have anti-diabetic effects [13].

The antimicrobial properties of herbs can effectively regulate the growth of spoilage and pathogenic bacteria in dairy products. Phenolic compounds are the main antimicrobial compounds found in herbs, and they can be used as effective replacements for artificial antimicrobial agents used in food production. Some pathogenic bacteria (*Salmonella enteritidis, Listeria monocytogenes*, and *Staphylococcus aureus*) and fungi have been found to be inhibited by phenolic compounds such as tea catechins, coumaric acid, ellagic acid, oleuropein, and ferulic acid [15]. Furthermore, the essential oils present in various herbs contains bioactive compounds which shows antimicrobial properties in addition to anti-inflammatory, anticarcinogenic, and a variety of other beneficial health promoting activities [16]. The use of synthetic chemical additives in food processing pose several health risks and these essential oils may be used to substitute these synthetic additives **Table 2** [17].

4. Application of herbs in milk and other functional dairy products

4.1 Milk

Recently the demand for milk fortified with herbs and spices has increased due to their therapeutic effects and health benefits. Kumar Gaur et al. reported that herbal milk containing tulsi juice, turmeric powder and ginger juice) was rich in antioxidants and total phenolic content which enhanced the shelf life of the product in addition to imparting the typical herbal flavor, improved sensory quality and consumer acceptability due to their various potential health benefits such as anticarcinogenic. Cardio-protective, anti-inflammatory and anti-microbial [18]. Pathur et al. reported that tulsi flavored herbal milk has improved sensory attributes and overall acceptability, enhanced keeping quality with good antioxidant properties when compared with normal milk [19]. Jankar et al. developed ready-to-serve turmeric-flavored milk by combining milk and turmeric powder. Turmeric is high in antioxidants and has anti-inflammatory, anticarcinogenic, immunomodulant along with several other medicinal, and nutritional properties. Turmeric blended milk relieves cough and cold symptoms, as well as headache and wound pain [20].

Kamble et al. [21] formulated flavored milk with different varieties of piper betel leaves. *Piper betel* leaves popularly known as Paan in India, are dark green heart-shaped aromatic leaves of the Piperaceae family. The leaves, which are widely used for mastication, are rich in aromatic volatile oils, phenols, and the alkaloid arakene, which act as a stimulant for muscular and mental efficiency. Piper betel leave flavored milk was reported to have good consumer acceptability [21]. Pugazhenthi and Jothylingam developed dietetic herbal flavored milk with 5% aloe vera pulp extract and artificial sweeteners such as aspartame and sucralose. The physico-chemical properties of dietetic herbal flavored milk were within the standard ranges, with a small rise in protein content when aspartame was added. Furthermore, the content of almost all minerals increased slightly, which could be due to minerals found in aloe vera pulp [22]. Kishore et al. tested medicinal herbs like fennel, tulsi, and lemongrass oil in herbal-flavored milk. They reported several functional health benefits of this flavored herbal milk due to tulsi, which decreases the risk of heart disease, soothes fever, headache, and sore throat; and fennel, which aids in blood purification, improves eyesight, lowers blood pressure, and reduces fiber, while lemongrass oil has antioxidant, anti-bacterial, and gastric ulcer-prevention properties [23].

Sawale et al. developed *Pueraria tuberosa* added herbal milk. The content of hydroxy methyl furfural (HMF), ethanol stability, and lightness of the herbal milk decreased, whereas the functional properties of milk, redness and yellowness, and antioxidant activity increased. They reported that the inclusion of *Pueraira tuberosa* may be ideal for the preparation of low heat-treated functional dairy food products [24]. Similarly, Vaquil et al. formulated a flavored milk with wheat grass juice added at a 12:1 milk-to-juice ratio in double toned milk with good quality characteristics and acceptability. The study indicated that, adding wheat grass juice increased the chlorophyll content and extended the shelf life by up to 15 days [25]. Rathod et al. prepared flavored milk by the inclusion of ginger juice which increased total solids, acidity, solid not fat, and ash content, while protein, fat, moisture, and pH decreased as the amount of ginger juice increased. On the basis of overall acceptability and sensory qualities, it was determined that flavored milk made with 96 parts milk and 4 parts ginger juice with 5% sugar was the most appropriate [26].

4.2 Yoghurt, Dahi and Lassi

Herbal supplemented yoghurts were formulated with potential multifunctional health benefits to consumers. Chowdhury et al. developed herbal yoghurts with a variety of herbal leaves, including tulsi (*Ocimum sanctum*), pudina (*Mentha arvensis*), and coriander (*Coriandrum sativum*). The yoghurt was made by combining pretreated herbal leaves with uniform milk containing *L. acidophilus* and *L. plantarum* strains (1:1 v/v) and incubating at 40°C for 6 hours. They observed that the presence of herbs in yoghurt did not affect the probiotic population and there was not any significant difference in total titratable acidity and in pH during storage. However, as compared to control yoghurt without any herbs, herbal yoghurt had higher -D-galactosidase enzymatic activity. They reported maximum β-D-galactosidase activity in tulsi incorporated yoghurt [27]. Similarly, Ghosh observed that tulsi extract and beetroot extract (level of 5%) with yoghurt had more nutritional benefits than natural yoghurt. They reported that folic acid and riboflavin content were improved in the yoghurt by the addition of tulsi and beetroot. Moreover, tulsi shows better antiradical properties in yoghurt [28].

There is growing experimental evidence for the use of aloe vera as nutraceutical and functional attributes as it contains important nutrients and essential minerals, bioactive compounds with several health benefits and immune modulating effects. Incorporation of aloe vera gel in yoghurt improves the functional properties and therapeutic values. In a study conducted by Govindammal et al. reported that adding 15% aloe vera gel to yoghurt increased overall acceptability based on sensory evaluation. When compared to plain yoghurt, the addition of aloe vera gel increased protein, fiber content, phytonutrients (such as steroids, anthroquinones, saponins, and phlabotannins) and showed an improvement in vitamin C. Aloe vera also served as a stabilizer, lowering the syneresis value of aloe vera yoghurt and improving the texture [29].

The effect of garlic (*Allium sativum*) and cinnamon (*Cinnamomum verum*) in three types of milk (cow, goat, and camel) on the growth and activity of Lactic Acid Bacteria and proteolytic activity during yoghurt fermentation was investigated by Shori and Salihin [30]. The presence of herbs increased the amount of lactic acid bacteria and proteolytic activity in cow, goat, and camel milk yoghurt during fermentation, according to the report. In another study, cinnamon powder fortified yoghurt was found to contain phenolic acids, flavonols, and cinnamaldehyde. The cinnamon-fortified yoghurt contains just 34.7 percent of the total phenolic compounds found in the cinnamon yoghurt water, with the remaining compounds bound to milk proteins. The *in vitro* digestion of cinnamon-fortified yoghurt resulted in the release of phenolic compounds from milk proteins, resulting in a higher amount of phenolic compounds recovered in the cinnamon-fortified yoghurt at the end of the digestion. Furthermore, adding cinnamon to yoghurt increases its radical scavenging behavior significantly. The yoghurt matrix also improves gastrointestinal stability and cinnamon polyphenol bio-accessibility. These findings demonstrate that cinnamon-fortified yoghurt can be a valuable source of dietary bioavailable polyphenols [31].

Azizkhani and Parsaeimehr indicated that addition of essential oils extracted from herbs such as peppermint, basil and zataria in probiotic yoghurt increases the antioxidant activity, antiradical activity and consumer acceptability [32]. Similarly, yoghurt made with *Rosmarinus officinalis* oil (0.14, 0.21, 0.29, and 0.36 g/L) was found to have improved flavor and texture in addition to microbiological and physicochemical properties [33]. Herbs like ginger and beet root, which contain high antioxidant properties and are beneficial to human health. In another study, the antioxidant role of herbal yoghurt was investigated by Srivastava et al. who observed that adding ginger or beet root extracts (2%) to the goat, cow and buffalo milk yoghurt modified the antioxidant properties of the herbal yoghurt. The highest antioxidant properties were found in ginger rhizome goat milk yoghurt and beet root extract goat milk yoghurt, followed by cow and buffalo milk herbal yoghurt [34]. Herbal yoghurt made by fortification with peppermint (*Mentha piperita*), dill (*Anethum graveolens*), and basil herbal extracts (*Ocimum basilicum*) were found to be rich in antioxidant activity, proteolytic activity, bioactive compounds, and improved angiotensin-1 converting enzyme inhibition (ACE) [35]. Among these herbs, peppermint yoghurt had the strongest inhibitory impact on ACE activity and proteolytic activity during fermentation and storage of yoghurt [35].

Addition of *Moringa oleifera* leaves powder (1.0–1.5% w/v) to yoghurt improved the nutritional profile of the yoghurt indicated by increased protein, fat and total solids content of the herbal yoghurt over the plain yoghurt [36]. However, the overall acceptability of the moringa enriched yoghurt was lesser than the plain yoghurt might be due to bitterness of the moringa leaves [36]. In another study conducted by Elbagory et al., it was observed that pomegranate peel extract and *Moringa oleifera* leaves extract could be used to improve the antibacterial, functional, and nutritional properties of yoghurt. During the storage times, it was discovered that a concentration of 2% of both pomegranate peels and *Moringa oleifera* leaves had the greatest inhibitory effect against the E.coli O111:H2 (EHEC O111:H2) population. They concluded that ethanolic extracts of pomegranate peels and *Moringa oleifera* leaves could be used to preserve yoghurt and enhance its consistency [37]. Similarly, addition of roselle extract to goat milk based yoghurt had significant antimicrobial activity of probiotic in yoghurt which enhanced the ability to inhibit both gram negative and gram positive bacteria due to the presence of peptides [38].

Labneh a concentrated yoghurt, is a traditional Middle Eastern food. According to studies, adding 0.2 ppm of thyme, marjoram, and sage essential oils to labneh increased its shelf life at 5°C. When stored at 5°C, the control Labneh (without essential oil) showed the presence of yeast and mold from the 14th day onwards [39]. Zaky et al. observed that adding 2 μL/100 ml milk of dill and caraway essential oils to labneh enhanced the flavor, shelf life, and organoleptic properties, especially taste and odor. Dill and caraway essential oils are both antioxidant and antimicrobial agents that are safe to use. The use of these essential oils aided in the development of total volatile fatty acids (TVFAs), which gradually increased in treated samples during storage. Furthermore, the contents of acetaldehyde and diacetyl in treated samples reached their highest levels after 14 days of storage, then gradually decreased until the end of the storage period. El-Sayed et al. investigated the antimicrobial properties of *Moringa oleifera* oil-fortified labneh. They observed that *Moringa oleifera* oil has a high percentage of oleic acid, antioxidant activity, and phenol content, and that it has greater antimicrobial activity against Gram-positive bacteria (*Bacillus cereus, Staphylococcus aureus* and *Bacillus subtilis*), Gram-negative bacteria (*Escherichia coli, Yersinia enterocolitica, Salmonella typhimurium, Listeria monocytogenes and Pseudomonas aeruginosa*), Yeast (*Saccharomyces cerevisiae*) and other three fungal strains. According to the study, adding *Moringa oleifera* oil to labneh increased total solid, fat, total volatile fatty acid, DPPH scavenging activity, tocopherols, and total lactic acid bacterial counts. The sensory properties of labneh samples improved and received higher scores as the ratios of *Moringa oleifera* oil were increased. With the addition of *Moringa oleifera* oil, however, the protein, ash, acidity, and water soluble vitamins content of labneh decreased concomitantly [40].

Dahi and lassi are traditional fermented milk beverages that have gained widespread popularity in India and several other countries. Many studies have found that supplementing lassi and dahi with aloe vera (*Aloe barbadensis Miller*) improves immuno-protective properties, improves growth of a probiotic strain and increases health benefits [41]. Similarly, lassi fortified with ginger (2%), turmeric (1%), and carrot extracts (15%) (v/v) helps to deliver phytochemicals and other nutrients for health benefits in our nutrition food system. The functional benefits of lassi are enhanced by the inclusion of probiotic microorganisms and antioxidant-rich herbal juices, which are the body's primary defense system for neutralizing free radicals and preventing damage [42].

4.3 Butter and ghee

The addition of herbal extract to ghee was influenced by growing customer understanding of food ingredients. Foods fortified with herbs that have inherent antioxidant properties are used in particular for people who suffer from Cardio Vascular Diseases (CVDs) [43]. The most commonly used extracts in ghee, according to Ozcan et al. are Sage (*Salvia officinalis*) and Rosemary (*Rosmarinus officinalis*). Antioxidant properties are higher in sage and rosemary extracts than in synthetic antioxidants [44]. According to Najgebauer et al. adding 2 percent dried herbs (sage or rosemary) to butter made from sour cream improved oxidative stability by delaying lipolysis in butter during storage [45]. Furthermore, Farag et al. observed that butter infused with thyme and cumin essential oils was more effective than the synthetic antioxidant butylated hydroxyl toluene in preventing its oxidation when kept at room temperature [46]. Similarly, Merai et al. found that adding 0.6 percent tulsi (*Ocimum sanctum*) leaf powder to creamery butter ghee resulted in ghee with equal stability to ghee containing 0.02 percent butylated hydroxyl anisole for one week at high storage temperature. Tulsi leaves are also thought to have the potential to extend the oxidative stability of ghee [47].

The effects of sage, rosemary, and oregano extracts on butter stability were investigated by Ahmet et al. They came to the conclusion that these extracts were more effective than BHA at stabilizing butter against oxidation. When stored at 5°C, sage extracts at 0.02–0.05 percent proved to be the most effective in stabilizing butter samples [48]. Renata et al. tested the oxidative stability of butter with added phenolics from rosemary herbs. The study found that rosemary alcoholic extract has the highest antioxidant properties measured in both DPPH radical inhibition and malondialdehyde (MDA) quantification assays, as well as no cytotoxicity. This suggests that using rosemary alcoholic extract as a natural antioxidant is effective, as it achieved the highest oxidative stability of butter when applied to butter at temperatures of 60 and 110°C, with a concentration of 400 mg of phenolic compounds per kg of butter. This reflected at the lowest formation of degraded peroxides from lipids [49].

Currently, the herbs incorporated ghee is advertised as medicinal ghee in India and around the world. In a clinical study conducted by Rajanikant and Patil, it was discovered that incorporating functional attributes of *Terminalia arjuna* in ghee provides beneficial effects against cardiovascular diseases, and that this product had excellent potentiality to act as a free radical scavenger, as well as improved the shelf life of ghee when compared to traditional ghee [50]. According to Parmar and Khamrui's research, combining 7% arjuna alcoholic extract with ghee made from creamery buffalo butter yielded the highest phytosterol content and sensorial properties [51]. The vasa ghee, which helps to reduce the risk of asthma, is another health-promoting herbal ghee. Vasa ghee is made with the aid of the Malabar nut or vasa (*Adhatoda vasica*). The anti-asthmatic effects of vasa ghee are due to a component called vasicinone, which is an anti- asthmatic agent found in this plant [52].

Using the carotene bleaching assay, DPPH assay, and Rancimat procedure, Nilkanth et al. evaluated the antioxidant activities of ashwagandha (*Withania somnifera*), vidarikand (*Pueraria tuberosa*), and shatavari (*Asparagus racemosus*) extracts in both aqueous and ethanolic forms and compared them to BHA. The phenolic content and antioxidant activities of ethanolic extracts of herbs were found to be higher than those of their aqueous extracts. The ethanolic extracts of the herbs were more effective than the aqueous extracts in preventing the growth of the peroxide value and conjugated diene in ghee. Free radical scavenging activity was improved when ghee was combined with an ethanolic extract of herbs. Vidarikand's ethanolic extract had the highest antioxidant activity of all the plants, followed by ashwagandha and shatavari. Herbs may thus be used as a natural antioxidant because they have health benefits as well as the ability to preserve food [53].

4.4 Ice cream

Trivedi et al. reported that incorporating *Ocimum sanctum* leaf juice extract or freeze dried leaf powder in ice cream mix resulted in very high market acceptability due to potential functional properties. Furthermore, adding basil juice or powder to ice cream had no effect on the amount of overrun [54]. Kumar et al. conducted research to produce ice cream with various levels (2–4%) of tulsi extract. When tulsi extract is added, fat, protein, reducing sugars, non-reducing sugars, and total solids all decrease proportionately but the herbal ice cream has good acceptability among the consumers [55].

In order to exploit the medicinal and functional health benefits of aloe vera, particularly fir diabetic patient, Ankush Verma standardized the process of development of ice cream with various levels of aloe vera and mint. The reported that 90 percent of ice cream mix, 10% aloe vera, and 0.05 percent mint extract earned the highest sensory ranking, with the best chemical characteristics (maximum total solids, acidity, protein, carbohydrate, and ash), and the best microbial analysis (SPC and negative in coli type test), suggesting that ice cream has good storage stability [56].

Pinto et al. [57] prepared ginger ice cream with 4, 6, and 8% ginger shreds in the ice cream mix and compared it to a control made with vanilla flavoring. The addition of ginger shreds resulted in a decrease in compositional attributes such as fat, protein, sugars, total solids, and pH, as well as an increase in acidity, which was particularly true at higher levels of shred addition. However, at higher levels of ginger shred addition, acidity, viscosity of ice cream mixes, and melting resistance of ice cream all increased significantly. Among different recipes, 4 percent ginger shredded ice cream had the best appropriate body and texture score as well as the highest acceptability score [57]. Gabb et al. developed ice cream with ginger rhizomes, which were converted into juice, pulp, candy, and powder before being added to the ice cream during the freezing process. The ginger paste and juice reduced fat, total solids, protein, and overrun while increasing antioxidant activity and phenols, while the ginger candy and powder increased solids, crude fiber, antioxidant activity, and phenols while lowering fat and overrun [58].

Sensory evaluation of curcumin (turmeric) powder as natural color for butterscotch flavor ice cream was investigated by Manoharan et al. Turmeric is a bright yellow colorant produced from the roots of the herb *Curcuma longa*, with pigments including curcuminoids, curcumin, and related compounds responsible for the yellow color. As a result, it's used as a natural colorant in butterscotch ice cream. According to the study, the use of curcumin powder at 0.5 percent in ice cream preparation achieved the highest scores for sensory qualities and overall acceptability [59].

Mint incorporated herbal ice cream had an increased protein and acidity levels and decreased fat and overrun levels. Herbal menthol at 0.5 percent of the ice-cream mix generated the strongest results for the mint flavored ice cream, providing a cooling sensation without altering the sensory and physical properties of the dessert [60]. Similarly, Jana et al. investigated the development of herbal ice cream with 3.50 percent and 2.50 percent lemon grass distillate and curry leaf distillate, respectively and lemongrass powder and curry leaf powder at 0.75 percent and 0.70 percent, respectively. They reported that, the herbal ice cream made with herbal distillates and, especially lemon grass distillate was due to its highest sensory score than herbal ice creams made with herbal powders [61].

4.5 Cheese

Mohamed et al. reported an improved shelf life and consistency of cream cheese (an acid-curd soft cheese with a short shelf life) on addition of *Moringa oleifera* ethanol extract at different ratios of 2.00, 3.00, and 4.00 g/100 g skimmed UF-retentate. According to the findings, the ethanolic extract of *M. oleifera* had the high total phenols and antioxidant activities, as well as a broad range of antimicrobial properties against various pathogenic strains and the largest inhibition region. The ethanolic extract was found to be more effective against gram positive, gram negative, and fungi strains. Furthermore, raising the concentration of *M. oleifera* extract resulted in an increase in probiotic strains and counts, especially with *Lactobacillus plantarum* and improved taste, odor, acidity, total solids, fat/dry matter, soluble nitrogen/total nitrogen, diacetyl, acetaldehyde, total volatile fatty acid, total phenol content, and antioxidant activity. The result suggested the use of *M. oleifera* extract as a natural preservative for cream cheese [62].

Bakheit and Foda developed spicy Mudaffara cheese by adding three different spices (clove, black cumin, and black pepper) with good consumer acceptability. The results suggested that, spicy Mudaffara cheese could be stored at room temperature for 4 to 6 weeks with good taste, depending on the spices used, while its shelf life increased to 8 weeks when kept refrigerated. Clove Mudaffara cheese, on the other hand, had the highest antioxidant activity, followed by black cumin and black pepper cheese [63]. Similarly, Hamid and Abdel developed traditional herbal Sudanese white cheese called Gibna cheese by adding 0.02 percent fenugreek, cinnamon, and cardamon powder to coagulated goat's milk curd. Adding spices to cheese significantly increased fat, protein, and ash content during storage, but total solids and acidity were not affected. The flavor, odor, and consistency of goat's milk cheese were all enhanced by using these spices [64]. Marinho et al. tested semi-hard cheese made from pasteurized and raw Holstein cow milk, coating it with and without lard and rosemary, and ripening it for 60 days. The cheese made from raw milk and coated with lard and rosemary was found to be the most acceptable, giving the final products a higher moisture content, as well as preferred color and texture characteristics [65].

The properties of fresh and ripened herby cheese samples were investigated by Zekai et al. Herby cheese, also known as Otlu peynir – a traditional cheese of eastern Turkey, is made from sheep milk, is widely produced and consumed. Herby cheese is made with around 25 different types of herbs, such as Allium spp., Thymus spp., Ferula spp., Anthriscus nemorosa, and so on. Coskun and Tuncturk also investigated the impact of the herb Allium sp. on biochemical changes in Turkish herby cheese. They observed that, by growing the herb ratios up to 3%, the herby cheese after ripening greatly raises the levels of lipolysis, Water-soluble Nitrogen, TCA-soluble Nitrogen, and PTA-soluble Nitrogen, which are indicators of proteolysis degrees [66].

Shan et al. [15] observed that cinnamon stick, oregano, clove, pomegranate peel, and grape seed extracts were effective against three foodborne pathogens in cheese (*Listeria monocytogenes, Staphylococcus aureus, and Salmonella enterica* in cheese at room temperature (23°C)). Treatment with these extracts reduced lipid oxidation and improved cheese stability. Clove extract had the strongest antioxidant and antibacterial properties among all the extracts tested and recommended to be used as natural preservatives [15]. These results were in conformity with the findings of Vrinda Menon and Garg, who reported that investigated the clove oil at 1% concentration in cheese can effectively prevent *Listeria monocytogenes* growth in food at both at 30°C and 7°C temperatures [67].

Hassanien et al. [68] found that supplementing cheese with 0.1 percent or 0.2 percent black cumin seed oil, w/w, has important inhibitory effects against certain pathogenic bacteria (*Escherichia coli ATCC 8739, Listeria monocytogenes Scott A, Salmonella enteritidis PT4* and *Staphylococcus aureus ATCC 6538*). The addition of black cumin seed oil to cheese has an antimicrobial effect during cold storage [68].

Josipović et al. developed a new herbal cottage cheeses with fresh or dried parsley, dill, pepper, garlic, and rosemary. The herbal cottage cheeses had optimal sensory properties, improved biological value, and extended shelf life. Foodborne pathogens such as *E. coli, Staphylococcus aureus, Salmonella typhimurium,* and *Listeria monocytogenes* were effectively minimized by the herbal extracts tested *in vitro* and *in situ*. Due to high mass fractions of flavones and phenolic diterpenes, as well as high mass fractions of caffeic and rosmarinic acids, dry rosemary had the highest antioxidant and antibacterial activity among these herbs. Consumers prefer fresh plants, but according to this study, dry plants contribute more to biological benefit and antioxidant properties. As a result, these plant extracts have the ability to serve as natural preservatives and antioxidants [69].

4.6 Shrikhand

Ashwagandha herb powder (0.5%) enriched shrikhand (an Indian dairy product made from lactic fermented curd) was developed by Landge et al. They observed that adding ashwagandha powder to shrikhand improved the organoleptic properties, consistency and extended the shelf life of the product to 52 days when kept refrigerated [70]. Nidhi Ojha investigated the effects of tulsi and turmeric powder in herbal shrikhand. They reported that adding 0.4 percent tulsi powder and 0.5 percent turmeric powder on the basis of Chakka in Shrikhand improved the product's sensory, microbiological activity, and nutritional value [71]. Similarly, Himanshu et al. developed tulsi extract (0.9%) incorporated functional herbal shrikhand without compromising the physicochemical properties of the product [72].

4.7 Other dairy products

Neethu et al. developed Origanum vulgare (also known as oregano, Spanish thyme and wild marjoram) incorporated in paneer made from malic acid coagulated milk. The sensory acceptability of malic acid was higher when it was combined with oregano spiced paneer. In comparison to industrial paneer, the growth of microorganisms was found to be less in this herbal paneer [73]. Shweta et al. reported that 0.6 percent turmeric can be used as a preservative to prolong the shelf life of paneer. When stored at 7 ± 1°C the shelf-life of the herbal paneer was increased to 12 days, compared to 7 days for control paneer [74]. Similarly, Bullerman and Gourma claimed that the compound Oleuropein, derived from the olive tree, can inhibit the

Dairy products	Herb(s) and spice(s) used	Targeted functional benefits	References
Milk	Tulsi juice (25%), ginger juice (3%) and turmeric powder (0.1%).	Anti-carcinogenic. Cardio-protective, anti-inflammatory. Anti-pyretic and anti-microbial.	Gaurav Kumar [18]
	Tulsi	Good antioxidant and iron-chelating properties	Palthur et al.
	Turmeric powder	Immunity booster.	Jankar [20]
	Piper betel leaves	Stimulant for muscular and mental efficiency, carminative, an antiseptic and an expectorant.	Kamble et al. [21]
	Aloe vera pulp (5%)	It is nutrient-dense and aids in the prevention of the several diseases.	Pugazhenth and Jothylingam [22]
	Fennel, tulsi and lemon grass oil	Lowers blood pressure, reduces the risk of heart disease, relieves fever, headaches, and sore throats, helps in blood purification. It also has antioxidant, anti-bacterial, and ulcer-prevention properties.	Kishore [23]
	Pueraria tuberosa	High antioxidant activity	Sawale et al. [24]
	Wheat grass juice	Anti-inflammatory, anti-oxidant, and antibacterial properties.	Vaquil et al. [25]
	Ginger juice	Antioxidant. Improve sensory and keeping quality.	Rathod et al. [26]
Yoghurt	Tulsi leaf	Greater β-D-galactosidase enzymatic activity.	Chowdhury et al. [27]
	Tulsi extract and beet root extract	Antiradical properties	Ghosh [28]
	Aloe vera gel	Antiviral, antimicrobial activity, adjuvant cancer care, ulcer remedy.	Govindammal et al. [29]
	Essential oils from peppermint, basil and zataria	Antioxidant activity	Azizkhani and Parsaeimehr [32]
	Moringa olifera leaf powder	Antimicrobial.	Kabuo et al. [36]
	Beet root and ginger extract	Higher antioxidant properties	Srivastava et al. [34]
	Garlic, cinnamon and peppermint	Antimicrobial and proteolytic activity	Bakrm and Salihin [30]
	Cinnamon powder	Intensify gastro intestinal stability	Ahmed Helala and Davide Tagliazcchi [31]
	Rosmarius officinalis oil	Improved functional properties	Ghalem and Zouaoui [33]
	Peppermint, dill and basil	Enhances inhibition of ACE activity.	Amirdivani and Baba [35]

Dairy products	Herb(s) and spice(s) used	Targeted functional benefits	References
Labneh	Thyme, marjoram and sage essential oils	Deliver phytochemicals and other nutrients for health benefits	Otaibi and Demerdash [39]
	Dill and caraway essential oil	Antioxidant and antimicrobial activity	Zaky et al. [79]
	Moringa oliefera oil	Antimicrobial activity	El-Sayed et al. [40]
Lassi	Ginger, turmeric and carrot extract	Rich in antioxidant and provides nutrients	Soma Maji et al. [42]
Shrikhand	Ashwagandha powder.	Respiratory stimulant activities and immuno-stimulating effect	Landge et al. [70]
	Turmeric and tulsi powder	Increased functional properties	Nidhi Ojha [71]
	Tulsi extract	Increased flavor and health benefits	Himanshu et al. [72]
Butter	Sage and rosemary	Increases oxidative stability.	Najgebauer et al. [45]
	Sage rosemary and oregano extracts	Increases oxidative stability.	Ahmet et al. [48]
	Rosemary extracts	Increases oxidative stability.	Renata et al. [49]
	Thyme and cumin essential oils.	Prevent deterioration of butter	Farag et al. [46]
	Rosemary	High antioxidant properties	Santos et al. [49]
Ghee	Sage and rosemary	High antioxidant properties	Ozcan [44]
	Terminalia arjuna	Protective against cardiovascular diseases	Rajanikant and Patil [50]
	Tulsi leaf powder	Increases oxidative stability	Merai et al. [47]
	Vidarikand	Antioxidant properties	Nilkanth Pawar [53]
Ice cream	Basil juice and freeze dried powder	Anti-stress, antioxidant, antibacterial, anti-fungal, antiviral and immuno-stimulant activities.	Trivedi et al. [54]
	Aloe vera and mint	anti-inflammatory gastro protective, antimicrobial and improve storage stability	Ankush Verma [56]
	Shredded ginger	Improves melting resistance	Pinto et al. [57]
	Curcumin powder	Improves sensory attributes and health benefits	Manoharan et al. [59]
	Pudina	Cooling sensation	Patil et al. [60]
	Lemon grass and distillate	Improves flavor and sensory attributes	Janu Atanu et al. [61]

Dairy products	Herb(s) and spice(s) used	Targeted functional benefits	References
Cheese	Cinnamon stick, oregano and clove	Effective against food borne pathogens. (Antimicrobial)	Shan et al. [15]
	Clove oil	Antimicrobial	Vrinda and Garge [67]
	Lard and rosemary	Flavor, color and texture	Marinho et al. [65]
	Black cumin seed	Inhibit food borne pathogens (Antimicrobial)	Hassanien et al. [68]
	Rosemary	High antioxidant property	Josipovic et al. [69]
	Moringa oliefera	High total phenolic content and antioxidant activities	Mohamed et al. [62]
	Black pepper	High antioxidant property	Bakcheit and Foda [63]
	Fenugreek, cinnamon and cardamom powder	Enhance flavor, color and consistency	Hamid and Abdelrahman [64]
	Oregano, thyme	Antimicrobial	Govaris et al. [80]
	Garlic	Antimicrobial	Shan et al. [15]
	Black cumin seed oil	Antimicrobial	Hassanien et al. [68]
	Rosemary essential oil	Antimicrobial	Moro et al. [81]
Paneer	Origanum vulgare	Reduction in asthma, diarrhea and indigestion.	Neethu et al. [73]
	Turmeric powder	Improved texture and keeping quality	Shweta Bunch et al. [74]
Peda	Ginger powder	Increases texture and flavor	Desale et al. [77]
Burfi	Stervia powder and safed musli powder	Superior in physic-chemical, microbial and quality attributes	Goyal and Samsheer [78]

Table 3.
List of some herbal dairy products formulated by incorporating different herbs for their functional and medicinal health benefits.